Phytochemicals as an Epigenetic Modifier in Cancer Prevention

AF858967

Online at: https://doi.org/10.1088/978-0-7503-5252-9

Phytochemicals as an Epigenetic Modifier in Cancer Prevention

Edited by
Nidhi Puranik
Department of Life Science, Yeungnam University, Gyeongsan 38541, South Korea

Deepa Yadav
Department of Zoology, Jiwaji University, Gwalior, Madhya Pradesh 474001, India

Sangeeta Shukla
Chaudhary Charan Singh University, Meerut, Uttar Pradesh 250001, India

IOP Publishing, Bristol, UK

ISBN 978-0-7503-5252-9 (ebook)
ISBN 978-0-7503-5250-5 (print)
ISBN 978-0-7503-5253-6 (myPrint)
ISBN 978-0-7503-5251-2 (mobi)

DOI 10.1088/978-0-7503-5252-9

Version: 20231101

IOP ebooks

British Library Cataloguing-in-Publication Data: A catalogue record for this book is available from the British Library.

Published by IOP Publishing, wholly owned by The Institute of Physics, London

IOP Publishing, No.2 The Distillery, Glassfields, Avon Street, Bristol, BS2 0GR, UK

US Office: IOP Publishing, Inc., 190 North Independence Mall West, Suite 601, Philadelphia, PA 19106, USA

Dedicated to The Almighty, who gave us the strength to complete this work.

Contents

Acknowledgments

All contributors to the respective chapters in this book are thankfully acknowledged by the editors. Their honest efforts, hard work, and analytical approach have been well appreciated and recognized. Dr Nidhi Puranik is thankful to Yeungnam University, Gyeongsan, South Korea, Dr Deepa Yadav is thankful to Jiwaji University, Gwalior, India, and Professor Sangeeta Shukla is thankful to Chaudhary Charan Singh University, Meerut, Uttar Pradesh, India for providing infrastructure facilities and all relevant assistance.

Editor biographies

Dr Nidhi Puranik

Dr Nidhi Puranik is a Research Assistant Professor in the Department of Life Science at Yeungnam University in Gyeongsan, South Korea. She did her PhD at Defence Research and Development Establishment-DRDO (Research Center) and her degree was awarded from Bharathair University, Coimbatore, Tamil Nadu, India. She has more than 10 years of research and teaching experience in the field of disease therapeutics and diagnostics. Her current research is focused on the screening and development of plant-based drugs for various diseases. She has been awarded the prestigious GATE, CSIR-NET, ICAR-NET, DRDO Junior research fellowship, MPCST Young Scientist award, MPCST Young Scientist training fellowship (National), and Young Investigator award (International). She has worked in various prestigious institutes of India—ICMR-NIREH, Bhopal, ICAR-IISR, Indore, Jiwaji University, Gwalior, and Barkatullah University, Bhopal. She has published over 40 research articles with high citation scores and one edited book with IOP and one Indian patent. The overall relevance and importance of her research work to human clinician medicine in the treatment and diagnosis of diseases cannot be underestimated.

Dr Deepa Yadav

Dr Deepa Yadav (PhD Biotechnology) from UNESCO Trace Element Satellite Centre, Jiwaji University Gwalior, Madhya Pradesh served as Research Associate at Biosensor Development Test and Evaluation Division, Defence Research Development and Establishment-DRDO, Jhansi Road, Gwalior, Madhya Pradesh and Counselor at UNESCO Trace Element Satellite Centre, Jiwaji University Gwalior, Madhya Pradesh. Dr Yadav has nine years of research experience with expertise in Pharmacognosy and Quality assessment of plants, metal toxicity, and toxicology DNA barcoding of herbal plants. She has published more than ten papers in national and international journals and also has one book published with Lambert's publishers entitled T cell signaling mechanisms. She has been awarded 39th Gold Medal from the Society of Toxicology, India, the National PD Shetty Memorial Award for HPTLC and Pharmacognosy, 32nd MPCST Young Scientist Award with other awards and achievements. Her research interest is the assessment and identification of biomolecules from native plant species using FTIR, HPTLC, HPLC, GCMS, and LCMS. The overall relevance and importance of her research work to human clinician medicine in the treatment of a variety of human cancers cannot be underestimated.

Professor (Dr) Sangeeta Shukla

Professor Sangeeta Shukla (PhD; DSc), Vice Chancellor, Chaudhary Charan Singh University, Meerut, Uttar Pradesh, Vice President for Asian Continent of TEU (UNESCO Trace Element Satellite Centre), India (former, Vice Chancellor, Jiwaji University, Gwalior, Madhya Pradesh). Professor Shukla has 35 years of teaching and research experience in toxicology and pharmacology, cancer prevention, metabolism of drugs, contraception, and metal toxicity. Professor Shukla has published 52 full-length research publications in National and 74 articles in International Journals of Sci Index with 11 books, 11 patents, and more than 1 Crores grant from projects (ICMR, DST, UGC, CCRUM, MPCST, UGC-SAP, DRDE, and DST-FIST) are her big achievements. As regards human resource and development, she has mentored more than 55 research scholars for PhD, MPhil, Wos-A scientist, Wos-B Scientist, Research Associate, Senior Research Fellow, Post Doc Students.

List of contributors

Divya Bisht
Biochemistry Discipline, School of Sciences, Indira Gandhi National Open University, New Delhi 110068, India

Gresh Chander
School of Biotechnology, Shri Mata Vaishno Devi University, Katra (J&K) 182320, India

Pallavi Singh Chauhan
Amity Institute of Biotechnology, Amity University Madhya Pradesh, Gwalior 474005 (M.P.), India

Narayanan Ganesh
Department of Research, Jawaharlal Nehru Cancer Hospital and Research Centre, Idgah Hills, Bhopal, India

Sagarkumar Joshi
Department of Microbiology and Biotechnology, School of Science, Gujarat University, Ahmedabad, Gujarat 380009, India
and
Darshan Institute of Science, Darshan University, Rajkot 363650, India

Pankaj Keshari
School of Life Sciences, Jawaharlal Nehru University, New Delhi 110067, India

Rahul Kumar
Department of Zoology, Sheodeni Sao College, Magadh University, Kaler 824127, India
and
University Department of Zoology, Vinoba Bhave University, Hazaribagh 825301, India
School of Life Sciences, Jawaharlal Nehru University, New Delhi 110067, India

Yashaswee Mishra
School of Life Sciences, Jawaharlal Nehru University, New Delhi 110067, India

Sumana Pal
School of Biotechnology, KIIT University, India

Deena Prakash
Biochemistry Discipline, School of Sciences, Indira Gandhi National Open University, New Delhi 110068, India

Nidhi Puranik
Department of Life Science, Yeungnam University, Gyeongsan 38541, South Korea

Bijendra Rai
Department of Chemistry, Government Holkar Science College, Indore, M.P., India

Alibha Rawat
Department of Research, Jawaharlal Nehru Cancer Hospital and Research Centre, Idgah Hills, Bhopal, India

Nidhi Saxena
Department of Microbiology, Faculty of Science, Atmiya University, Rajkot 360005, India

Arvind Kumar Shakya
Assistant Professor, Biochemistry Discipline, School of Sciences, Indira Gandhi National Open University, New Delhi 110068, India

Minseok Song
Department of Life Science, Yeungnam University, Gyeongsan 38541, South Korea

Amit Sonkar
Department of Biochemistry, All India Institute of Medical Sciences, Guwahati, India

Priyanka Sonkar
Department of Biosciences, Bharathiar University, Coimbatore, India

Anushree Sharma
Department of Biochemistry and Genetics, Barkatullah University, Bhopal 462026, India

Ajay Kumar Sharma
University Department of Zoology, Vinoba Bhave University, Hazaribagh 825301, India

Neha Sharma
Amity Institute of Biotechnology, Amity University Madhya Pradesh, Gwalior 474005 (M.P.), India

Pramod Kumar Singh
Department of Biosciences, Netaji Subhas University, Jamshedpur, Jharkhand, India

Rohit Kumar Singh
Agricultural Research Organization, Volcani Institute, Israel

Uday Suryakant
School of Biotechnology, KIIT University, India

Rajesh Singh Tomar
Amity Institute of Biotechnology, Amity University Madhya Pradesh, Gwalior 474005 (M.P.), India

Smarti Verma
Department of Zoology, Government Veerangana Jhalkari Bai Girls College, Gwalior (M.P.), India

Dhananjay Yadav
Department of Life Science, Yeungnam University, Gyeongsan, Gyeongbuk 38541, Republic of Korea

Shiv Kumar Yadav
Department of Botany, Government Lal Bahadur Shastri PG College, Sironj, Madhya Pradesh 464228, India

Chapter 1

Phytochemicals and cancer: an overview

Nidhi Puranik and Minseok Song

Cancer is one of the leading causes of death worldwide, with millions of new cancer cases and deaths worldwide every year. Cancer chemoprevention is the use of artificial, organic, or biological substances to reduce the risk of developing cancer in people who are otherwise healthy. Chemopreventive drugs either prevent DNA damage, which results in malignancy, or they stop or reverse the division of premalignant cells with DNA damage, which inhibits the growth of cancer. Clinical trials for breast, prostate, and colon cancer have shown the value of this strategy. There is an obvious need for an alternate strategy given the ongoing rise in cancer incidence, the ineffectiveness of traditional chemotherapies to control cancer, and the excessive toxicity of chemotherapies. Numerous difficulties have been presented by conventional cancer therapy, such as toxicity, medication resistance, and cost. Contrarily, plant-based diets that make use of phytochemicals have recently attracted more attention due to their capacity to influence a wide range of molecular pathways in a less harmful way. We discuss phytochemicals and the mechanisms underlying the chemopreventive and anti-cancer actions of several phytochemicals in this chapter.

1.1 Introduction

Cancer is one of the most common causes of death and a major global public health issue (Siegel *et al* 2023). As a direct and indirect result of oncogenic mutations, tumorigenesis is dependent on the reprogramming of cellular metabolism. The capacity of cancer cells to obtain essential nutrients from frequently nutrient-deficient environments and use these nutrients to both sustain viability and create new biomass is a common characteristic of cancer cell metabolism. Cancer-related metabolic reprogramming can affect intracellular and extracellular metabolites, which can have a significant impact on gene expression, cellular differentiation, and the tumor microenvironment (Pavlova and Thompson 2016). The intricacy of cancer

doi:10.1088/978-0-7503-5252-9ch1

has always made cancer research difficult. In terms of genetic changes, organ involvement, prognosis, and therapeutic administration, various cancer kinds can show significant variations. Although there are several therapy options, their effectiveness depends on the disease's nature and stage. Careful surgical removal of cancerous tissues or tumors, radiation therapy, chemotherapy, and immunotherapy are typically used as treatment options. Surgery and radiotherapy have localized effects, whereas chemotherapy and targeted therapy have systemic effects. Whether such therapies are employed alone or in conjunction with other treatments depends on the type and stage of the cancer. Chemotherapy and small-molecule targeted treatment are two therapeutic modalities used to treat cancer with chemical substances. Chemotherapy medications often have cytotoxic effects and disrupt several cell cycle phases. Their use is justified by the fact that cancer cells typically divide more quickly than healthy cells do, rendering them more vulnerable to chemotherapeutic drugs (Naeem *et al* 2022).

Chemoprevention involves the use of substances that can stop, stop the spread of, or delay cancer. It has been claimed that a number of phytochemicals derived from edible plants can obstruct a particular step in the carcinogenic process. Numerous studies have shown that phytochemicals can act as a chemopreventative agent against human cancer by reversing the cancer cell cycle, reducing tumor growth, and triggering apoptosis. It has been shown that dietary phytochemicals can be employed appropriately in chemoprevention and that consuming them regularly is a promising new approach to prevent carcinogenesis, considering both the cancer epidemiology and trial findings.

Traditional natural products have been employed to control numerous diseases, even to develop new agents with high efficiency and low side effects. Vitamins are an important component of nutrition and one of the emerging therapeutic drugs to prevent cancer. The role of various vitamins as an anti-cancer drug is discussed in chapter 2. Flavonoids, polyphenols, terpenoids, alkaloids, saponins, coumarins, and other phytochemicals that are potentially found in natural plants and target a variety of signaling pathways may be an effective strategy to stop the spread of cancer and the development of resistance to chemotherapy.

Phytochemicals inhibit the growth of cancer in a number of ways, including programmed cell death, senescence, and inhibition of cell migration. This is because the majority of medications derived from plants have a cytotoxic activity that targets multiple molecular pathways rather than specific signals. They also modulate a number of signaling pathways, decreasing oncogenes while enhancing tumor suppressor genes, and regulating related upstream and downstream mediators to halt the progression of cancer. Phytochemicals can also be created in a way that boosts their low water solubility, advances their anti-cancer activity, and lowers cancer's chemoresistance.

In order to boost the anti-cancer efficiency of phytochemicals and delay the generation of cancer cells that are resistant to them, the numerous processes by which they can prevent cancer have come into focus. Malignant cancer also activates a number of molecular pathways, with cell death being the main one. When apoptotic processes are disturbed, different strategies may be considered as a way to significantly slow the growth of cancer (Zheng *et al* 2022).

An effort has been made in this book chapter to introduce dietary phytochemicals, their beneficial effects on preventing cancer, as well as their mechanisms of action (Meybodi *et al* 2017).

1.2 Hallmarks of cancer

A group of diseases known as cancers can affect any organ in the body. They share a number of traits, such as the development from healthy cells, the proliferation outside the boundaries of normal tissue, the loss of differentiation, and the *in situ* invasion of nearby tissues that causes extravasation and metastases to other parts of the body (Floor *et al* 2012).

The term 'Hallmarks of Cancer' describes a collection of functional skills that human cells obtain as they move from stages of healthy growth to neoplastic growth states, with a focus on skills that are crucial for the growth of malignant tumors. Although we subsequently raised this to eight, our original concept called for the complimentary engagement of six separate signature talents. This formulation was influenced by the knowledge that human tumors are the product of multistep processes and that the growth of these functional skills may be connected in some manner to the many stages of tumor pathogenesis.

There are undoubtedly a wide range of aberrations (and, consequently, acquired abilities and characteristics) in the malignant pathogenesis, which encompasses a variety of tumor types and an increasing number of subtypes. These aberrations are caused by tissue-specific barriers that must be overcome during particular tumorigenesis pathways. While recognizing the relevance of such specialized processes, we limited the hallmarks designation to parameters indicating extensive interaction throughout the spectrum of human malignancies (Hanahan 2022).

In their 2000 research publication, The Hallmarks of Cancer (henceforth referred to as Hallmarks I), Hanahan and Weinberg attempted to divide the complicated biology of cancer into six major hallmarks. These characteristics include the ability to produce enough growth signals on its own, insensitivity to anti-growth signals, evasion of apoptosis, infinite capacity for replication, persistent angiogenesis, and tissue invasion and metastasis. Ten years later, follow-up research (henceforth referred to as Hallmarks II) added two additional hallmarks: reprogramming energy metabolism and avoiding immune response, as well as two enabling traits: genomic instability and mutation, and tumor-promoting inflammation (Hanahan 2011, Fouad and Aanei 2017). The hallmarks of cancer are represented in figure 1.1.

1.3 Phytochemicals and cancer

Plants include phytochemicals, which are non-nutritive compounds with anti-disease properties. To prove fruits and vegetables' health-promoting qualities, different epidemiological studies that initially found a consistent link between high consumption and a reduced risk of contracting a number of diseases, including various types of cancer, have historically been employed. Following an investigation,

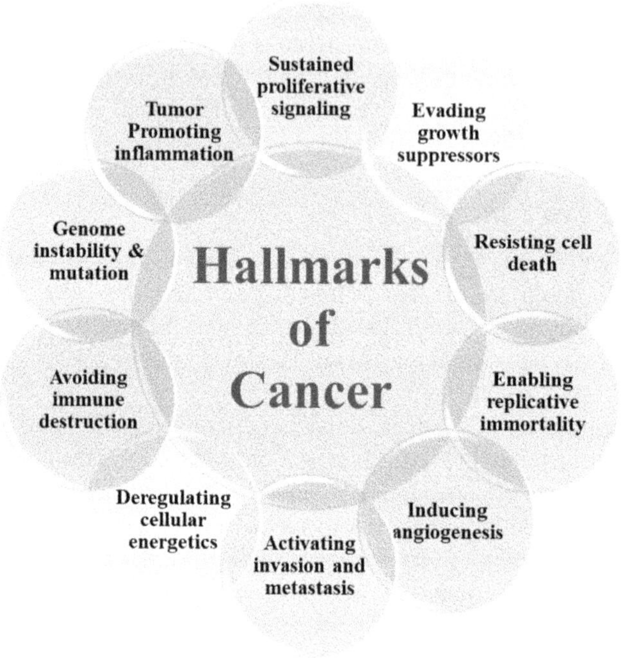

Figure 1.1. A summary of various phytochemicals and their mechanism of action as anticancer agents studied in previously published papers.

specific dietary phytochemicals with anti-cancer properties were found (González-Vallinas *et al* 2013).

Phytochemicals are metabolites found in all plants, including grains, fruits, vegetables, and plants. Most of them contain active ingredients. Numerous studies have demonstrated the health benefits of regularly consuming these bioactive substances as supplements or dietary ingredients (Liu 2013). Based on their chemical makeup and pharmacological characteristics, these phytochemicals can be grouped into the following five higher-order classes: carotenoids, phenols, alkaloids, organic nitrogen and sulfur compounds, and others (Vargas-Mendoza *et al* 2022) as shown in figure 1.2. Numerous natural phytochemicals and dietary compounds may have chemopreventive properties, according to epidemiological and preclinical data. Additionally, *in vitro* and animal studies suggest that these substances may alter signaling pathways involved in cell proliferation and apoptosis in transformed cells, boost the host immune system, and make malignant cells more susceptible to cytotoxic agents (Kotecha *et al* 2016). Numerous case-control and epidemiological studies have demonstrated a negative correlation between dietary intake of phytochemicals and the incidence of breast, colon, lung, pancreatic, and prostate cancer. Among the cellular and molecular processes controlled by these chemopreventive phytochemicals are apoptosis, cell cycle, cell proliferation, DNA repair, differentiation, carcinogen activation/detoxification by xenobiotic metabolizing enzymes, functional inactivation/activation of oncogenes and tumor-suppressor

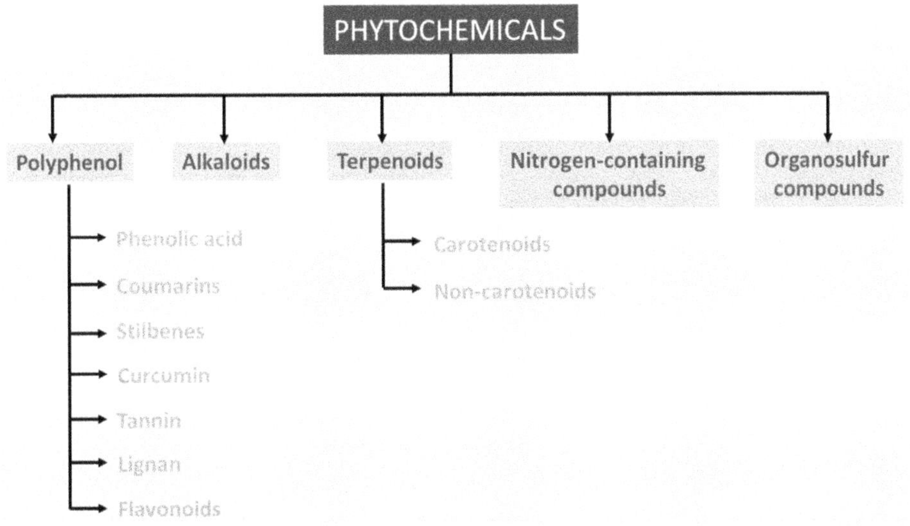

Figure 1.2. Broad classification of phytochemicals.

genes, by preventing DNA damage caused by oxidative stress, angiogenesis, and metastasis. The decrease of oxidative stress-mediated carcinogenesis is another way that phytochemicals can exert their anti-cancer potential (George *et al* 2021). Furthermore, *in vitro* and *in vivo* studies show that a number of phytochemicals increase oxidative stress in cancer cells, which increases the efficiency of chemotherapy treatments. In the context of cancer chemoprevention and treatment, numerous researchers have looked into the role of dietary phytochemicals like curcumin, epigallocatechin gallate, resveratrol, phenethyl isothiocyanate, sulforaphane, hesperidin, quercetin, and 2'-hydroxyflavanone in regulating oxidative stress and associated signaling pathways (Chikara *et al* 2018, Biswas *et al* 2022).

To date, various research studies revealed the role of phytochemicals as a chemotherapeutic agent for the treatment and management of various cancers, as shown in figure 1.3. The role of dietary natural food as a therapeutic drug to prevent lung cancer is discussed in chapters 4 and 5 in detail.

1.3.1 Polyphenols

Polyphenols, which are essentially defined by containing two or more phenol units, are the most prevalent organic molecules generated in plants. A classification of natural polyphenols into five classes is possible using their chemical makeup. Flavonoids, phenolic acids, lignans, stilbenes, and other polyphenols are among these groups. Flavonoids and phenolic acids comprise about 60% and 30%, respectively, of all naturally occurring polyphenols, making them the two most frequent polyphenol subgroups (Zhou *et al* 2016).

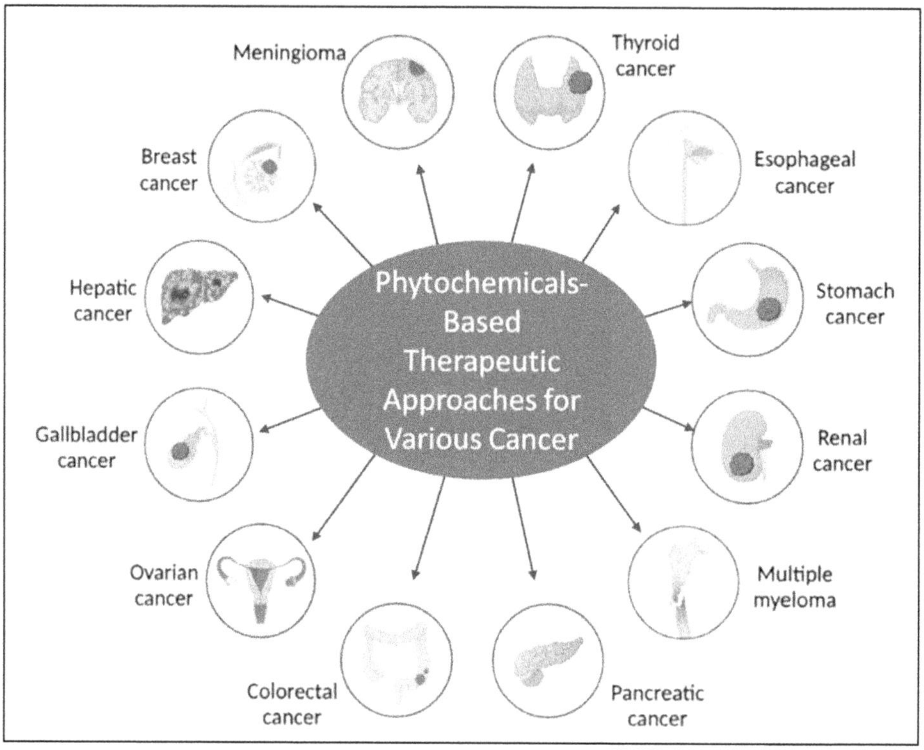

Figure 1.3. Role of phytochemicals as a chemotherapeutic agent for the treatment and management of various cancer (created with BioRender.com).

In order to learn more about polyphenols' potential health benefits, including protection against oxidative stress, diabetes, cardiovascular disease, neurodegenerative disease, and aging, several studies have been done on the topic. These polyphenols can inhibit cell cycle processes, change signaling pathways, and trigger apoptosis, among other cancer prevention strategies. Additionally, polyphenols regulate the activities of enzymes required for the development of cancerous cells. Natural polyphenols may prevent cancer through a number of mechanisms, including DNA interaction, anti-angiogenic actions, and others, according to recent studies (Bhosale *et al* 2020).

Through the activation of cellular defense mechanisms such as antioxidant and detoxifying enzyme systems, phenolic compounds have an impact on the growth of cancer. Additionally, they interfere with signaling pathways that control cell proliferation and inflammation, which results in cell cycle arrest and/or cellular death. The fact that polyphenols can alter the epigenome of cancer cells strongly suggests that they have anti-cancer capabilities. Apoptosis, cell cycle arrest, antioxidant enzyme activity, cell cycle alteration, and anti-cancer drug elimination are just a few of the mechanisms through which naturally occurring polyphenolic compounds present in the diet can exert their anti-cancer effects (Briguglio *et al* 2020).

Polyphenols and their metabolites playing a crucial role as molecular regulators at the epigenetic level in cancer protection is discussed in more detail in chapter 6, however, the role of the flavonoids class of polyphenol is separately discussed in chapter 7 as an epigenetic regulator in cancer treatment and management.

1.3.2 Alkaloids

The highly complex chemical class of alkaloids has a ring structure that contains nitrogen atoms (Khattak and Khan 2016). Under basic and neutral conditions, alkaloids can dissolve in lipids; in acidic conditions, they can dissolve in water. Natural alkaloids are solids with a small molecular weight. They are widely dispersed in plants and make up around 20% of the secondary metabolites. Alkaloids can be broadly grouped according to their source and method of production. The alkaloids are divided into three categories based on their sources: real alkaloids, proto-alkaloids, and pseudoalkaloids. The real alkaloids have heterocyclic rings with nitrogen and are derived from amino acids. Alkaloids are essential in the fight against cancerous cells. They inhibit the function of the topoisomerase enzyme, which is involved in a number of cellular activities, including DNA replication, and cause death in addition to changing other intracellular targets and signaling cascades (Rampogu *et al* 2022).

A variety of pharmacological effects, including antibacterial, antimalarial, antifungal, and anti-cancer properties, are also present in many alkaloids (Debnath *et al* 2018). In reality, the US Food and Drug Administration has approved a number of alkaloids derived from plants for use as chemotherapeutic drugs, including camptothecin, a well-known powerful topoisomerase I inhibitor (Tilaoui *et al* 2021) and vinblastine, interacts with tubulin to disrupt the cell cycle (Choudhari *et al* 2020). Alkaloids such as colchicine, vinblastine, vincristine, vindesine, vinorelbine, and vincamine have potential antitumor action (Dhyani *et al* 2022). Numerous alkaloids have cytotoxic effects on human colon cancer cells and possess anti-colon cancer capabilities. The most intriguing chemicals appear to be those that can affect DNA replication and division at the level of the checkpoints that are present throughout the G1/S and G2/M transitions. The therapeutic potential of these alkaloids for the successful treatment of colon cancer is enormous (Khan *et al* 2022).

The oral administration of the compounds is difficult due to the alkaloids' poor water solubility and low bioavailability. By using a semi-synthetic and biochemical transformation strategy, we can produce molecules with higher water solubility and hence boost bioavailability. Similar methods have been used to make various alkaloids more potent and water-soluble. A few rutaecarpine derivatives with an amine function have better anti-cancer efficacy against HeLa cells and water solubility than the original molecule (Huang *et al* 2017, Mondal *et al* 2019).

1.3.3 Terpenoids

The main components of plant resin and essential oils are 'terpenes,' a combination of isomeric hydrocarbons with the molecular formula C10H16. Terpenoids are a class of hydrocarbons with the general formula (C5H8)n that are formed from plants, including their oxygenated, hydrogenated, and dehydrogenated derivatives. The letter 'n' represents the number of isoprene units. The four primary subgroups of terpenoids are mono, di, oligo, and polyterpenes. Terpenoids are used in the chemical, pharmaceutical, fragrance, and flavor sectors and are made up of about 25 000 distinct chemical structures. Terpenoids may act as an antiproliferative agent against a range of cancer types, according to *in vitro*, *in vivo*, and human epidemiological research (Sharma *et al* 2017).

The roots, vegetative tissues, and other portions of the plant all contain terpenoids, the largest and most diversified class of chemicals generated by plants. Terpenoids are divided into subclasses based on their isoprene structural units, and they include the following: hemiterpenoids (acyclic, monocyclic, bicyclic), sesquiterpenoids (acyclic, monocyclic, bicyclic, tricyclic, lactones), diterpenoids (acyclic, monocyclic, bicyclic, tricyclic, tetracyclic, macrocyclic), and sesterterpenoids (Chopra *et al* 2021).

Terpenoids come in a variety of forms, and their pharmacological and possibly anti-cancer properties have garnered interest. Among other things, certain terpenoids have an anti-cancer effect by triggering cell cycle arrest, delaying cancer cell differentiation, and activating apoptosis to suppress the early stages of carcinogenesis. Some terpenoids can inhibit angiogenesis and metastasis at an advanced stage of cancer growth by altering a number of intracellular signaling pathways (Rabi and Gupta 2008, Kamran *et al* 2022).

Nuclear factor kappa B (NF-kB), a transcription factor, is one of the main inducible proteins in mammals that are known to regulate gene expression in many crucial physiological processes, including oxidative stress, inflammation, etc. NF-kB's significance in the etiology of cancer has also been demonstrated. A variety of terpenoids block the NF-kB signaling cascade via phosphorylating IkB, binding to DNA, translocating p65, and other mechanisms (Jain *et al* 2016).

Recently, natural terpenoids have drawn increased interest as a possible therapy for melanoma. They unquestionably outperform conventional chemotherapeutic drugs due to their decreased cytotoxicity. Plant terpenoids have been demonstrated to exhibit dose-dependent cytotoxicity, induce apoptosis, necrosis, or autophagy, increase ROS production, oxidative stress, and induce ER stress, cause cell cycle arrest, induce DNA damage, decrease the expression and activity of proteins involved in melanogenesis, interfere with cell signaling pathways that control cell growth, proliferation, migration, adhesion, and invasion, and decrease the expression and activity of melanoma (Kłos and Chlubek 2022).

1.3.4 Organosulfur compounds (OSCs)

Organosulfur-containing substances are widely dispersed in both the environment and human bodies. There are two primary groups of vegetables that contain OSCs and have distinctive properties. Garlic, onion, shallot, leek, and chives are a few popular allium species that contain S-alkyl-l-cysteine sulfoxides (Bommareddy *et al* 2016). Rucola (rocket salad) is a member of the Eruca genus, which is a subfamily of the Brassicaceae, which also includes cabbage, cauliflower, Brussels sprouts, kale, and other cruciferous vegetables (Goncharov *et al* 2016).

Organosulfur compounds have been shown to have a wide range of biological effects, including the induction of carcinogen detoxification, inhibition of tumor cell proliferation, antimicrobial activity, free radical scavenging, inhibition of DNA adduct formation, induction of cell cycle arrest, induction of apoptosis, and many more. According to some research, these chemicals may act as chemopreventive agents through a combination of the aforementioned routes. Strong data from epidemiological and experimental carcinogenesis lends credence to the notion that people who consume a lot of organosulfur in their diet have a lower risk of contracting various cancers. Test animals' skin, lungs, mammary glands, esophagus, breast, and other organs have shown OSCs to have anti-carcinogenic effects. Together, these studies show a strong correlation between ingesting organosulfur compounds in any form and cancer prevention. Because the protective effects of all these phytochemicals are the consequence of additives and synergistic combination, additional research is required to fully understand the chemopreventive activity of organosulfur compounds and to establish an effective dose that has no toxicity in humans (Moriarty *et al* 2007). Recent studies have shown that several naturally occurring OSC analogs can prevent the development of cancer cells both in culture and *in vivo*. Changes in the cell cycle and the start of G2/M phase arrest are frequently associated with OSC-induced changes in cancer cell proliferation. It has been demonstrated that the OSC can trigger apoptosis by altering the proportion of the Bcl-2 family of proteins in both *in vitro* and *in vivo* situations. Additionally, it has been demonstrated that OSC made from garlic has anti-angiogenic effects (Herman-Antosiewicz *et al* 2007).

Organosulfur compounds, especially allyl derivatives, have also been shown to prevent the development of cancer in the lung, mammary gland, esophagus, stomach, and other organs of experimental animals, which have been connected to the anti-carcinogenic capabilities (Omar and Al-Wabel 2010). Experimental animal and laboratory studies have shown that garlic and several of its organosulfur constituents are highly powerful inhibitors of a variety of malignancies and cancer cells in culture, including those of the breast, colon, skin, uterus, esophagus, and lung. Which special garlic component(s) underpins the specific cellular and molecular pathways that regulate the anti-cancer effects is not known with certainty. Depending on the conditions of its growth, garlic can include at least 33 distinct organosulfur compounds in addition to amino acids, vitamins, and minerals. Allicin, water-soluble S-allyl mercapto cysteine (SAMC), oil-soluble diallyl disulfide (DADS), and diallyl sulfide (DAS) are among the allyl sulfur compounds produced by enzymatic activity when garlic is minced or crushed that are thought to be responsible for the majority of these anti-cancer effects (Xiao *et al* 2005). Garlic's anti-carcinogenic properties have been related to a variety of its chemical elements, but most research has focused on some of its thioallyl constituents. The anti-cancer properties of the garlic components appear to be mediated through a variety of routes, including prevention of mutagenesis, modification of enzyme activity, suppression of DNA adduct, and impacting the intrinsic pathway for apoptotic cell death and cell cycle machinery (Omar and Al-Wabel 2010). They also have been found to stimulate the breakdown of carcinogens and block the covalent binding of carcinogens to DNA. There is renewed interest in studying the medical potential of garlic, particularly in terms of cancer prophylaxis and prevention, as a result of the wide spectrum of effects of garlic and its chemical constituents. Multiple mechanisms working together produce the anti-carcinogenic effects seen in laboratory studies in a range of experimental systems (Das 2002).

Researchers have investigated the efficacy of various nanoformulations of chemicals derived from garlic in treating various cancers, including those of the skin, ovary, prostate, gastric, breast, lung, colorectal, liver, oral, and pancreatic (Pandey *et al* 2023).

According to the detailed mechanism of anti-cancer activity from *in vitro*, preclinical, and clinical research, phytochemicals target apoptosis proteins, such as anti-apoptotic proteins and apoptotic proteins, which stop cell cycle and proliferation. By, for example, decreasing the expression and activity of cyclins and CDKs or boosting the expression of CDKs inhibitors, they alter the expression of growth-related genes. By regulating the expression of MMP-2, 8 and 9, Wnt/-catenin, PARP, oxidative markers, including Nrf-2, antioxidant-related gene, and inhibiting the formation of mammospheres, it prevents metastasis and angiogenesis. It also controls inflammation by modulating TNF-, NF-B, IB kinase, COX-2, IL-1, TNF-, phospho-Akt, and phosphor-p65. Additionally, controlling cell signaling (NF-B, PI3K/Akt, MAPK/ERK, p-mTOR, Wnt, Notch-1, hedgehog), controlling epigenetics (regulating DNA methylation and histone modification), and activating the immune system (NK cell, CD8+ T, CD4+ T, and cytokines like IL-9 and IL-13) in BC cell lines are also important (Sohel *et al* 2023).

1.3.5 Nitrogen-containing compounds

To create active biological chemicals, medicinal chemists are concentrating on nitrogen-containing heterocyclic compounds such as pyrrole, pyrrolidine, pyridine, imidazole, pyrimidines, pyrazole, indole, quinoline, oxadiazole, azole, benzimidazole, etc. According to FDA records, about 60% of novel small-molecule medicines include nitrogen-based heterocycles in their pharmacological design. Axitinib, Bosutinib, Cediranib, Dasatanib (Sprycel®), Erlotinib (Tarceva®), Gefitinib (Iressa®), Imatinib (Gleevec®), Lapatinib (Tykerb®), Linifanib, Sorafenib (Nexavar®), Sunitinib (Sutent®), and Tivozanib (Lang *et al* 2020).

1.4 Different mechanism of phytochemicals as an anti-cancerous agent

The multi-target mechanism of action of phytochemicals, which includes anti-mutagenic, antioxidant, and antiproliferative actions, is primarily responsible for their anti-cancer effects. They may also alter the host immunological response to cancer, lowering inflammatory levels and boosting lymphocyte activity. Multiple signaling pathways are involved in carcinogenesis, which makes multi-targeted medicines like

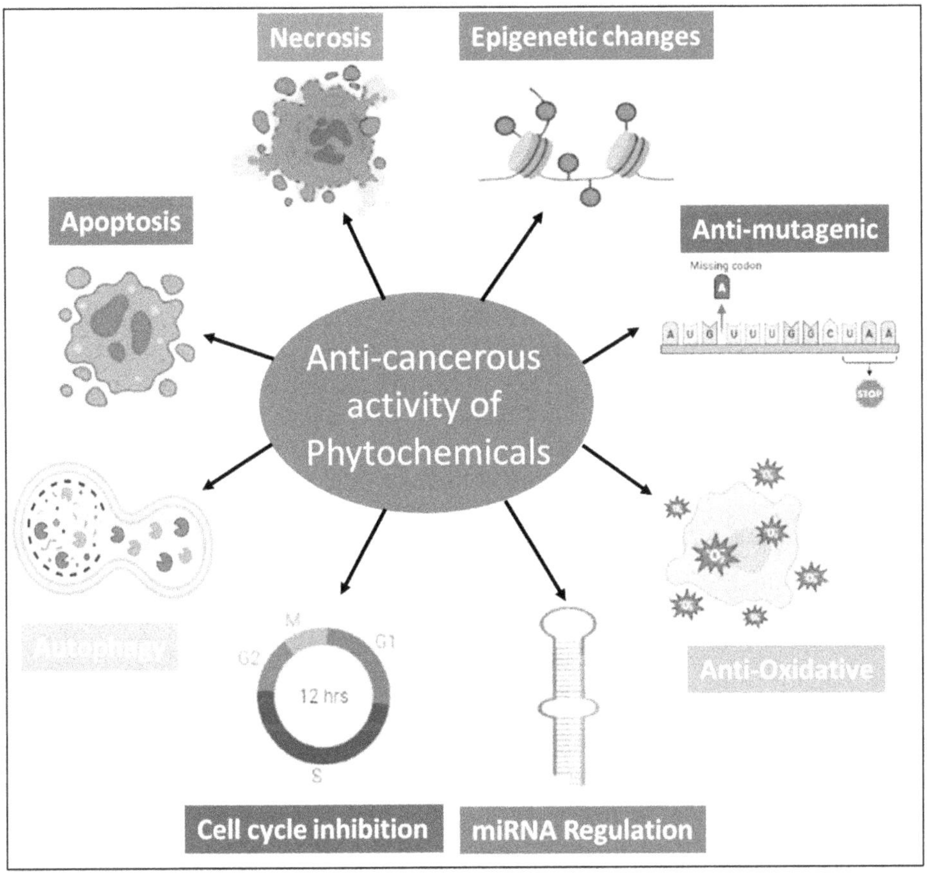

Figure 1.4. Different anti-cancer activity of phytochemicals (created with BioRender.com).

phytochemicals potentially effective anti-cancer treatments (Catalano 2016). Preclinical and clinical research is accumulating evidence that phytochemicals can influence the genesis and progression of cancer by favorably modulating a number of signaling pathways (Rizeq *et al* 2020). The most common and known mechanism of phytochemicals as anti-cancer agents is represented in figure 1.4 and discussed in detail further.

1.4.1 Anti-oxidants

An imbalance between reactive oxygen species (ROS) and antioxidants, as well as increased oxidative stress, are characteristics of cancer (Luo *et al* 2022). Reactive oxygen species (ROS) generation and cellular antioxidant capacity are out of balance, which leads to oxidative stress. During mitochondrial oxidative phosphorylation, ROS, including superoxide anion (O_2^-), hydrogen peroxide (H_2O_2), and hydroxyl radicals (OH), are continuously created in aerobic cells. Moreover, ROS are produced by a variety of activities, including inflammation, infection, mechanical and chemical stressors, as well as exposure to UV and ionizing radiation.

A cell's proliferative, survival, apoptotic, differentiational, immunological, motile, and stress-responsive pathways are all triggered by basal levels of ROS. On the other hand, elevated amounts of ROS cause DNA, protein, and lipid damage that, if left unrepaired, results in mutations and supports the development of cancer. However, excessive ROS generation causes significant permanent DNA damage, including single-strand breaks, double-strand breaks, base alterations, and DNA cross-links, which ultimately result in cell death. As a result, controlling cellular ROS is essential for preserving cellular homeostasis. Phytochemicals have been demonstrated to affect a number of ROS-mediated signaling pathways, the dysregulation of which favors carcinogenesis (Chikara *et al* 2018).

A master switch in cellular antioxidant signaling, nuclear transcription factor erythroid 2-related factor 2 (NRF2) is a transcription factor that is essential for the adaptive survival response to ROS-induced oxidative stress. NRF2 is momentarily activated when the cellular redox balance is disturbed, however severe oxidative stress can overpower this. As a result, it's important to keep the NRF2-mediated antioxidant defense capacity functioning at its best. This review covers the possible chemopreventive effects of natural NRF2 inducers/activators in humans, particularly those found in plant-based diets. Certain phytochemicals obtained from the diet have been demonstrated to activate NRF2, defending cells and tissues from oxidative stress-induced carcinogenesis (Chun *et al* 2021).

The oxidative stress-responsive genes can be silenced by phenolic phytochemicals with antioxidant activity, which in turn inhibits the development of cancer cells. However, phenolic phytochemicals and another class of phytochemicals known as isothiocyanates can cause the production of H_2O_2 to cause cancer cells to experience an excessive amount of oxidative stress. The stress genes are turned on as an immediate reaction. Key biological components like DNA, however, are irreparably harmed once the necessary threshold for cancer cells to handle the induced oxidative stress has been achieved. Genes that start cell cycle arrest and/or apoptosis are simultaneously activated. In order to prevent the growth of cancer cells, phytochemicals can either remove the inherent H_2O_2 or, ironically, produce more H_2O_2 (Loo 2003).

By stimulating GST (a phase II metabolizing enzyme) and quinine reductase, curcumin (diferuloylmethane) reduces ROS produced by chemical carcinogens. Curcumin can both use ROS production to kill cancer cells and scavenge ROS by inducing ROS-scavenging enzymes such GST, hemeoxygenase-1, and redox-sensitive inducible enzymes. Through the upregulation of tumor suppressor p53 and the downregulation of anti-apoptotic proteins NF-kB and COX-2, it has been discovered that curcumin generates ROS over the threshold level required to cause apoptosis. By boosting the expression of proapoptotic proteins (BAX, Cytochrome C, p53, and p21), Caspase 3, and decreasing the mitochondrial membrane potential, curcumin causes apoptosis in colon cancer. Additionally, curcumin suppresses proinflammatory enzymes including inducible NOS (iNOS) and tumor necrosis factor (TNF) to exert its anti-cancerous effects. Additionally, Curcumin can reduce the expression of hypoxia-inducible factor-1 (HIF-1) to decrease hypoxia-induced ROS in hepatic carcinoma cells (HCCs) (Fatma *et al* 2023).

By lowering the free radical burden in cancer cells, curcumin demonstrated its capacity to alter a number of signaling pathways. One such signaling molecule, extracellular signal-regulated protein kinase (ERK1/2), is implicated in inhibiting ROS generation, tumor invasion, and migration. In response to the ERK1/2 pathway, NF-kB is also activated in cancer cells. In order to combat free radical imbalance in the cells, endogenous enzymes including catalase (CAT), superoxide dismutase (SOD), and hemeoxygenase-1 are crucial. By changing the levels of the enzymes matrix metalloproteinase (MMPs), vascular endothelial growth factor (VEGF), and protein kinase (PKC), phenolic substances may be able to limit the generation of ROS in numerous organs and prevent metastases (George *et al* 2021).

1.4.2 Cell cycle inhibition

Effects of a number of organosulfur compounds on colon cancer cells' ability to proliferate and the activation of apoptosis. Additionally, the results of the present investigation indicate that the growth inhibition, G2-M cell cycle arrest, and induction of apoptosis that are brought about by these two compounds may be significantly influenced by an active allyl moiety connected to a disulfide moiety. As a result, synthetic organosulfur compounds or the allyl sulfides found in garlic may prove to be potent cancer preventative and/or treatment agents. A novel anti-cancer compound's identification and/or manufacture may benefit from this structure-function association. Additionally, the synthetic organosulfur chemical tritylcys is a novel inducer of apoptosis and a highly effective inhibitor of the proliferation of colon cancer cells. These findings imply that this substance and other substances that are structurally similar may offer a fresh chemical class of potent anti-cancer medicines (Xiao *et al* 2005). Targeting the foremost molecular signaling pathways regulating tumor development with phytochemicals is discussed in detail in chapter 8.

1.4.3 Autophagy

There has been a thorough examination of the function of autophagy in cancer. An important regulator of cell survival and homeostasis, autophagy has also been linked to tumor suppression in previous studies. However, a theory that autophagy promotes carcinogenesis has been linked to a decrease in its capacity to respond to stress, which has a significant impact on cell metabolism and survival processes. Compared to other cells, cancer cells are more dependent on autophagy (Chirumbolo *et al* 2018). According to additional research, phytochemicals influence autophagy and apoptosis, two critical cellular processes involved in the pathobiology that underlies the genesis and management of cancer. In order to augment traditional cancer chemotherapy, pharmacological targeting of autophagy and apoptotic signaling utilizing phytochemicals is a promising technique (Rahman *et al* 2021).

1.4.4 Necrosis and apoptosis

Through the mitochondrial pathway or death receptor pathway, apoptosis is the process by which contaminated, cancerous, and functionally non-essential cells are eliminated. Membrane channels and apoptogenic proteins play an important role in the regulation of the apoptotic process. Through the course of the cell cycle, apoptosis maintains cellular homeostasis within the human body. Loss of apoptotic regulation extends cancer cell survival and permits the buildup of mutations that can encourage angiogenesis, boost cell proliferation, disturb differentiation, and increase invasiveness throughout tumor progression. As a possible pharmacological target for the treatment of cancer, the apoptotic pathway has received substantial research. Drugs' off-target behaviors, however, as well as their detrimental effects, have long been a source of worry. Numerous cancer cell lines have been examined for phytochemicals' effectiveness both singly and in combination (Wani *et al* 2023).

Nitric Oxide (NO), a crucial signaling molecule that controls cancer and both promotes and inhibits it, is produced by NO synthases (NOS). Since elevated NO levels are lethal to cancer cells, NOS is a crucial target in the fight against cancer. In the current work, the phytochemicals quercetin, sulforaphane, genistein, and epigallocatechin-3-gallate were revealed to have modulatory effects on the NO pathway and apoptosis in HeLa cervical cancer cells (Sundaram *et al* 2020).

1.4.5 Epigenetic regulator

In the field of epigenetics, changes in gene expression or cell phenotypic that are reversible but heritable but don't involve changes in the DNA sequence are studied. Epigenetic changes have emerged as interesting therapeutic targets for cancer prevention due to their reversible nature and early occurrence throughout the course of cancer formation. DNA methylation, modifications in the chromatin structure caused by post-translational modification of histones and some non-histone proteins, and miRNAs, which can either degrade mRNAs or regulate their translation process, are the main epigenetic mechanisms for the regulation of gene expression. These epigenetic processes help the cell adapt to environmental changes like dietary changes or exposure to chemicals, radiation, and hormones. They are crucial for the regulation of the cell's normal functions at all stages, including development and differentiation. Changes in epigenetic targets, however, can potentially result in a number of illnesses, including cancer (Thakur *et al* 2014).

Numerous studies have been conducted on the role of dietary phytochemicals as epigenetic modifiers in cancer and their impact on gene expression and signaling pathways. Common dietary substances can influence the human genome either directly or indirectly by changing the structure or expression of genes; some dietary substances also have an impact on post-translational processes. Inhibitors of histone deacetylases (HDACs) and histone acetyltransferases (HATs) can be used to target the acetylation of histones and non-histone proteins, which has been proven to alter cell metabolism. As seen in figure 1.5, natural substances derived from broccoli,

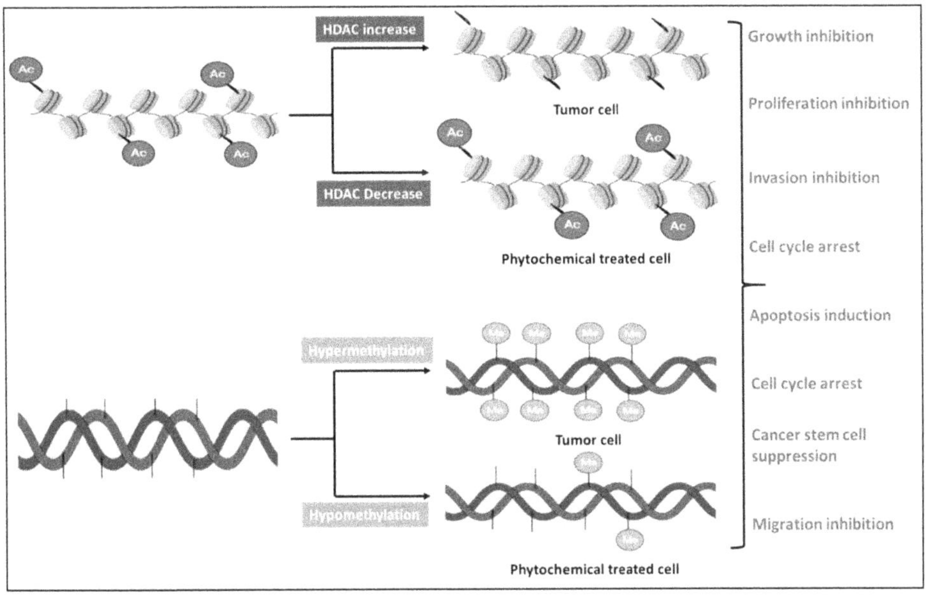

Figure 1.5. DNA methylation and histone modification are reversed by phytochemicals and inhibit tumor progression (created with BioRender.com).

garlic, and curcumin are thought to have inhibitory effects on HDACs and HATs through their influence on epigenetic processes for normalizing the dysregulated metabolism of cancer cells (Pehlivan 2021). Many research-based studies have revealed that phytochemicals play a crucial role as epigenetic modifiers, a detailed study is provided in chapter 3 in tabular form, however, chapter 12 provides an illustrative account of some of the most important and popular methods used to study different epigenetic signatures associated with a particular cell or tissue.

1.4.6 Anti-mutagenic

Punica granatum contains the bioactive compounds punicalagin (PC) and ellagic acid (EA), which prevent DNA adducts caused by BP and have potent anti-mutagenic and antiproliferative properties (Zahin *et al* 2014). Because of the chemoprotective properties of tomatoes, lycopene, and tomato-based products in the reduction of carcinogenesis, lycopene exerts anti-mutagenic effects (Polívková *et al* 2010). In addition to perhaps acting as a chemopreventive agent in carcinogenesis in both cancer patients and medical professionals handling anti-cancer medications, lipoic acid (LA) has anti-mutagenic properties (Unal *et al* 2013). We showed that extracts from *Acacia salicina* including phenols, total flavonoids, and sterols considerably reduced the mutagenicity brought on by sodium azide (SA) and 4-nitro-o-phenylenediamine (Chatti *et al* 2011). According to one study, the plant extract from the leaves of *Accacia salicina* contains anti-mutagenic and antioxidant properties (Boubaker *et al* 2011). According to a study by Rashid and colleagues, the mint plant, *Mentha arvensis*, has the greatest phenolic content and demonstrated significant anti-mutagenic action (Rashid *et al* 2023). According to Sharma *et al*, *Glycyrrhiza glabra* root extract possesses anti-mutagenic behavior (Sharma *et al* 2014). The isolated chemicals from *Ajuga bracteosa* have been tested on mice models and have shown anti-mutagenic action, making them potential sources for the development of cancer drugs (Ganaie *et al* 2018).

1.4.7 miRNA regulation

MicroRNAs are short non-coding RNAs (ncRNAs) of about 22 nucleotides in length that post-transcriptionally regulate the expression of genes, particularly mRNAs, by binding between the 5' end (also known as the 'seed') of the miRNA and complementary sequences in target RNAs. They are involved in a number of cellular biological processes (Cai *et al* 2009, Slack and Chinnaiyan 2019). By attaching to the 3′ untranslated region of the primary transcript mRNA, miRNAs can control gene expression at the post-transcriptional stage. The original transcript is cut apart, mRNA degradation is induced, and translational repression occurs as a result of the complementarity between miRNA and mRNA through base pairing (Samec *et al* 2019).

A cancer's ability to spread and become resistant to treatment is fundamentally impacted by the aberrant control of miRNA expression, which is also linked to metastases. Furthermore, cancer stem cells (CSCs), which are multipotent cells with stem-like characteristics, are thought to be regulated by miRNAs. Additionally, in several experimental *in vivo*/*in vitro* research as well as in clinical trials, the protective effects of phytochemicals such as curcumin, resveratrol, sulforaphane, epigallocatechin-3 gallate, genistein, ellagic acid, and indole-3 carbinol were highlighted. In order to increase the efficacy of cancer treatment, phytochemicals are predicted to have therapeutic applications in conjunction with conventional medicine. On the other hand, several phytochemicals and vital minerals with possible cancer-promoting effects can control specific pathways promoting carcinogenesis by upregulating oncomiRNAs. Human diets typically contain these organic substances and dietary elements linked to the development of cancer. It is, therefore, necessary to learn how they interact with epigenetic mechanisms, such as miRNAs that express themselves abnormally (Samec *et al* 2019). Effects of various phytochemicals as miRNA regulators in cancer are discussed in chapter 3 in more detail.

A summary of various phytochemicals and their mechanism of action as anti-cancer agents studied in published papers is listed in table 1.1.

Chapter 9 focuses on the evolution in the role of different phytochemicals as anti-cancer agents from the past as well as current contribution to the treatment of cancer.

1.5 Purification of anti-cancer phytochemicals

The quality and amount of the active phytoconstituents determine the therapeutic efficacy of any medicinal plant. A plant's many components may have varying degrees of pharmacological action. The pharmacological action could not be caused by the purified component but rather by the combined or synergistic effects of the

Table 1.1.

Class	Phytochemical	Cancer	target	Result	References
Polyphenol	EGCG	Prostate cancer	Androgen receptor	Block AR-regulated gene expression and cell growth in human PCa cells	Siddiqui *et al* (2011)
	Resveratrol	Prostate cancer	miRNA	Down-regulated oncogenic miRs and up-regulated tumor suppressor miRs in PCa cells	Dhar *et al* (2011)
	Quercetin	Colorectal or PPC1 prostate cancer cells	p^{53}	Synergistically potentiated the antiproliferative activity of DNA-damaging drugs	Samuel *et al* (2012)
	Quercetin, apigenin, emodin, rhein	Leukaemia	caspases 3, 8 and 9	inhibition of cell proliferation, cell cycle arrest and induction of apoptosis.	Mahbub *et al* (2015)
	Curcumin	Acute myeloid leukemia	DNA	DNA damage, cell viability, cell cycle, and apoptosis	Papież (2013)
	Fisetin, quercetin, and (−)-catechin	Breast cancer	DNA	Potent ATR/ATM inhibition	Kuo *et al* (2016)
	Fisetin	Osteosarcoma	Cell cycle regulator	Cell cycle arrest	Ferreira de *et al* (2018)
Alkaloids	Bisbenzylisoquinoline	Ovarian cancer	Caspases 3/7	Cytotoxicity effects and apoptosis induction	Uche *et al* (2016)
	Cathachunine	Leukemia	Intrinsic apoptotic pathway	Induction of apoptosis	Wang *et al* (2016)
	Rohitukine	A549 cell line (Lung cancer)	p53, caspase9 and Bcl-2 protein	Induction of apoptosis	Safia *et al* (2015)
	Trisphaeridine and pretazettine	Tumor cell	P-glycoprotein	Induction of apoptosis	Zupko *et al* (2009)
	Cryptolepine	Tumor cell	Topoisomerase II and microtubule	Induce cytotoxicity in tumor cell	Laryea *et al* (2009)

(*Continued*)

Table 1.1. (*Continued*)

Class	Phytochemical	Cancer	target	Result	References
	Cryptolepine	Lung cancer	p53 and p21	Cell cycle alteration and cell death in	Zhu and Gooderham (2006)
	Brucine	LoVo cells	Cell cycle kinase and factors	Induces G1 phase arrest and apoptosis	Zheng *et al* (2013)
	Monoterpene bisindole	Colon cancer	Apoptotic factors	Apoptosis inducers	Mansoor *et al* (2013)
	scutebarbatine A	Lung cancer	Apoptotic factors	Mitochondria-mediated apoptosis	Yang *et al* (2014)
	Oxymatrine	Breast cancer	Bax and Bcl-2	Mitochondria-mediated apoptosis.	Lin *et al* (2016)
	Oxymatrine	Lung cancer	Bax and Bcl-2	Inhibited cell proliferation by inducing apoptosis	Wang *et al* (2015)
	Jerantinine B	Cancer	Polo-like kinase 1	Significantly arrested cells at the G2/M cell cycle phase, potently inhibiting tubulin polymerization	Qazzaz *et al* (2016)
Terpenoids	Auraptene	Cervical and Ovarian Cancer	Matrix Metalloproteinasas 2 and 9 Activity	Inhibits Migration and Invasion of tumor cell	Jamialahmadi *et al* (2018)
	Citrus auraptene	Colorectal	Aberrant crypt foci (ACF) and β -catenin-accumulated crypt	Lowered cell proliferation activity and increased apoptotic cells	Hayashi *et al* (2007)
	D-limonene	Leukemia	bcl-2, p53 and bax	Inhibit cell growth and induce apoptosis	Guo *et al* (2006)
	Carvacrol	Colon cancer	MMP-2 and MMP-9	Inhibits proliferation and induces apoptosis	Fan *et al* (2015)
	β-Elemene	Melanoma	Plasminogen activator, receptor MMP-2, and MMP-9	Inhibits proliferation and induces apoptosis	Shi *et al* (2014)
	β-Caryophyllene	Melanoma	CCL19/21-CCR7 axis	Inhibits solid tumor growth	Jung *et al* (2015)
	Sesquiterpene Lactones	leukemia	Anti-apoptotic Bcl-2, caspase and cytochrome c	Induce cell apoptosis in tumor cell	Estévez-Sarmiento *et al* (2020)
	Oleanolic acid Ursolic	Melanoma	Cell cycle factors	Anti-proliferative activity	Caunii *et al* (2017)

Organosulfur compounds	Sulforaphane	Breast cancer	Epigenetic Repression of hTERT Expression	Significantly inhibits the viability and proliferation	Meeran, *et al* (2010)
	Isothiocyanates	Colorectal cancer	miRNA-155, miR-23b, miR-27b	Inhibit development of CRC i	Slaby *et al* (2013)
	Sulforaphane	Cervical cancer	DNMT3B and HDAC1	Inhibit tumor development	Khan *et al* (2015)
	Sulforaphane	Liver cancer	Histone deacetylases enzyme	Cell cycle arrest, apoptosis, DNA damage, and suppression of proliferation	Dos Santos *et al* (2020)
	Crucifera sulforaphane	Nasopharyngeal carcinoma	DNA methyltransferase 1 (DNMT1)/Wnt inhibitory factor-1 (WIF1) axis	Inhibits the growth of tumor	Chen *et al* (2019)
	Diallyl disulfide	Osteosarcoma	miR-134	Suppresses cell proliferation and invasion	Li *et al* (2019)
	Diallyl thiosulfinate	Multiple myeloma	miR-127–3p	Inhibit the proliferation of side population cells	He *et al* (2021)
	Diallyl disulfide	Gastric cancer	miR-22 and miR-200b	Suppresses proliferation and induces apoptosis	Tang *et al* (2013)
	Benzyl isothiocyanate	Bladder cancer	miR-99a	Prevent cancer progression	Tsai *et al* (2020)
	Phenethyl isothiocyanate	Prostate cancer	P21 promoter & histone deacetylases	Induces growth arrest and apoptosis in tumor cell	Wang *et al* (2008)
Nitrogen-containing compounds	Podophyllotoxin derivatives	Tumor cell	Cell cycle	Effective inhibitory activity in tumor cell	Yin *et al* (2023)
	Pyrazole and pyrazolo [1,5-a] pyrimidine	—	CDK2	Apoptotic activity	Ali *et al* (2019)
	Thieno [2,3-d] pyrimidine derivatives	Cancer cell	Topoisomerase II	Arrest the cell cycle, and induce apoptosis	El-Metwally *et al* (2020)
	Thieno[2,3-d] pyrimidine analogs	Tumors	Purine nucleotide biosynthesis pathway	Inhibit the growth of tumor cell	Wallace-Povirk *et al* (2021)
	4-Amino-thieno [2, 3-d] pyrimidine-6-carboxylates	Breast cancer	Tyrosine kinase receptors	Antiproliferative activity	Mavrova *et al* (2022)

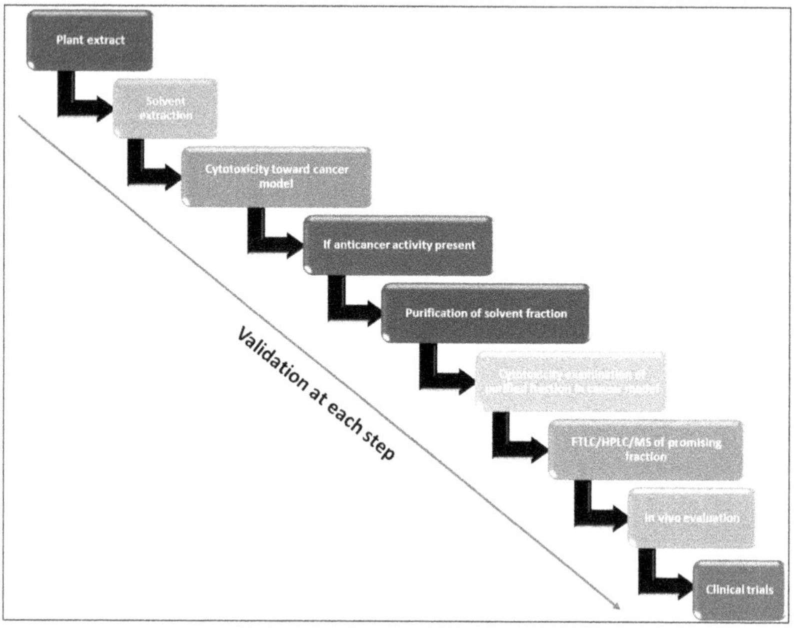

Figure 1.6. A schematic representation of phytochemical extraction, purification, evaluation for anti-cancer activity, and clinical trial.

bioactive phytoconstituents. It takes a lot of work to develop these bioactive phytoconstituents into anti-cancer therapeutics. Purification methods for these phytochemicals with pharmacological activity are numerous. These include bio-assay-guided fractionation, combinatorial chemistry, and isolation and assay. The separation of bioactive phytochemicals from a mixture of substances using various analytical techniques based on biological activity testing is known as bioassay-guided fractionation. Testing of a natural extract with known bioactivity kicks off the procedure. The active extract is separated on the appropriate matrices, the eluted fractions are checked for bioactivity, and the active fractions are then investigated using a variety of analytical methods. A schematic representation of phytochemical extraction, purification, evaluation for anti-cancer activity, and clinical trial is shown in figure 1.6. Molecule(s) must first be purified before being tested *in vivo* for anti-cancer properties. If the molecule successfully kills a tumor, other factors, such as safety and side effects, dose concentration, pharmacokinetics, medication interactions, etc, must be investigated for the drug molecule (Singh *et al* 2016). An overview of phytochemicals under clinical trials for various cancers is discussed in chapter 10 and how to screen the possible phytochemicals against cancer by structure-based docking studies is provided in chapter 11.

1.6 Conclusion and future prospective

These physiologically active substances are categorized into five main groups: phenolics, carotenoids, organosulfur compounds, compounds containing nitrogen, and alkaloids. They are well-known for their potential health advantages in the prevention of numerous diseases, including cancer. Numerous epidemiological studies in several cancers, the majority of which were based on a diet high in plants, have demonstrated the potent anti-cancer effect of phytochemicals. However, because of toxicity and bioavailability restrictions, the powerful anti-cancer potential seen in a number of *in vitro* studies cannot be replicated *in vivo* in humans (Rudzińska *et al* 2023). As specifics were disputed in this investigation, the emphasis was solely on finding new anti-cancer medications or inventive treatment tactics and regimens against distinct malignancies. In order to evaluate the specific structural kinds and mechanistic action for the development of novel anti-cancer drugs, a variety of naturally occurring bioactive chemicals and metabolites can be researched and explored. There is no substitute for green cancer medicines that don't have any side effects, even if the process of discovering new pharmaceuticals, which comprises chemical isolation, characterization, and biological activity determination as well as preclinical and clinical trials, is time-consuming and expensive.

This review's objective is to call attention to the potency of plants as anti-cancer agents and to draw the conclusion that most research in this field never moves past the first phases, failing to realize the full potential of these plants and their therapeutic importance at the molecular level. Only a few researchers are now conducting clinical trials as well as *in vivo* tests. Some individuals are concerned about the toxicity and safety of medicinal and herbal plants despite the fact that they provide a wide range of important benefits. In other cases, a plant may have certain parts that are poisonous but others that are edible, making some medicinal plants potentially harmful to sensitive persons or causing allergies. As a result, any medicinal or herbal plant must undergo a toxicological study in order to detect potential adverse effects and determine the maximum exposure levels at which they are likely to appear. Major detrimental health impacts could result from underestimating the toxicological challenges brought on by taking drugs made from medicinal plants (Rizwanullah *et al* 2018). Now, several methods have been created to work past these limitations. According to recent studies, chemically modifying phytochemicals can boost their efficiency while reducing some of their downsides. It has been shown that several combinations of phytochemical compositions are more potent than traditional treatments. Additionally, it has been asserted that phytochemicals delivered as nanoparticles are substantially more efficient. A thorough analysis of their utility, method of action in pathway regulation, application, and associated challenges is required. Combining phytochemicals with chemotherapeutic medicines is a novel and promising treatment strategy that tries to target crosstalk between multiple signals cascades to limit chemoresistance and reduce carcinogenic features (Zheng *et al* 2022). A significant obstacle to currently available chemotherapeutic treatments is drug-associated toxicity. However, using natural substances to prevent cancer may lessen the related harm. However, the main issue with the majority of naturally occurring chemopreventive drugs is their bioavailability (Ranjan *et al* 2019).

To more effectively treat and manage cancer, medication and drug delivery system development is being pushed by nanotechnology. The development of phytochemical-based drug delivery by various kinds of nanomaterials is discussed in chapter 13 in detail and the potential role of nano-phytochemical in breast cancer treatment is provided in chapter 14.

Acknowledgments

The author thanks their organization for providing infrastructure facilities for writing this chapter.

References

Ali G M, Ibrahim D A, Elmetwali A M and Ismail N S 2019 Design, synthesis and biological evaluation of certain CDK2 inhibitors based on pyrazole and pyrazolo [1,5-a] pyrimidine scaffold with apoptotic activity *Bioorg. Chem.* **86** 1–4

Bhosale P B, Ha S E, Vetrivel P, Kim H H, Kim S M and Kim G S 2020 Functions of polyphenols and its anticancer properties in biomedical research: a narrative review *Transl. Cancer Res.* **9** 7619

Biswas P *et al* 2022 A comprehensive analysis and anti-cancer activities of quercetin in ROS-mediated cancer and cancer stem cells *Int. J. Mol. Sci.* **23** 11746

Bommareddy A, VanWert A L, McCune D F, Brozena S L, Witczak Z and Singh S V 2016 The role of organosulfur compounds derived from Allium vegetables in cancer prevention and therapy *Critical Dietary Factors in Cancer Chemoprevention* (Cham: Springer) pp 111–52

Boubaker J, Mansour H B, Ghedira K and Chekir-Ghedira L 2011 Antimutagenic and free radical scavenger effects of leaf extracts from *Accacia salicina Ann. Clin. Microbiol. Antimicrob* **10** 1–0

Briguglio G, Costa C, Pollicino M, Giambo F, Catania S and Fenga C 2020 Polyphenols in cancer prevention: new insights *Int. J. Funct. Nutr.* **1** 1

Cai Y, Yu X, Hu S and Yu J 2009 A brief review on the mechanisms of miRNA regulation *Genom. Proteom. Bioinform* **7** 147–54

Catalano E 2016 Role of phytochemicals in the chemoprevention of tumors *arXiv Preprint* arXiv:1605.04519

Caunii A *et al* 2017 Effects of ursolic and oleanolic on SK-MEL-2 melanoma cells: *in vitro* and *in vivo* assays *Int. J. Oncol.* **51** 1651–60

Chatti I B, Boubaker J, Skandrani I, Bhouri W, Ghedira K and Ghedira L C 2011 Antioxidant and antigenotoxic activities in *Acacia salicina* extracts and its protective role against DNA strand scission induced by hydroxyl radical *Food Chem. Toxicol.* **49** 1753–8

Chen L *et al* 2019 Crucifera sulforaphane (SFN) inhibits the growth of nasopharyngeal carcinoma through DNA methyltransferase 1 (DNMT1)/Wnt inhibitory factor 1 (WIF1) axis *Phytomedicine.* **63** 153058

Chikara S, Nagaprashantha L D, Singhal J, Horne D, Awasthi S and Singhal S S 2018 Oxidative stress and dietary phytochemicals: role in cancer chemoprevention and treatment *Cancer Lett.* **413** 122–34

Chirumbolo S, Bjørklund G, Lysiuk R, Vella A, Lenchyk L and Upyr T 2018 Targeting cancer with phytochemicals via their fine tuning of the cell survival signaling pathways *Int. J. Mol. Sci.* **19** 3568

Chopra B, Dhingra A K, Dhar K L and Nepali K 2021 Emerging role of terpenoids for the treatment of cancer: a review *Mini Rev. Med. Chem.* **21** 2300–36

Choudhari A S, Mandave P C, Deshpande M, Ranjekar P and Prakash O 2020 Phytochemicals in cancer treatment: from preclinical studies to clinical practice *Front. Pharmacol* **10** 1614
Chun K S, Raut P K, Kim D H and Surh Y J 2021 Role of chemopreventive phytochemicals in NRF2-mediated redox homeostasis in humans *Free Radical Biol. Med.* **172** 699–715
Das S 2002 Garlic—a natural source of cancer preventive compounds *Asian Pac. J. Cancer Prev.* **3** 305–11
Debnath B, Singh W S, Das M, Goswami S, Singh M K, Maiti D and Manna K 2018 Role of plant alkaloids on human health: a review of biological activities *Mater. Today Chem.* **9** 56–72
Dhar S, Hicks C and Levenson A S 2011 Resveratrol and prostate cancer: promising role for microRNAs *Mol. Nutr. Food Res.* **55** 1219–29
Dhyani P *et al* 2022 Anticancer potential of alkaloids: a key emphasis to colchicine, vinblastine, vincristine, vindesine, vinorelbine and vincamine *Cancer Cell Int.* **22** 1–20
Dos Santos P W, Machado A R, De Grandis R A, Ribeiro D L, Tuttis K, Morselli M, Aissa A F, Pellegrini M and Antunes L M 2020 Transcriptome and DNA methylation changes modulated by sulforaphane induce cell cycle arrest, apoptosis, DNA damage, and suppression of proliferation in human liver cancer cells *Food Chem. Toxicol.* **136** 111047
El-Metwally S A, Khalil A K and El-Sayed W M 2020 Design, molecular modeling and anticancer evaluation of thieno [2, 3-d] pyrimidine derivatives as inhibitors of topoisomerase II *Bioorg. Chem.* **94** 103492
Estévez-Sarmiento F, Saavedra E, Ruiz-Estévez M, León F, Quintana J, Brouard I and Estévez F 2020 Chlorinated guaiane-type sesquiterpene lactones as cytotoxic agents against human tumor cells *Int. J. Mol. Sci.* **21** 9767
Fan K, Li X, Cao Y, Qi H, Li L, Zhang Q and Sun H 2015 Carvacrol inhibits proliferation and induces apoptosis in human colon cancer cells *Anti-Cancer Drugs* **26** 813–23
Fatma H, Jameel M and Siddique H R 2023 An update on phytochemicals in redox homeostasis:'virtuous or evil' in cancer chemoprevention? *Chemistry* **5** 201–22
Ferreira de Oliveira J M, Pacheco A R, Coutinho L, Oliveira H, Pinho S, Almeida L, Fernandes E and Santos C 2018 Combination of etoposide and fisetin results in anti-cancer efficiency against osteosarcoma cell models *Arch. Toxicol.* **92** 1205–14
Floor S L, Dumont J E, Maenhaut C and Raspe E 2012 Hallmarks of cancer: of all cancer cells, all the time? *Trends Mol. Med.* **18** 509–15
Fouad Y A and Aanei C 2017 Revisiting the hallmarks of cancer *Am. J. Cancer Res.* **7** 1016
Ganaie H A, Ali M N, Ganai B A and Bashir S 2018 Antimutagenic activity of compounds isolated from *Ajuga bracteosa* wall ex. benth against EMS-induced mutagenicity in mice *Toxicol. Rep.* **5** 108–12
George B P, Chandran R and Abrahamse H 2021 Role of phytochemicals in cancer chemoprevention: insights *Antioxidants.* **10** 1455
Goncharov N, Orekhov A N, Voitenko N, Ukolov A, Jenkins R and Avdonin P 2016 Organosulfur compounds as nutraceuticals *Nutraceuticals* (New York: Academic) pp 555–68
González-Vallinas M, González-Castejón M, Rodríguez-Casado A and Ramírez de Molina A 2013 Dietary phytochemicals in cancer prevention and therapy: a complementary approach with promising perspectives *Nutr. Rev.* **71** 585–99
Guo X M, Lu Q, Liu Z J, Wang L F and Feng B A 2006 Effects of D-limonene on leukemia cells HL-60 and K562 *in vitro Zhongguo Shi Yan Xue Ye Xue Za Zhi* **14** 692–5
Hanahan D and Weinberg R A 2011 Hallmarks of cancer: the next generation *Cell* **144** 646–74

Hanahan D 2022 Hallmarks of cancer: new dimensions *Cancer Discov.* **12** 31–46

Hayashi K, Suzuki R, Miyamoto S, Shin-Ichiroh Y, Kohno H, Sugie S, Takashima S and Tanaka T 2007 Citrus auraptene suppresses azoxymethane-induced colonic preneoplastic lesions in C57BL/KsJ-db/db mice *Nutr. Cancer* **58** 75–84

He W, Fu Y, Zheng Y, Wang X, Liu B and Zeng J 2021 Diallyl thiosulfinate enhanced the anti-cancer activity of dexamethasone in the side population cells of multiple myeloma by promoting miR-127-3p and deactivating the PI3K/AKT signaling pathway *BMC Cancer* **21** 1–0

Herman-Antosiewicz A, Powolny A A and Singh S V 2007 Molecular targets of cancer chemoprevention by garlic-derived organosulfides 1 *Acta Pharmacol. Sin.* **28** 1355–64

Huang G, Drakopoulos A, Saedtler M, Zou H, Meinel L, Heilmann J and Decker M 2017 Cytotoxic properties of the alkaloid rutaecarpine and its oligocyclic derivatives and chemical modifications to enhance water-solubility *Bioorgan. Med. Chem. Lett.* **27** 4937–41

Jain H, Dhingra N, Narsinghani T and Sharma R 2016 Insights into the mechanism of natural terpenoids as NF-κB inhibitors: an overview on their anticancer potential *Exp. Oncol.* **38** 158–68

Jamialahmadi K, Salari S, Alamolhodaei N S, Avan A, Gholami L and Karimi G 2018 Auraptene inhibits migration and invasion of cervical and ovarian cancer cells by repression of matrix metalloproteinasas 2 and 9 activity *J. Pharmacopuncture* **21** 177

Jung J I *et al* 2015 β-Caryophyllene potently inhibits solid tumor growth and lymph node metastasis of B16F10 melanoma cells in high-fat diet–induced obese C57BL/6N mice *Carcinogenesis* **36** 1028–39

Kamran S, Sinniah A, Abdulghani M A and Alshawsh M A 2022 Therapeutic potential of certain terpenoids as anticancer agents: a scoping review *Cancers* **14** 1100

Khan H, Alam W, Alsharif K F, Aschner M, Pervez S and Saso L 2022 Alkaloids and colon cancer: molecular mechanisms and therapeutic implications for cell cycle arrest *Molecules* **27** 920

Khan M A *et al* 2015 Sulforaphane reverses the expression of various tumor suppressor genes by targeting DNMT3B and HDAC1 in human cervical cancer cells *Evid. Based Complement. Alternat. Med.* **2015** 412149

Khattak S and Khan H 2016 Anti-cancer potential of phyto-alkaloids: a prospective review *Curr. Cancer Therap. Rev.* **12** 66–75

Kłos P and Chlubek D 2022 Plant-Derived Terpenoids: a promising tool in the fight against melanoma *Cancers* **14** 502

Kotecha R, Takami A and Espinoza J L 2016 Dietary phytochemicals and cancer chemo-prevention: a review of the clinical evidence *Oncotarget* **7** 52517

Kuo C Y, Zupkó I, Chang F R, Hunyadi A, Wu C C, Weng T S and Wang H C 2016 Dietary flavonoid derivatives enhance chemotherapeutic effect by inhibiting the DNA damage response pathway *Toxicol. Appl. Pharmacol.* **311** 99–105

Lang D K, Kaur R, Arora R, Saini B and Arora S 2020 Nitrogen-containing heterocycles as anticancer agents: an overview *Anti-Cancer Agents Med. Chem. (Formerly Current Medicinal Chemistry-Anti-Cancer Agents)* **20** 2150–68

Laryea D, Isaksson A, Wright C W, Larsson R and Nygren P 2009 Characterization of the cytotoxic activity of the indoloquinoline alkaloid cryptolepine in human tumour cell lines and primary cultures of tumour cells from patients *Invest. New Drugs* **27** 402–11

Li Y, Wang Z, Li J and Sang X 2019 Diallyl disulfide suppresses FOXM1-mediated proliferation and invasion in osteosarcoma by upregulating miR-134 *J. Cell. Biochem.* **120** 7286–96

Lin B, Li D and Zhang L 2016 Oxymatrine mediates Bax and Bcl-2 expression in human breast cancer MCF-7 cells *Pharmazie* **71** 154–7

Liu R H 2013 Health-promoting components of fruits and vegetables in the diet *Adv. Nutr.* **4** 384S–92S

Loo G 2003 Redox-sensitive mechanisms of phytochemical-mediated inhibition of cancer cell proliferation *J. Nutr. BioChem.* **14** 64–73

Luo M, Zhou L, Huang Z, Li B, Nice E C, Xu J and Huang C 2022 Antioxidant therapy in cancer: rationale and progress *Antioxidants.* **11** 1128

Mahbub A A, Le Maitre C L, Haywood-Small S L, Cross N A and Jordan-Mahy N 2015 Polyphenols act synergistically with doxorubicin and etoposide in leukaemia cell lines *Cell Death Dis.* **1** 1–2

Mansoor T A, Borralho P M, Dewanjee S, Mulhovo S, Rodrigues C M and Ferreira M J 2013 Monoterpene bisindole alkaloids, from the African medicinal plant Tabernaemontana elegans, induce apoptosis in HCT116 human colon carcinoma cells *J. Ethnopharmacol.* **149** 463–70

Mavrova A, Dimov S, Sulikovska I, Yancheva D, Iliev I, Tsoneva I, Staneva G and Nikolova B 2022 Design, cytotoxicity and antiproliferative activity of 4-amino-5-methyl-thieno [2,3-d] pyrimidine-6-carboxylates against MFC-7 and MDA-MB-231 breast cancer cell lines *Molecules* **27** 3314

Meeran S M, Patel S N and Tollefsbol T O 2010 Sulforaphane causes epigenetic repression of hTERT expression in human breast cancer cell lines *PLoS One* **5** e11457

Meybodi N M, Mortazavian A M, Monfared A B, Sohrabvandi S and Meybodi F A 2017 Phytochemicals in cancer prevention: a review of the evidence *Iran. J. Cancer Prev.* **10** e7219

Mondal A, Gandhi A, Fimognari C, Atanasov A G and Bishayee A 2019 Alkaloids for cancer prevention and therapy: current progress and future perspectives *Eur. J. Pharmacol.* **858** 172472

Moriarty R M, Naithani R and Surve B 2007 Organosulfur compounds in cancer chemoprevention *Mini Rev. Med. Chem.* **7** 827–38

Naeem A, Hu P, Yang M, Zhang J, Liu Y, Zhu W and Zheng Q 2022 Natural products as anticancer agents: current status and future perspectives *Molecules* **27** 8367

Omar S H and Al-Wabel N A 2010 Organosulfur compounds and possible mechanism of garlic in cancer *Saudi Pharm.* J **18** 51–8

Pandey P, Khan F, Alshammari N, Saeed A, Aqil F and Saeed M 2023 Updates on the anticancer potential of garlic organosulfur compounds and their nanoformulations: plant therapeutics in cancer management *Front. Pharmacol.* **14** 1154034

Papiez M A 2013 The influence of curcumin on the action of etoposide in a rat acute myeloidleukemia cell line *Folia Med. Crac.* **53** 61–72

Pavlova N N and Thompson C B 2016 The emerging hallmarks of cancer metabolism *Cell Metab.* **23** 27–47

Pehlivan F E 2021 Diet-Epigenome interactions: epi-drugs modulating the epigenetic machinery during cancer prevention *Epigenetics to Optogenetics: A New Paradigm in the Study of Biology* (London: IntechOpen)

Polívková Z, Šmerák P, Demová H and Houška M 2010 Antimutagenic effects of lycopene and tomato purée *J. Med. Food* **13** 1443–50

Qazzaz M E, Raja V J, Lim K H, Kam T S, Lee J B, Gershkovich P and Bradshaw T D 2016 In vitro anticancer properties and biological evaluation of novel natural alkaloid jerantinine B *Cancer Lett.* **370** 185–97

Rabi T and Gupta S 2008 Dietary terpenoids and prostate cancer chemoprevention *Front. Biosci: A J. Virtual Libr.* **13** 3457

Rahman M A, Hannan M A, Dash R, Rahman M H, Islam R, Uddin M J, Sohag A A, Rahman M H and Rhim H 2021 Phytochemicals as a complement to cancer chemotherapy: pharmacological modulation of the autophagy-apoptosis pathway *Front. Pharmacol.* **12** 639628

Rampogu S, Balasubramaniyam T and Lee J H 2022 Phytotherapeutic applications of alkaloids in treating breast cancer *Biomed. Pharmacother.* **155** 113760

Ranjan A, Ramachandran S, Gupta N, Kaushik I, Wright S, Srivastava S, Das H, Srivastava S, Prasad S and Srivastava S K 2019 Role of phytochemicals in cancer prevention *Int. J. Mol. Sci.* **20** 4981

Rashid W, Asim S, Rashid S, Rafique S, Aziz R S, Iftikhar S, Rashid M and Arfat Y 2023 Antioxidant and anti-mutagenic potential of mint (*Mentha arvensis*) and its chemical characterization by HPLC *Pakistan J. Med. Health Sci.* **17** 514

Rizeq B, Gupta I, Ilesanmi J, AlSafran M, Rahman M M and Ouhtit A 2020 The power of phytochemicals combination in cancer chemoprevention *J. Cancer* **11** 4521

Rizwanullah M, Amin S, Mir S R, Fakhri K U and Rizvi M M 2018 Phytochemical based nanomedicines against cancer: current status and future prospects *J. Drug Target.* **26** 731–52

Rudzińska A, Juchaniuk P, Oberda J, Wiśniewska J, Wojdan W, Szklener K and Mańdziuk S 2023 Phytochemicals in cancer treatment and cancer prevention—review on epidemiological data and clinical trials *Nutrients* **15** 1896

Safia K M, Jadiya P, Sheikh S, Haque E, Nazir A, Lakshmi V and Mir S S 2015 The chromone alkaloid, rohitukine, affords anti-cancer activity via modulating apoptosis pathways in A549 cell line and yeast mitogen activated protein kinase (MAPK) pathway *PLoS One* **10** e0137991

Samec M *et al* 2019 The role of dietary phytochemicals in the carcinogenesis via the modulation of miRNA expression *J. Cancer Res. Clin. Oncol.* **145** 1665–79

Samuel T, Fadlalla K, Mosley L, Katkoori V, Turner T and Manne U 2012 Dual-mode interaction between quercetin and DNA-damaging drugs in cancer cells *Anticancer Res.* **32** 61–71

Sharma S H, Thulasingam S and Nagarajan S 2017 Terpenoids as anti-colon cancer agents–A comprehensive review on its mechanistic perspectives *Eur. J. Pharmacol.* **795** 169–78

Sharma V, Agrawal R C and Shrivastava V K 2014 Assessment of median lethal dose and anti-mutagenic effects of *Glycyrrhiza glabra* root extract against chemically induced micronucleus formation in Swiss albino mice *Int. J. Basic Clin. Pharmacol.* **3** 292–7

Shi H, Liu L, Liu L, Geng J, Zhou Y and Chen L 2014 β-Elemene inhibits the metastasis of B16F10 melanoma cells by downregulation of the expression of uPA, uPAR, MMP-2, and MMP-9 *Melanoma Res.* **24** 99–107

Siddiqui I A, Asim M, Hafeez B B, Adhami V M, Tarapore R S and Mukhtar H 2011 Green tea polyphenol EGCG blunts androgen receptor function in prostate cancer *FASEB J.* **25** 1198

Siegel R L, Miller K D, Wagle N S and Jemal A 2023 Cancer statistics, 2023 *CA: Cancer J. Clin.* **73** 17–48

Singh S, Sharma B, Kanwar S S and Kumar A 2016 Lead phytochemicals for anticancer drug development *Front. Plant Sci.* **7** 1667

Slaby O *et al* 2013 Identification of microRNAs regulated by isothiocyanates and association of polymorphisms inside their target sites with risk of sporadic colorectal cancer *Nutr. Cancer* **65** 247–54

Slack F J and Chinnaiyan A M 2019 The role of non-coding RNAs in oncology *Cell* **179** 1033–55

Sohel M, Aktar S, Biswas P, Amin M A, Hossain M A, Ahmed N, Mim M I, Islam F and Mamun A A 2023 Exploring the anti-cancer potential of dietary phytochemicals for the patients with breast cancer: a comprehensive review *Cancer Med.* **12** 14556–83

Sundaram M K, Khan M A, Alalami U, Somvanshi P, Bhardwaj T, Pramodh S, Raina R, Shekfeh Z, Haque S and Hussain A 2020 Phytochemicals induce apoptosis by modulation of nitric oxide signaling pathway in cervical cancer cells *Eur. Rev. Med. Pharmacol. Sci.* **24** 11827–44

Tang H, Kong Y, Guo J, Tang Y, Xie X, Yang L, Su Q and Xie X 2013 Diallyl disulfide suppresses proliferation and induces apoptosis in human gastric cancer through Wnt-1 signaling pathway by up-regulation of miR-200b and miR-22 *Cancer Lett.* **340** 72–81

Thakur V S, Deb G, Babcook M A and Gupta S 2014 Plant phytochemicals as epigenetic modulators: role in cancer chemoprevention *AAPS J.* **16** 151–63

Tilaoui M, Ait Mouse H and Zyad A 2021 Update and new insights on future cancer drug candidates from plant-based alkaloids *Front. Pharmacol.* **12** 719694

Tsai T F, Chen P C, Lin Y C, Chou K Y, Chen H E, Ho C Y, Lin J F and Hwang T I 2020 Benzyl isothiocyanate promotes miR-99a expression through ERK/AP-1-dependent pathway in bladder cancer cells *Environ. Toxicol.* **35** 47–54

Uche F I, Drijfhout F P, McCullagh J, Richardson A and Li W W 2016 Cytotoxicity effects and apoptosis induction by bisbenzylisoquinoline alkaloids from *Triclisia subcordata Phytother. Res.* **30** 1533–9

Unal F, Taner G, Yuzbasioglu D and Yilmaz S 2013 Antigenotoxic effect of lipoic acid against mitomycin-C in human lymphocyte cultures *Cytotechnology* **65** 553–65

Vargas-Mendoza N *et al* 2022 Phytochemicals and modulation of exercise-induced oxidative stress: a novel overview of antioxidants *Am. J. Transl. Res.* **14** 8292

Wallace-Povirk A *et al* 2021 Discovery of 6-substituted thieno [2,3-d] pyrimidine analogs as dual inhibitors of glycinamide ribonucleotide formyltransferase and 5-aminoimidazole-4-carboxamide ribonucleotide formyltransferase in de novo purine nucleotide biosynthesis in folate receptor expressing human tumors *Bioorg. Med. Chem.* **37** 116093

Wang B, Han Q and Zhu Y 2015 Oxymatrine inhibited cell proliferation by inducing apoptosis in human lung cancer A549 cells *Bio-Med. Mater. Eng.* **26** S165–72

Wang L G, Liu X M, Fang Y, Dai W, Chiao F B, Puccio G M, Feng J, Liu D and Chiao J W 2008 De-repression of the p21 promoter in prostate cancer cells by an isothiocyanate via inhibition of HDACs and c-Myc *Int. J. Oncol.* **33** 375–80

Wang X D *et al* 2016 Induction of apoptosis in human leukemia cells through an intrinsic pathway by cathachunine, a unique alkaloid isolated from *Catharanthus roseus Phytomedicine* **23** 641–53

Wani A K *et al* 2023 Targeting apoptotic pathway of cancer cells with phytochemicals and plant-based nanomaterials *Biomolecules* **13** 194

Xiao D, Pinto J T, Gundersen G G and Weinstein I B 2005 Effects of a series of organosulfur compounds on mitotic arrest and induction of apoptosis in colon cancer cells *Mol. Cancer Ther.* **4** 1388–98

Yang X K, Xu M Y, Xu G S, Zhang Y L and Xu Z X 2014 *In vitro* and *in vivo* antitumor activity of scutebarbatine A on human lung carcinoma A549 cell lines *Molecules* **19** 8740–51

Yin M *et al* 2023 Synthesis and anticancer activity of podophyllotoxin derivatives with nitrogen-containing heterocycles *Front. Chem.* **11** 1191498

Zahin M, Ahmad I, Gupta R C and Aqil F 2014 Punicalagin and ellagic acid demonstrate antimutagenic activity and inhibition of benzo [a] pyrene induced DNA adducts *BioMed Res. Int.* **2014** 467465

Zheng L, Wang X, Luo W, Zhan Y and Zhang Y 2013 Brucine, an effective natural compound derived from nux-vomica, induces G1 phase arrest and apoptosis in LoVo cells *Food Chem. Toxicol.* **58** 332–9

Zheng Z, Zhang L and Hou X 2022 Potential roles and molecular mechanisms of phytochemicals against cancer *Food Funct.* **13** 9208–25

Zhou Y, Zheng J, Li Y, Xu D P, Li S, Chen Y M and Li H B 2016 Natural polyphenols for prevention and treatment of cancer *Nutrients* **8** 515

Zhu H and Gooderham N J 2006 Mechanisms of induction of cell cycle arrest and cell death by cryptolepine in human lung adenocarcinoma A549 cells *Toxicol. Sci.* **91** 132–9

Zupko I, Rethy B, Hohmann J, Molnár J, Ocsovszki I and Falkay G 2009 Antitumor activity of alkaloids derived from *Amaryllidaceae* species *In vivo* **23** 41–8

IOP Publishing

Nidhi Puranik, Deepa Yadav and Sangeeta Shukla

Chapter 2

Vitamins: an emerging natural therapeutic drug to prevent cancer

Anushri Sharma, Shiv Kumar Yadav and Nidhi Puranik

The second most common cause of death in the world is cancer. In recent years, conventional methods including surgery, chemotherapy, and radiotherapy have been the primary cancer treatment. On the basis of clinical results of the impacts of dietary sources included in cancer patients' diets, numerous experts from around the world have been examining a substantial correlation between damage caused by oxidation and cancer over the last few decades. Various scientific reports reported that vitamins C, D, and E are mostly responsible for reducing adverse effects from chemotherapy and radiation treatment for malignancies of the lungs, stomach, prostate, colon, gastric, head, and neck. Nowadays, while receiving cancer treatment, people take vitamins as a supplement; some do so to avoid cancer. In this chapter, we discuss the emerging therapeutic drugs to prevent cancer and the most important aspect of vitamins related to cancer prevention and treatment, their natural sources, their roles in the body, and vitamins as important nutrition components.

2.1 Introduction

According to WHO, cancer is a leading cause of death worldwide, accounting for nearly 10 million deaths in 2020 (WHO 2022). Lung, prostate, colon, stomach, and liver cancer are the most common cancers in men, however, breast, colon, lung, cervical, and thyroid cancers occur in women commonly. An estimated 9.6 million people died of cancer worldwide in 2018. 400 000 children are diagnosed with cancer each year, but 30%–50% of these cancers are preventable. Cancer is a set of disorders characterized by unchecked cell growth and proliferation (Yadav *et al* 2022, Kim *et al* 2023). In healthy organisms, cells divide, differentiate, and eventually die in order. The loss of control of cellular growth and development leads to excessive

doi:10.1088/978-0-7503-5252-9ch2

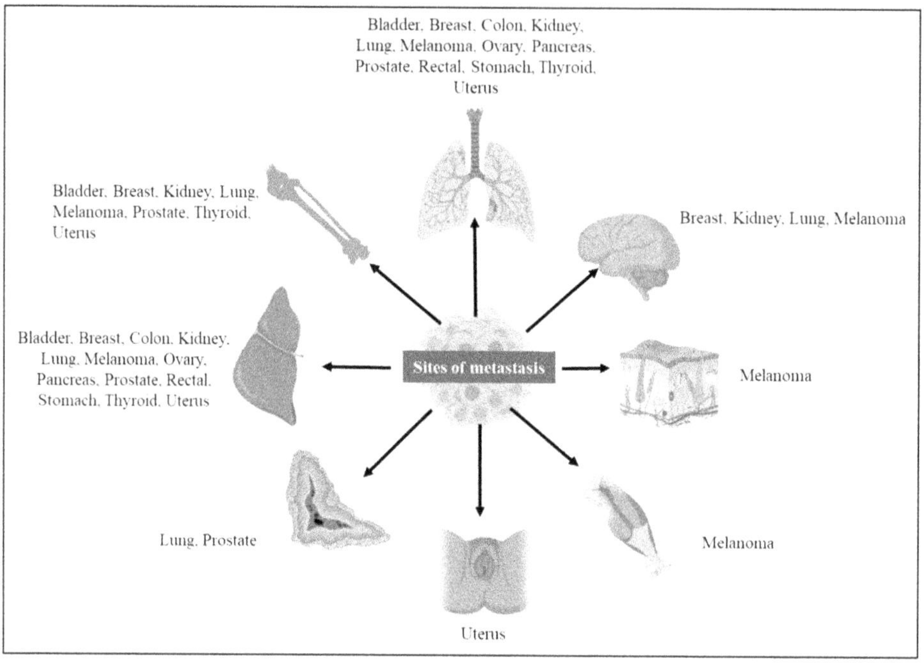

Figure 2.1. Cancer and their major sites of metastasis (organ) (created with BioRender.com).

Table 2.1. Comparison between benign and malignant tumors.

Characteristics	Benign tumors	Malignant tumors
Differentiation	Well-differentiated	Lack differentiation
Growth rate	Slow	Fast
Invasiveness	Absent	Present
Metastasis	Absent	Present

proliferation and spread of cells causing tumors and leads to cancer. Cancer that spreads to parts of the body far from where it started is called metastatic cancer. The most typical locations of metastasis, excluding lymph nodes, for a few prevalent tumors are listed below (figure 2.1).

Tumors are basically of two types—benign tumors and malignant tumors (Ohshika *et al* 2021). A basic comparison of benign and malignant tumors is given in table 2.1. They are often benign tumors that continue to be encased in a layer of connective tissue and increase via expansion. They do not have cancer. Benign tumors can grow anywhere in the body. They have different names depending on their origin, e.g. adenoma is a tumor on or in the gland; lipoma is the most common type of benign tumor where a lipoma forms from fat cells that grow below the skin;

Table 2.2. A list of common anti-cancer drugs and their chemical nature.

S. No.	Anti-cancer drug	Chemical nature
1	Methotrexate	Folic acid analog
2	6-Mercaptopurine	Purine analog
3	Actinomycin-D	Antibiotic
4	Vinblastine and Vincristine	Alkaloids
5	Cisplatin	Platinum compound
6	6-Thioguanine	Purine analog
7	Mitomycin C	Antibiotic

myoma benign tumors grow from smooth muscle, however, leiomyomas often grow in the uterus (or uterine fibroids) or in the digestive tract. Tumors can be diagnosed by CT scan, MRI, mammogram, and x-ray. Surgeries are commonly performed to remove benign tumors. Malignant tumors, unchecked cell proliferation, and metastasis, or the spread of cells to different parts of the body, are characteristics of malignant tumors (Martin *et al* 2013). The list of cancers and the main sites of metastasis are given (figure 2.1). Malignant tumors can develop anywhere on or in the body such as carcinomas including breast, prostate, bladder, lung, and malignant neoplasms of the skin, lung, colon, and rectum. Sarcoma in connective tissue such as bone, cartilage, and tendon. Myeloma is in plasma cells of bone marrow. Leukemia is also called blood cancer. They are cancers of bone marrow. Lymphomas develop in the glands or nodes of the lymphatic system. Surgery, chemotherapy, and radiation therapy are some of the useful methods for the treatment of malignant tumors.

In recent years precautionary measures have been advised to prevent or slow cancer growth. Antioxidants prevent the formation and detoxification of existing free radicals. Antioxidants assist the body to detoxify different carcinogens and boost immunological function. The majority of fruits and vegetables are high in antioxidants. It is advised to increase consumption to avoid cancer.

Vitamins are crucial elements for human metabolism, acting as coenzymes or enzymes in numerous activities that are necessary for the body to function normally. Numerous research that looked at this association over the past few years has shown that vitamins are essential for human health and disease. Today, it is understood that vitamins can play a significant part in both the prevention and treatment of cancer (Mamede *et al* 2011). Among them, some have biochemical perspectives such as antioxidants, namely Vit E, beta-carotene, and Vit C. Table 2.2 shows the list of the most common anti-cancer drugs and their chemical nature.

2.2 Vitamins

Vitamins are organic compounds that the human body requires in a minute amount. The majority of vitamins must be ingested from food due to the fact that the body either does not produce them or manufactures very little of them. For example, humans must get vitamin C from food while dogs can produce all the vitamin C they need. A person does not have enough vitamin D in their diet. The human body synthesizes the vitamin in sunlight and that is the best source of vitamin D. Various vitamins have diverse functions in the human body, and it is essential to consume the appropriate amount of each vitamin to maintain optimal health. There are 15 major vitamins that have diverse biochemical functions.

They are classified on the basis of the solubility of vitamins, vitamins are classified as fat-soluble (A, D, E, and K) vitamins and water-soluble (C and B) vitamins. Table 2.3 represents the basic type, general name, and requirements on a daily basis for normal growth of cells. Vitamin A serves as a controller of cell and tissue expansion and distinction. Vitamin D imitates hormones, controlling mineral metabolism in bones and other organs. The B-complex vitamins function as enzyme coenzyme helpers or their precursors. Vitamins C and E work as antioxidants (Bender 2003). Both underdose and overdose of vitamins may potentially produce medically relevant illness, although it is less likely with an overdose of water-soluble vitamins.

2.3 Vitamins and cancer

It is thought that diet is responsible for nearly a third of all preventable cancers, which is comparable to the amount caused by smoking. Inadequate intake of essential vitamins may explain why those who consume low quantities of fruit and vegetables have elevated chances of cancer occurrence. As such, better dietary choices, taking multivitamins and mineral supplements, and encouraging food fortification to increase vitamin intake may assist in preventing cancer and other chronic conditions. The possibility that high vitamin consumption may offer cancer protection has received a lot of attention in recent years. The cellular mechanisms involved in carcinogenesis are significantly influenced by vitamin A and its equivalents. A large intake of preformed vitamin A does not appear to be relevant for the prevention of cancer, while blood vitamin A levels are closely regulated. In addition to their ability to trap free radicals, the antioxidant vitamins C, E, and beta-carotene may also engage in other biological processes that contribute to their ability to prevent cancer (Van Poppel and Van den Berg 1997). A meta-analysis confirmed that low doses of vitamins A, C, and E can significantly reduce the risk of gastric cancer (Kong *et al* 2014).

2.3.1 Vitamin A and cancer

Retinoids are derivatives of vitamin A and these compounds are composed of four isoprene units and are differentially named depending on the terminal functional group, e.g. retinol (OH), retinal (CHO), and retinoic acid (CO_2H) (Wada 2021). Vitamin A and retinol derivatives have a significant physiological impact on a variety of biological processes, including cell differentiation, proliferation, and death. They play a significant role in oxidative stress and cancer formation as potent antioxidants (Kim *et al* 2021). Animal meals are the source of retinol

Table 2.3. Vitamins and their basic characteristics.

Vitamins	Solubility	RDA	Deficiency disease	Syndrome	Food source
A Retinol Retinal (Vit A aldehyde) Retinoic acid Beta-carotene (provitamin A)	Fat-soluble vitamin	0.7 mg/1 mg	Night blindness Hyperkeratosis keratomalacia	Hypervitaminosis A (dermatitis, enlargement of the liver, decalcified bone, loss of weight, and loss of hair	Egg yolk, liver, kidney, milk, cheese, liver oils, butter, fish, yellow and green vegetables, fruits, carrots, spinach, and pumpkin
B1 Antineuritic Thiamine	Water-soluble vitamin	1–1.5 mg in adults and 0.7–1.2 mg in children	Beri Beri, Wernickle-korsakoff syndrome	Loss of appetite, peripheral neuropathy, Nausea	Pork, whole meal grains, and brown rice green leafy vegetables, yeast, potatoes, liver, eggs
B2 Flavin Riboflavin monophosphate (FNM)	Water-soluble vitamin	1.2 mg/1.7 mg	Ariboflavinosis	Cheilosis, that is, fissures at the corner of the mouth, Glottis	Milk and milk products, cereals, fruits, and fish
B3 Nicotinic acid	Water-soluble vitamin	15 mg/20 mg	Pellegra dementia dermititis	Inflammation of skin, anxiety, irritability	Meat, fish, eggs, and vegetables
B5 Pantothenic acid Panthenol Pantethine	Water-soluble vitamin	5–10 mg	Paresthesia	Peripheral neuropathy 'burning feet syndrome'	Egg, liver, meat, yeast, and milk

(*Continued*)

Table 2.3. (*Continued*)

Vitamins	Solubility	RDA	Deficiency disease	Syndrome	Food source
B_6 Pyridoxine Pyridoxal Pyridoxamine	Water-soluble vitamin	2–2.2 mg/day	Neurological symptoms anemia	Wilson's disease, rheumatoid arthritis	Wheat, corn, cabbage, roots, and tubers
B_7 Vitamin H Anti-egg white injury factor Biotin	Water-soluble vitamin	100–300 mg	Dermatitis, glottis	Anemia, loss of appetite, nausea and may also result in depression, hallucination, and muscle pain	Liver, kidney, yolk, milk, and tomatoes
B_9 Folic acid	Water-soluble vitamin	10–12 mg	Megaloblastic anemia	Neural defects in pregnant women, Abnormally large red blood cells	Whole grains, cereals, liver, kidney, yeast, and eggs
B_{12} Cyanocobalamine Adenosylcobalmine	Water-soluble vitamin	4 μg/days	Pernicious anemia	Autoimmune destruction of gastric parietal calls, dietary deficiency, neural degeneration, and demyelination of the nervous system	Curd, eggs, fish, pork, milk
C Ascorbic acid	Water-soluble vitamin	60–70 mg	Scurvy (pirates' disease)	Stomach pain, diarrhoea	Many fruits and vegetables, liver
D_1	Fat-soluble vitamin	5 mg		Renal rickets Hypervitaminosis D	Exposure to sunlight, Consumption of natural food

Ergocalciferol and cholecalciferol			Rickets (children) osteomalacia (adults)		
E Tocopherols and tocotrienols	Fat-soluble vitamin	8 mg/10 mg	Deficiency is very rare; mild hemolytic anemia in newborn infants	Possible increased incidence of congestive heart failure	Wheat germ oil, seed, peanut oil, sunflower oil, meat, butter, and egg
$\mathbf{K_1}$ Phylloquinone Phytonadione	Fat-soluble vitamin	0.14 mg	Faulty absorption, diarrheal disease, and intestinal flora	Hemolytic anemia and jaundice in infants	Leafy green food such as spinach
$\mathbf{K_2}$ Menaquinon	Fat-soluble vitamin	0.14 mg	Lack of active prothrombin	Increased breakdown of red blood cells	Poultry, beef, pork, and fish

(Doldo *et al* 2015). It was studied that retinoids could suppress the development and progression of various tumors such as skin, lung, bladder, and breast cancer (Niles 2004, Bryan *et al* 2011). Gloria and group demonstrate how lycopene and beta-carotene can reduce cell growth, stop the cell cycle at certain points, and boost apoptosis in breast cancer cell lines. The study conclude that the effect was cell-type-dependent and that carotenoids are potential biologically active cancer-interfering agents (Gloria *et al* 2014). Hou *et al* studied the level of vitamin A in the serum of breast cancer patients and found that early breast cancer patients did not have lower serum vitamin A levels. Particularly in women with metastatic liver cancer, the serum vitamin A levels were dramatically reduced in the metastatic breast cancer group ($P < 0.05$). Patients with metastatic breast cancer may benefit from post-operative vitamin A supplementation (Hou *et al* 1998). This type of study was also performed in the Korean population and the result found that there is a negative correlation between serum antioxidant vitamins and the risk of breast cancer in Korea, suggesting that antioxidant vitamins—serum α-tocopherol, carotenoids, and retinol—may offer breast cancer protection (Kim *et al* 2001). A longitudinal study of breast cancer patients to evaluate patients' pre- and post-radiotherapy serum levels of vitamin A and their connection to the breast cancer stage was studied by Matos *et al*. The study concluded that adequate serum concentrations of retinol and beta-carotene suppress the negative effects of radiation (Matos *et al* 2014). Another study also revealed that retinoids most likely exert their chemopreventive effects at the tumor promotion stage of carcinogenesis. By reducing proliferation, causing apoptosis, inducing differentiation, or a combination of these effects, retinoids prevent the propagation of tumors (Niles 2000).

Various experimental studies demonstrated that retinoids have a lot of potential for use in the chemoprevention and treatment of bladder cancer (Tratnjek *et al* 2021). Meta-analysis findings by Huang and their group suggest that high consumption of vitamin A, carotene, beta-carotene, and lycopene may be associated with a low risk of developing pancreatic cancer (Huang *et al* 2016). Another meta-analysis study revealed that increased intake of retinol and vitamin A may greatly lower the risk of breast cancer (Fulan *et al* 2011). It was observed that cell proliferation, growth, and differentiation of human breast cancer cell lines are regulated by retinol (He *et al* 2018) and RA inhibits the growth of estrogen receptor-positive in human breast cancer cell lines (Zhao *et al*1995, Ribeiro *et al* 2014).

2.3.2 Vitamin B complex and cancer

Vitamin B complex contains eight different kinds of vitamins that are essential for the life of cells (Peterson *et al* 2020). One of the major functions of the vitamin B complex (niacin, folate, pantothenic acid, pyridoxine, biotin, riboflavin, and thiamine) is to act as a coenzyme for various enzymatic reactions (Zastre *et al* 2013). They have various other functions for the normal functioning of cells and to maintain the homeostasis of cells.

2.3.2.1 Thiamin and cancer

Thiamine deficiency, on the other hand, can arise in cancer patients and lead to catastrophic conditions like Wernicke's encephalopathy that call for parenteral thiamine supplementation. Thiamine has a growth-inhibitory effect on cancer when given in extremely high doses (Lu'o'ng and Nguyễn 2013). Another study revealed that a high dose of thiamine reduces cancer cell proliferation by a mechanism similar to dichloroacetate which is the inhibition of pyruvate dehydrogenase kinases (PDKs) (Hanberry *et al* 2014). Thus, understanding the significance of enzyme cofactors in cancer cell metabolism will provide important dietary strategies and new molecular targets to reduce disease progression (Lonsdale and Marrs 2020). The amount of thiamin is low in many cancer patients and deficiency might cause delirium in cancer patients (Onishi *et al* 2018, Onishi *et al* 2021). It inhibits the breast cancer cell growth. (Liu *et al* 2018). Liu *et al* 2018 and the group study the effect of thiamin on breast cancer cell line MCF7 and found that a high thiamine dose decreased MCF7 cell proliferation but had no effect on apoptosis or the cell-cycle profile It inhibits cell proliferation by increasing pyruvate dehydrogenase activity and by reducing cell acidification.

2.3.2.2 Riboflavin and cancer

Riboflavin deficiency is commonly defined as a cancer risk factor, although there are conflicting data on this point (Powers 2003). A meta-analysis of 27 studies of about 50 000 cases and more than 1.2 million individual people analyzing riboflavin and other B vitamins concluded that B2 may decrease the cancer of breast cancer, but was of borderline significance (Zeng *et al* 2020). Another meta-analysis examining components of one-carbon metabolism and kidney cancer risk found no significant correlation between B vitamins and cancer risk (Clasen *et al* 2020). Serum riboflavin levels are diminished in patients with esophageal squamous cell carcinoma compared with healthy people (Li *et al* 2019). Riboflavin may reduce the risk of colorectal cancer in women, possibly through her FAD-dependent methylenetetrahydrofolate reductase. The study of riboflavin and ovarian cancer threat found no relationship (de Vogel *et al* 2008). In non-smoking women, increased riboflavin intake has a relationship with reduced lung cancer risk (Takata *et al* 2012).

2.3.2.3 Niacin and cancer

'Nicotinic acid' and 'nicotinamide', in tandem called 'niacin', are the dietary messenger of the bioactive products 'nicotinamide adenine dinucleotide (NAD) and NAD phosphate (NADP)'. NAD and NADP are imperative cofactors for most cellular redox responses and are basic for keeping up cellular responses and breathing. NAD also works as a co-substrate for various ADP-ribosylating enzymes with diverse functions.

There is very limited research done on niacin and its supplements in cancer patients previously discovered to be niacin deficient (Inculet *et al* 1987). They found that only 40% of patients improved their niacin status with standard-dose intravenous vitamin B supplementation, and most responded effectively to double their recommended doses of riboflavin and niacin (Premkumar *et al* 2008). 'PARP-1 inhibitors' combined with mutagenic drugs may accelerate the elimination of other types of cancer cells, which increases the risk of acute damage to normal tissues such as bone marrow and secondary malignancies. It is not certain whether it is worthwhile, but most tumor tissues have adapted to some amount of instability, downregulating apoptotic signaling. Bone marrow cells may be more sensitive to this treatment than a few sorts of cancer cells (Kirkland 2009).

2.3.2.4 Biotin and cancer

A vitamin B complex supplement that the body needs in small amounts to operate and remain healthy. Biotin makes a difference in some enzyme change over substances within the body into vitality and boosts tissue advancement. It is found in yeast, whole grain, egg yolks, and liver and kidney. Biotin is water-soluble and should taken every day. Low biotin level can cause skin, nerve, and eye infections. Biotin is displayed in greater amounts in a few cancer tissues than in typical tissues. Controlled biotin substances utilized to treat a few sorts of cancer help discover cancer cells.

The biotin transporter is overexpressed in a number of aggressive cancer cell lines including ovarian, leukemia, colon (Colo-26), breast, renal, and lung cancer cell lines. As a result, the demand for biotin in rapidly expanding tumors is larger than that of normal tissues. Therefore, several cancer-targeting drugs are delivered through biotin conjugation and it is found that in comparison to normal cells, cancer cells that are biotin-positive exhibit higher amounts of cytotoxicity when exposed to biotin-linked drugs (Maiti and Paira 2018). Several studies revealed that an appealing and extremely creative method to increase the efficiency and efficacy of anti-cancer therapy and decrease its cytotoxicity is the conjugation of biotin with anti-cancer compounds (Yang *et al* 2009, Tripodo 2014, Lu *et al* 2019).

2.3.2.5 Pyridoxine and cancer

Vitamin B6 is one of the water-soluble vitamins that commonly acts as a cofactor for more than 100 biochemical reactions (Parra and Stahl 2018) and consists of three different sets of pyridine derivatives called 'pyridoxine, pyridoxal, pyridoxamine' (Wu and Lu 2012). Pyridoxal-5′-phosphate, the form of vitamin B6, acts as a group transfer intermediate in many enzymatic reactions and acts as an antioxidant molecule, decreasing food uptake or decreasing tissue or plasma levels. A case-control study on the effect of micronutrients on oral and pharyngeal cancer risk revealed that micronutrients including vitamin B6 have a protective effect against oral cancer (Negri *et al* 2006). Numerous studies have demonstrated that low vitamin B6 intake raises the chance of developing cancer (Merigliano *et al* 2018). Mocellin and their group conducted a systematic review on the role of vitamin B6 in cancer risk and an epidemiological-based research study revealed that vitamin B6 lowers the cancer risk and Pyridoxal-5′-phosphate could play an important role as a cancer screening biomarker, particularly for gastrointestinal malignancies (Mocellin *et al* 2017). Another meta-analysis study suggests that a high intake of vitamin B6 and a high concentration of blood pyridoxal phosphate (PLP) levels reduce the risk of pancreatic cancer (Peng *et al* 2019, Wei and Mao 2020). The meta-analysis study on the role of vitamin B on the risk of esophageal cancer provides credence to the idea that vitamin B may affect esophageal cancer development. Vitamin B12 indicated an increased risk of esophageal cancer, while vitamins B1, B3, B6, and B9 showed a decreased risk of esophageal cancer (Ma *et al* 2018).

2.3.2.6 Folic acid and cancer

Folic acid is a crucial water-soluble B vitamin found in foods such as green vegetables and dairy products. Folic acid may be a manufactured frame of the vitamin found in dietary supplements and fortified food products, i.e. grains and cereals. Folate serves as a coenzyme to transfer one-carbon units required for the formation of deoxy-thymidylate, purines, and other methylation processes making them essential to life as a component and catalyst for vital biochemical activities (Ebara 2017, Menezo *et al* 2022).

Several animal models have shown that a low-folate diet induces mutagenic properties, and 'some data from clinical trials suggest that folic acid supplementation may reduce the risk of progression of precancerous mucosal lesion' (MacFarlane *et al* 2015). Folic acid supplementation plays an important role in preventing colorectal carcinomas (Chen and Liu 2014). According to the dose-response meta-analysis, dietary folate consumption increased by 100 g/day lowered the estimated risk of esophageal cancer by 12%. These results imply that dietary and serum folate exert a preventative impact against the development of esophageal cancer (Zhao *et al* 2017). The impact of prophylactic treatment with folic acid was examined in patients included in the study with recurrent mild or moderate laryngeal dysplasia. '25% showed a reduction in affected area volume. In the control group, 67% showed no change and 25% showed disease progression with suspected malignant transformation' (Mesolella *et al* 2017). Folic acid is associated with diminished epidermal thickness and cell expansion, expression indicative of cell increases, lipid oxidation, decreased glutathione, and reduced carcinogenicity in the skin of mice (Koul *et al* 2018). 'In a meta-analysis assessing the risk of head and neck squamous cell carcinoma found that folic acid intake was associated with a reduction in the risk of squamous cell carcinoma of the head and neck region (OR 0.957, 95% CI 0.935–0.980)' (Fan *et al* 2017).

2.3.3 Vitamin C and cancer

Vitamin C is a water-soluble group, an antioxidant, and an important cofactor for collagen biosynthesis, carnitine and catecholamine metabolism, and dietary iron absorption. Humans cannot manufacture vitamin C, so it is obtained only through the intake of fruits and vegetables. Citrus fruits, berries, tomatoes, potatoes, and green leafy vegetables are excellent sources of vitamin C (Abdullah *et al* 2023). Vitamin C has diverse functions in the immune system as an antibacterial agent, promotes lymphocyte proliferation, and is rapidly consumed during infection (Carr and Maggini 2017).

The use of high-dose vitamin C in cancer patients is common among practitioners of complementary and alternative medicine in patients with cancer (Zasowska-Nowak *et al* 2021). Early-stage clinical trials have demonstrated the safety of vitamin C and shown that it is effective in eliminating tumor cells from a variety of cancer types. The multi-targeting properties of vitamin C have recently come to light, revealing a role as a cancer-specific pro-oxidative cytotoxic agent, anti-cancer epigenetic regulator, and immune modulator, reversing the epithelial-to-mesenchymal transition, inhibiting hypoxia, and oncogenic kinase signaling, and enhancing immune response (Böttger *et al* 2021).

A number of mechanisms have been studied to support vitamin C's role in cancer treatment and prevention including enhancing the activity of the immune system, stimulation of collagen synthesis, prevention of metastasis by inhibiting certain enzymatic reactions, and inhibition of tumor-causing viruses. Vitamin C deficiency is commonly associated with cancer patients, wound healing in cancer patients after surgery, improvement of chemosensitivity, reduction of chemotherapy toxicity, and neutralization of certain carcinogens (Dachs *et al* 2021). Exposure to high doses of Vitamin C halting tumor cell growth has been shown in various experiments (Chen *et al* 2005, Cabanillas 2010). A schematic representation of the cell death or growth inhibition by vitamin C is shown in figure 2.2. Administration of vitamin C constrains cytokine production associated with metastasis, tumor development, and inflammation, while also improving tumor containment and improving chemotherapy (Cha *et al* 2011, 2013). Some reports indicate that hypodermic injection increases vitamin C levels compared to oral administration, and therapeutic efficacy is inversely proportional to vitamin C excess (Magrì *et al* 2020). Ascorbic acid has anti-cancer properties, but most of the mechanisms behind this effect remain enigmatic. The biological roles and processes behind a number of intriguing and curious concepts provide a solid scientific basis for his use of vitamin C in cancer therapy. Due to its wide accessibility in nature, negligible harmfulness, and low impact, ascorbic acid may end up an imperative restorative alternative in the battle against cancer (Mastrangelo *et al* 2018). Ascorbic acid is linked to better side effects

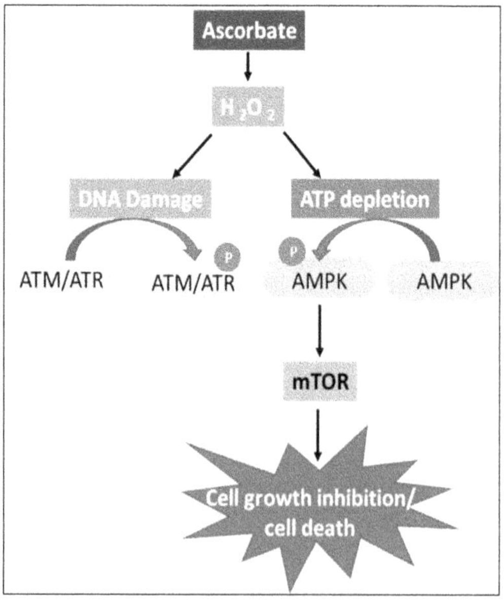

Figure 2.2. Vitamin C and tumor cell growth inhibition lead to cell death.

and tolerability of conventional therapy as well as tumor shrinkage in patients with advanced illness. These results lead us to the conclusion that larger-scale clinical trials are required to investigate the therapeutic advantages of ascorbic acid in colon cancer (El Halabi *et al* 2018).

2.3.4 Vitamin D and cancer

Vitamin D is a fat-soluble group that increases the absorption of calcium, magnesium, and phosphate in the digestive tract and has many other biological effects. In humans, the most important group are vitamin D3 (cholecalciferol) and vitamin D2 (ergocalciferol). A few foods naturally contain significant amounts of vitamin D, such as oily fish. Like many breakfast cereals, milk and plant-based milk replacers are fortified with vitamin D (Catharine 2011). Early epidemiological studies recommend that the rate and mortality of a few sorts of cancer are lower in individuals living in southern regions, where sun-oriented radiation is generally higher than in individuals living in northern regions. Since UV introduction from the sun advances vitamin D generation, the analysts hypothesized that fluctuations in vitamin D levels might play a part in this association. The main precursor form of vitamin D is present in nature and its functional form synthesis is shown in figure 2.3. Vitamin D is a hormone with anti-carcinogenic effects (Martin-Gorgojo *et al* 2021).

According to experimental evidence, getting enough vitamin D from the bloodstream and being exposed to sunlight can lower the risk of developing cancer. Numerous *in vitro* and *in vivo* research points to vitamin D as a supplement

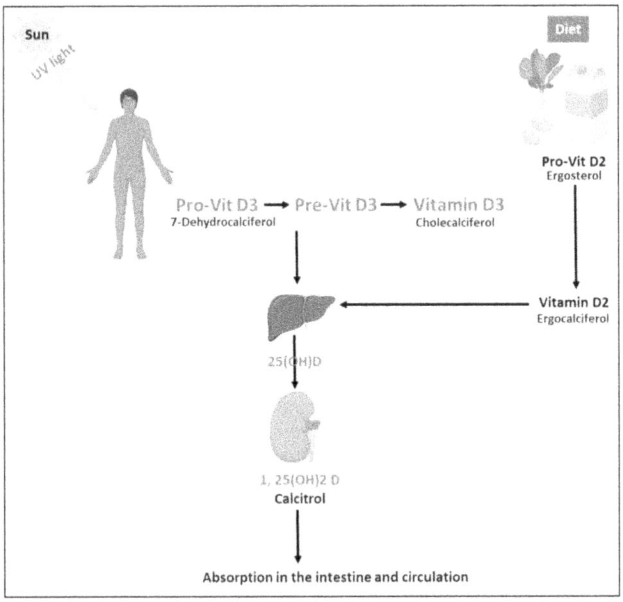

Figure 2.3. Synthesis of vitamin D (created with BioRender.com).

that may be useful for the treatment and prevention of cancer (Varghese *et al* 2021). According to the findings of this meta-analysis, a lack of vitamin D raises the risk of developing liver cancer. Compared to healthy controls, hepatocellular carcinoma (HCC) patients had reduced 25(OH)D3 levels. It would be advantageous to keep serum vitamin D levels at a healthy range to prevent liver cancer (Yi *et al* 2021). Experiments conducted *in vitro* and *in vivo* have shown that vitamin D has anti-tumor and immunomodulatory properties. The involvement of vitamin D in the inflammatory situations of the lung has been suggested by a number of lines of research. According to epidemiological research, having enough vitamin D may be essential for preventing lung cancer (Wang *et al* 2021). It was also seen that vitamin D was deficient in some breast cancer patients (Welsh 2021). According to the scientific research analyzed, increasing 25(OH)D concentrations through sensitive sun exposure and/or vitamin D supplementation to lower cancer risk and, in conjunction with standard care, to treat cancer (Nica-Badea *et al* 2021). Vitamin D exposure also helps to reduce the reduction of development of head and neck cancer (Pu *et al* 2021). Numerous epidemiological studies have shown that higher intakes or blood levels of vitamin D are associated with a lower risk of colorectal cancer (Gandini *et al* 2011, Ma *et al* 2011) and breast cancer (Bernhardt *et al* 2021).

The reduction of cancer cell survival and proliferation is caused by metabolic adjustments associated with the anti-cancer effects of vitamin D therapy of cells, which have been extensively researched in prostate cancer and other cancer cell lines. Calcium (calcitriol, 1,25-dihydroxycholecalciferol) is the compound that has been most thoroughly studied in cancer treatment. The following physiological properties of calcitriol are connected with inhibiting tumor growth.

1. Induction of caspase-dependent MAPK/ERK kinase (MEK) cleavage (Colston 2002, Johnson *et al* 2006).
2. Start of the p53 homolog (Johnson *et al* 2006).
3. Blockage of the formation of new blood vessels (Chung *et al* 2009, Miyata *et al* 2013).
4. Blockage of migration and invasion (Chen *et al* 2015, Hou *et al* 2016).
5. Start of differentiation (Koeffler *et al* 1985, Abe *et al* 1986).
6. Regulatory of expression of tumor-associated growth factors (Chen *et al* 2015, Irani *et al* 2015, Mohapatra *et al* 2015).

2.3.5 Vitamin E and cancer

Vitamin E is a fat-soluble vitamin group with several forms, but only α-tocopherol is utilized by the human body and its main function is to act as an antioxidant by scavenging free electrons that can damage cells. Vitamin E includes eight forms, including alpha, beta, gamma, and delta tocopherols and tocotrienols. However, only α-tocopherol is found in abundance and is maintained in blood plasma (Cho 2010, Rizvi *et al* 2014). Vitamin E supplements typically contain all isomers of α-tocopherol. Its existence has a minimum movement level of natural sources in the forms of tocopherol but only the α-form or equivalent has been measured for sufficient nutrition. The ability of vitamin E to prevent cancer has received a great deal of attention due to the role that oxidative stress plays in the development of cancer (Didier *et al* 2023). In certain intervention trials, supplementing populations with vitamin E showed beneficial effects in reducing cancer risk. Lower vitamin E intake or nutritional status has been linked to higher cancer risk (Yang *et al* 2020).

Cancer can be prevented by consuming vitamin E in the diet or through supplements that are high in γ- and α-tocopherols, but not by taking large amounts of α-tocopherol (Yang *et al* 2012). Supplementing with vitamin E was linked to a statistically significant decline in the incidence of prostate cancer but not to a decline in overall mortality, cancer incidence, or cancer mortality. Men who have a high chance of developing prostate cancer can utilize vitamin E to prevent the disease (Alkhenizan and Hafez 2007).

Vitamin E may also protect against cancer by blocking the formation of carcinogenic nitrosamines formed in the stomach from nitrites in food and boosting immune function. All forms of vitamin E show cancer-preventive function (Jiang 2017). This concept is consistent with many observations that dietary intake or plasma levels of α-tocopherol and other tocopherols are inversely associated with cancer risk, especially in smokers with greater oxidative stress (Mahabir *et al* 2008, Ju *et al* 2010). The highest anti-cancer actions are exhibited by γ- and α-tocotrienols, which also have the same molecular pathway that controls the cell cycle, induces apoptosis and autophagy, and inhibits invasion, metastasis, and angiogenesis (Constantinou *et al* 2020).

This extensive population study, which used information from cancer-specific genome-wide association study (GWAS) and a longitudinal biobank cohort, found reasonable non-causal relationships between circulating vitamin E and ten prevalent malignancies in the populations of Europe. It is necessary to conduct further research on ancestral diversity to confirm such causal relationships (Xin *et al* 2022). A randomized control trials-based study also concluded that it is challenging to get an agreement regarding the efficiency of Vitamin E in cancer therapies due to the heterogeneous outcomes (Donnelly *et al* 2022).

2.3.6 Vitamin K and cancer

Vitamin K is a group of fat-soluble vitamins. It is vital for blood clotting, bone and vascular well-being, and different physiological functions. Selected proteins including clotting factors undergo post-translational (carboxylation) which requires the vitamins K1 (phylloquinone) and K2 (menaquinones). Currently, these altered proteins are thought to play a role in a number of physiological and pathological processes, including cancer (Dahlberg *et al* 2017, Xv *et al* 2018). In observational studies, vitamin K intake has been shown to be negatively correlated with cancer incidence and mortality (Welsh *et al* 2022). Vitamin K exerts antiproliferative, proapoptotic, and autophagic effects and has been associated with a reduced risk of cancer (Popa *et al* 2021). Vitamin K induces non-apoptotic cell death along with autophagosome formation in the triple-negative breast cancer cell lines (Miyazawa *et al* 2020). It also initiates apoptotic, cell cycle progression, and metastasis-promoting signaling molecules in prostate cancer (Dasari *et al* 2018) and also inhibits prostate tumor by targeting androgen-dependent and androgen-independent growth (Samykutty *et al* 2013). It shows anti-cancer effects on gastric cancer cell lines (Tokita *et al* 2006), bladder cancer (Duan *et al* 2016), colon cancer (Orlando *et al* 2015), breast cancer (Beaudin *et al* 2019).

Vitamin K shows an anti-cancer effect by regulating the redox state. Vitamins C and K can alter the redox system of mitochondria and change the energy metabolism of cancer cells (Ivanova *et al* 2018). Vitamin K inhibits cancer cell growth by apoptosis, cell cycle arrest, autophagy, and manipulation of other transcription factors like Myc and Fos. There is potential for vitamin K and its derivatives as an adjuvant therapy when combined with other vitamins or chemotherapeutic medicines for prostate and other cancer (Dasari *et al* 2017). It was observed that vitamin K3 induces apoptosis in the MCF7 breast cancer cell line (Wellington *et al* 2020), and it generates cytotoxic reactive oxygen species to inhibit cancer cell growth (He *et al* 2015).

2.4 Conclusion and future prospective

Vitamins are the accessory food factor required in the diet. The point that a high intake of vitamins may give protection against cancer has drawn a lot of attention in the area of research and among individuals. Vitamin A (retinol) has an important role in cellular processes related to carcinogenesis, however, its high intake does not seem to have much relation to cancer prevention. Generally, vitamin A plays a major part in health and well-being. Vitamin B has an important factor that has an influence on oncogene expression. Vitamin B deficiencies are moderately uncommon in certain populations such as vegetarians, who may not have B12 in their diet. Generally, good calories that incorporate an assortment of nutrient-dense nourishments are the perfect way to guarantee satisfactory vitamin B ingestion. Vitamin C, vitamin E, and vitamin D have cancer-prevention properties but a higher intake of vitamin D can lead to skin or colon cancer due to its influence on cell proliferation. Vitamins are acting as an emerging therapeutic drug to prevent cancer and they can be consumed orally in the form of medicine, but the advice to have a rich diet in the form of fruit and vegetables will help to decrease the risk of cancer.

The scientific community has shown growing interested in vitamins recently, and it is now known that they are crucial to the genesis of many diseases, including cancer. More research is required to determine the true role of vitamins in cancer prevention and therapy because the scientific evidence regarding cancer that has been established so far is not conclusive but rather optimistic (Russo *et al* 2015). However, various meta-analysis studies revealed that vitamins have no or negligible effect on the prevention of cancer (Zhang *et al* 2014). Some studies show no significant associations between dietary vitamin intake and cancer prevention and management. Further research is, therefore, necessary to shed more light on this matter.

References

Abdullah M, Jamil R T and Attia F N 2023 *Vitamin C (Ascorbic Acid)* (Treasure Island, FL: StatPearls Publishing)

Abe J, Moriya Y, Saito M, Sugawara Y, Suda T and Nishii Y 1986 Modulation of cell growth, differentiation, and production of interleukin-3 by 1α,25-dihydroxyvitamin D3 in the murine myelomonocytic leukemia cell line WEHI-3 *Cancer Res.* **46** 6316–21

Alkhenizan A and Hafez K 2007 The role of vitamin E in the prevention of cancer: a meta-analysis of randomized controlled trials *Ann. Saudi Med.* **27** 409–14

Beaudin S, Kokabee L and Welsh J 2019 Divergent effects of vitamins K1 and K2 on triple-negative breast cancer cells *Oncotarget.* **10** 2292

Bender D A 2003 *Nutritional Biochemistry of the Vitamins* (Cambridge: Cambridge University Press)

Bernhardt S M, Borges V F and Schedin P 2021 Vitamin d as a potential preventive agent for young women's breast cancer *Cancer Prev. Res.* **14** 825–38

Böttger F, Vallés-Martí A, Cahn L and Jimenez C R 2021 High-dose intravenous vitamin C, a promising multi-targeting agent in the treatment of cancer *J. Exp. Clin. Cancer Res.* **40** 1–44

Bryan M, Pulte E D, Toomey K C, Pliner L, Pavlick A C, Saunders T and Wieder R 2011 A pilot phase II trial of all-trans retinoic acid (Vesanoid) and paclitaxel (Taxol) in patients with recurrent or metastatic breast cancer *Invest. New Drugs* **29** 1482–7

Cabanillas F 2010 Vitamin C and cancer: what can we conclude-1,609 patients and 33 years later? *P. R. Health Sci.* J. **29** 215–7

Carr A C and Maggini S 2017 Vitamin C and immune function *Nutrients* **9** 1211

Catharine R 2011 *Dietary Reference Intakes for Calcium and Vitamin D/Committee to Review Dietary Reference Intakes for Vitamin D and Calcium* (Food and Nutrition Board)

Cha J, Roomi M W, Ivanov V, Kalinovsky T, Niedzwiecki A and Rath M 2011 Ascorbate depletion increases growth and metastasis of melanoma cells in vitamin C deficient mice *Exp. Oncol.* **42** 55–64

Cha J, Roomi M W, Ivanov V, Kalinovsky T, Niedzwiecki A and Rath M 2013 Ascorbate supplementation inhibits growth and metastasis of B16FO melanoma and 4T1 breast cancer cells in vitamin C-deficient mice *Int. J. Oncol.* **42** 55–64

Chen J and Liu J 2014 The dual effect of folic acid supplementation in preventing colorectal carcinomas *Global J. Gastroenterol. Hepatol.* **2** 4–10

Chen P T, Hsieh C C, Wu C T, Yen T C, Lin P Y, Chen W C and Chen M F 2015 1α, 25-dihydroxyvitamin D3 inhibits esophageal squamous cell carcinoma progression by reducing IL6 signaling *Mol. Cancer Ther* **14** 1365–75

Chen Q, Espey M G, Krishna M C, Mitchell J B, Corpe C P, Buettner G R, Shacter E and Levine M 2005 Pharmacologic ascorbic acid concentrations selectively kill cancer cells: action as a pro-drug to deliver hydrogen peroxide to tissues *Proc. Natl Acad. Sci.* **102** 13604–9

Chen S, Zhu J, Zuo S, Ma J, Zhang J, Chen G, Wang X, Pan Y, Liu Y and Wang P 2015 1,25 (OH) 2D3 attenuates TGF-β1/β2-induced increased migration and invasion via inhibiting epithelial–mesenchymal transition in colon cancer cells *Biochem. Biophys. Res. Commun.* **468** 130–5

Cho S H 2010 Vitamin E: α-tocopherol and the other forms of vitamin E *J.Nutr. Health* **43** 304–14

Chung I, Han G, Seshadri M, Gillard B M, Yu W D, Foster B A, Trump D L and Johnson C S 2009 Role of vitamin D receptor in the antiproliferative effects of calcitriol in tumor-derived endothelial cells and tumor angiogenesis *in vivo Cancer Res.* **69** 967–75

Clasen J L, Heath A K, Scelo G and Muller D C 2020 Components of one-carbon metabolism and renal cell carcinoma: a systematic review and meta-analysis *Eur.J. Nutr.* **59** 3801–13
Colston K W 2002 Mechanisms implicated in the growth regulatory effects of vitamin D in breast cancer *Endocr.-Relat. Cancer* **9** 45–59
Constantinou C, Charalambous C and Kanakis D 2020 Vitamin E and cancer: an update on the emerging role of γ and δ tocotrienols *Eur. J. Nutr.* **59** 845–57
Dachs G U, Gandhi J, Wohlrab C, Carr A C, Morrin H R, Pullar J M, Bayer S B, Eglinton T W, Robinson B A and Vissers M C 2021 Vitamin C administration by intravenous infusion increases tumor ascorbate content in patients with colon cancer: a clinical intervention study *Front. Oncol.* **10** 600715
Dahlberg S, Ede J and Schött U 2017 Vitamin K and cancer *Scand. J. Clin. Lab. Invest.* **77** 555–67
Dasari S, Ali S M, Zheng G, Chen A, Dontaraju V S, Bosland M C, Kajdacsy-Balla A and Munirathinam G 2017 Vitamin K and its analogs: potential avenues for prostate cancer management *Oncotarget.* **8** 57782
Dasari S, Samy A L, Kajdacsy-Balla A, Bosland M C and Munirathinam G 2018 Vitamin K2, a menaquinone present in dairy products targets castration-resistant prostate cancer cell-line by activating apoptosis signaling *Food Chem. Toxicol.* **115** 218–27
de Vogel S, Dindore V, van Engeland M, Goldbohm R A, van den Brandt P A and Weijenberg M P 2008 Dietary folate, methionine, riboflavin, and vitamin B-6 and risk of sporadic colorectal cancer *J. Nutr.* **138** 2372–8
Didier A J, Stiene J, Fang L, Watkins D, Dworkin L D and Creeden J F 2023 Antioxidant and anti-tumor effects of dietary vitamins A, C, and E *Antioxidants* **12** 632
Doldo E, Costanza G, Agostinelli S, Tarquini C, Ferlosio A, Arcuri G, Passeri D, Scioli M G and Orlandi A 2015 Vitamin A, cancer treatment and prevention: the new role of cellular retinol binding proteins *BioMed Res. Int.* **2015** 624627
Donnelly J, Appathurai A, Yeoh H L, Driscoll K and Faisal W 2022 Vitamin E in cancer treatment: a review of clinical applications in randomized control trials *Nutrients.* **14** 4329
Duan F, Yu Y, Guan R, Xu Z, Liang H and Hong L 2016 Vitamin K2 induces mitochondria-related apoptosis in human bladder cancer cells via ROS and JNK/p38 MAPK signal pathways *PLoS One* **11** e0161886
Ebara S 2017 Nutritional role of folate *Congenit. Anom* **57** 138–41
El Halabi I, Bejjany R, Nasr R, Mukherji D, Temraz S, Nassar F J, El Darsa H and Shamseddine A 2018 Ascorbic acid in colon cancer: from the basic to the clinical applications *Int. J. Mol. Sci.* **19** 2752
Fan C, Yu S, Zhang S, Ding X, Su J and Cheng Z 2017 Association between folate intake and risk of head and neck squamous cell carcinoma: an overall and dose–response PRISMA meta-analysis *Medicine.* **96** 42
Fulan H *et al* 2011 Retinol, vitamins A, C, and E and breast cancer risk: a meta-analysis and meta-regression *Cancer Causes Control* **22** 1383–96
Gandini S, Boniol M, Haukka J, Byrnes G, Cox B, Sneyd M J, Mullie P and Autier P 2011 Meta-analysis of observational studies of serum 25-hydroxyvitamin D levels and colorectal, breast and prostate cancer and colorectal adenoma *Int. J. Cancer* **128** 1414–24
Gloria N F, Soares N, Brand C, Oliveira F L, Borojevic R and Teodoro A J 2014 Lycopene and beta-carotene induce cell-cycle arrest and apoptosis in human breast cancer cell lines *Anticancer Res.* **34** 1377–86

Hanberry B S, Berger R and Zastre J A 2014 High-dose vitamin B1 reduces proliferation in cancer cell lines analogous to dichloroacetate *Cancer Chemoth. Pharm* **73** 585–94

He J, Gu Y and Zhang S 2018 Vitamin A and breast cancer survival: a systematic review and meta-analysis *Clin. Breast Cancer* **18** e1389–400

He T, Hatem E, Vernis L, Lei M and Huang M E 2015 PRX1 knockdown potentiates vitamin K3 toxicity in cancer cells: a potential new therapeutic perspective for an old drug *J. Exp. Clin. Cancer Res.* **34** 1–3

Hou M F, Tsai L Y, Huang C J, Huang Y S, Hsieh J S, Huang T J, Chen H M and Wang J Y 1998 Serum vitamin A level in breast cancer patients *Kaohsiung J. Med. Sci.* **14** 673–8

Hou Y F, Gao S H, Wang P, Zhang H M, Liu L Z, Ye M X, Zhou G M, Zhang Z L and Li B Y 2016 1α, 25 (OH) 2D3 suppresses the migration of ovarian cancer SKOV-3 cells through the inhibition of epithelial–mesenchymal transition *Int. J. Mol. Sci.* **17** 1285

Huang X, Gao Y, Zhi X, Ta N, Jiang H and Zheng J 2016 Association between vitamin A, retinol and carotenoid intake and pancreatic cancer risk: evidence from epidemiologic studies *Sci. Rep.* **6** 38936

Inculet R I, Norton J A, Nichoalds G E, Maher M M, White D E and Brennan M F 1987 Water-soluble vitamins in cancer patients on parenteral nutrition: a prospective study *J. Parenter. Enter. Nutr.* **11** 243–9

Irani M, Seifer D B, Grazi R V, Julka N, Bhatt D, Kalgi B, Irani S, Tal O, Lambert-Messerlian G and Tal R 2015 Vitamin D supplementation decreases TGF-β1 bioavailability in PCOS: a randomized placebo-controlled trial. The *J. Clin. Endocrinol. Metab.* **100** 4307–14

Ivanova D, Zhelev Z, Getsov P, Nikolova B, Aoki I, Higashi T and Bakalova R 2018 Vitamin K: redox-modulation, prevention of mitochondrial dysfunction and anticancer effect *Redox Biol.* **16** 352–8

Jiang Q 2017 Natural forms of vitamin E as effective agents for cancer prevention and therapy *Adv. Nutr.* **8** 850–67

Johnson C S, Muindi J R, Hershberger P A and Trump D L 2006 The antitumor efficacy of calcitriol: preclinical studies *Anticancer Res.* **26** 2543–9

Ju J, Picinich S C, Yang Z, Zhao Y, Suh N, Kong A N and Yang C S 2010 Cancer-preventive activities of tocopherols and tocotrienols *Carcinogenesis* **31** 533–42

Kim J A, Jang J H and Lee S Y 2021 An updated comprehensive review on vitamin A and carotenoids in breast cancer: mechanisms, genetics, assessment, current evidence, and future clinical implications *Nutrients* **13** 3162

Kim M K, Ahn S H and Lee-Kim Y C 2001 Relationship of serum α-tocopherol, carotenoids and retinol with the risk of breast cancer *Nutr. Res.* **21** 797–809

Kim S J, Puranik N, Yadav D, Jin J O and Lee P C 2023 Lipid nanocarrier-based drug delivery systems: therapeutic advances in the treatment of lung cancer *Int. J. Nanomed.* 2659–76

Kirkland J B 2009 Niacin status and treatment-related leukemogenesis *Mol. Cancer Ther.* **8** 725–32

Koeffler H P, Hirji K and Itri L 1985 1,25-Dihydroxyvitamin D3: *in vivo* and *in vitro* effects on human preleukemic and leukemic cells *Cancer Treat. Rep.* **69** 1399–407

Kong P, Cai Q, Geng Q, Wang J, Lan Y, Zhan Y and Xu D 2014 Vitamin intake reduce the risk of gastric cancer: meta-analysis and systematic review of randomized and observational studies *PLoS One* **9** e116060

Koul A, Kaur N and Chugh N A 2018 Folic acid modulates DMBA/TPA-induced changes in skin of mice: a study relevant to carcinogenesis *J. Diet. Suppl.* **15** 72–87

Li S S *et al* 2019 The association between the whole blood riboflavin level and the occurrence, development and prognosis of esophageal squamous cell carcinoma *Zhonghua yu Fang yi xue za zhi [Chin. J. Prev. Med.]* **53** 1124–9

Liu X, Montissol S, Uber A, Ganley S, Grossestreuer A V, Berg K, Heydrick S and Donnino M W 2018 The effects of thiamine on breast cancer cells *Molecules.* **23** 1464

Lonsdale D and Marrs C 2020 The potential of lipid soluble thiamine in the treatment of cancer *AIMS Biophys* **7** 17–26

Lu R, Zhou L, Yue Q, Liu Q, Cai X, Xiao W, Hai L, Guo L and Wu Y 2019 Liposomes modified with double-branched biotin: a novel and effective way to promote breast cancer targeting *Bioorg. Med. Chem.* **27** 3115–27

Lu'o'ng K V and Nguyễn L T 2013 The role of thiamine in cancer: possible genetic and cellular signaling mechanisms *Cancer Genom. Proteom.* **10** 169–85

Ma Y, Zhang P, Wang F, Yang J, Liu Z and Qin H 2011 Association between vitamin D and risk of colorectal cancer: a systematic review of prospective studies *J. Clin. Oncol.* **29** 3775–82

Ma J L, Zhao Y, Guo C Y, Hu H T, Zheng L, Zhao E J and Li H L 2018 Dietary vitamin B intake and the risk of esophageal cancer: a meta-analysis *Cancer Manage. Res.* **5** 5395–410

MacFarlane A J, Behan N A, Field M S, Williams A, Stover P J and Yauk C L 2015 Dietary folic acid protects against genotoxicity in the red blood cells of mice *Mutat. Res./Fundam. Mol. Mech. Mutagen.* **779** 105–11

Magrì A *et al* 2020 High-dose vitamin C enhances cancer immunotherapy *Sci. Transl. Med.* **12** eaay8707

Mahabir S, Schendel K, Dong Y Q, Barrera S L, Spitz M R and Forman M R 2008 Dietary α-, β-, γ-and δ-tocopherols in lung cancer risk *Int. J. Cancer* **123** 1173–80

Maiti S and Paira P 2018 Biotin conjugated organic molecules and proteins for cancer therapy: a review *Eur. J. Med. Chem.* **145** 206–23

Mamede A C, Tavares S D, Abrantes A M, Trindade J, Maia J M and Botelho M F 2011 The role of vitamins in cancer: a review *Nutr. Cancer* **63** 479–94

Martin T A, Ye L, Sanders A J, Lane J and Jiang W G 2013 Cancer invasion and metastasis: molecular and cellular perspective *Madame Curie Bioscience Database [Internet]* (Landes Bioscience)

Martin-Gorgojo A, Gilaberte Y and Nagore E 2021 Vitamin D and skin cancer: an epidemiological, patient-centered update and review *Nutrients* **13** 4292

Mastrangelo D, Pelosi E, Castelli G, Lo-Coco F and Testa U 2018 Mechanisms of anti-cancer effects of ascorbate: cytotoxic activity and epigenetic modulation *Blood Cells Mol. Dis.* **69** 57–64

Matos A, Nogueira C, Franca C, Carvalho A, Vieira S L, Penna A and Ramalho A 2014 The relationship between serum vitamin A and breast cancer staging before and after radiotherapy *Nutr. Hosp.* **29** 136–9

Menezo Y, Elder K, Clement A and Clement P 2022 Folic acid, folinic acid, 5 methyl tetrahydrofolate supplementation for mutations that affect epigenesis through the folate and one-carbon cycles *Biomolecules* **12** 197

Merigliano C, Mascolo E, Burla R, Saggio I and Vernì F 2018 The relationship between vitamin B6, diabetes and cancer *Front. Genet.* **9** 388

Mesolella M, Iengo M, Testa D, Ricciardiello F and Iorio B 2017 Chemoprevention using folic acid for dysplastic lesions of the larynx *Mol. Clin. Oncol.* **7** 843–6

Miyata Y, Ohba K, Matsuo T, Watanabe S I, Hayashi T, Sakai H and Kanetake H 2013 Tumor-associated stromal cells expressing E-prostanoid 2 or 3 receptors in prostate cancer: correlation with tumor aggressiveness and outcome by angiogenesis and lymphangiogenesis *Urology* **81** 136–42

Miyazawa S, Moriya S, Kokuba H, Hino H, Takano N and Miyazawa K 2020 Vitamin K2 induces non-apoptotic cell death along with autophagosome formation in breast cancer cell lines *Breast Cancer* **27** 225–35

Mocellin S, Briarava M and Pilati P 2017 Vitamin B6 and cancer risk: a field synopsis and meta-analysis *J. Natl. Cancer Inst.* **109** djw230

Mohapatra S, Saxena A, Gandhi G, Koner B C, Singh T and Ray P C 2015 Does vitamin D mediate inhibition of epithelial ovarian cancer by modulating cytokines? *Clin Transl. Oncol.* **17** 590–5

Negri E, Franceschi S, Bosetti C, Levi F, Conti E, Parpinel M and La Vecchia C 2000 Selected micronutrients and oral and pharyngeal cancer *Int. J. Cancer* **86** 122–7

Nica-Badea D and Udristioiu A 2021 The relevance of supplemental vitamin D in malignancies *Anti-Cancer Agents Med. Chem.* **21** 1942–9

Niles R M 2000 Recent advances in the use of vitamin A (retinoids) in the prevention and treatment of cancer *Nutrition.* **16** 1084–9

Niles R M 2004 Signaling pathways in retinoid chemoprevention and treatment of cancer *Mutat. Res./Fund. Mol. Mech. Mutagen* **555** 97–105

Ohshika S, Saruga T, Ogawa T, Ono H and Ishibashi Y 2021 Distinction between benign and malignant soft tissue tumors based on an ultrasonographic evaluation of vascularity and elasticity *Oncol. Lett.* **21** 1

Onishi H, Ishida M, Uchida N, Sato I and Takahashi T 2018 The rate and treatment outcome of thiamine deficiency in cancer patients diagnosed with delirium: a preliminary study *J. Clin. Oncol.* **36** 205–5

Onishi H, Sato I, Uchida N, Takahashi T, Furuya D, Ebihara Y, Yoshioka A, Ito H and Ishida M 2021 High proportion of thiamine deficiency in referred cancer patients with delirium: a retrospective descriptive study *Eur. J. Clin. Nutr.* **75** 1499–505

Orlando A, Linsalata M, Tutino V, D'Attoma B, Notarnicola M and Russo F 2015 Vitamin K1 exerts antiproliferative effects and induces apoptosis in three differently graded human colon cancer cell lines *BioMed. Res. Int.* **2015** 296721

Parra M, Stahl S and Hellmann H 2018 Vitamin B6 and its role in cell metabolism and physiology *Cells* **7** 84

Peng J *et al* 2019 Single-cell RNA-seq highlights intra-tumoral heterogeneity and malignant progression in pancreatic ductal adenocarcinoma *Cell Res.* **29** 725–38

Peterson C T, Rodionov D A, Osterman A L and Peterson S N 2020 B vitamins and their role in immune regulation and cancer *Nutrients* **12** 3380

Popa D S, Bigman G and Rusu M E 2021 The role of vitamin k in humans: implication in aging and age-associated diseases *Antioxidants* **10** 566

Powers H J 2003 Riboflavin (vitamin B-2) and health *The Am. J. Clin. Nutr.* **77** 1352–60

Premkumar V G, Yuvaraj S, Shanthi P and Sachdanandam P 2008 Co-enzyme Q10, riboflavin and niacin supplementation on alteration of DNA repair enzyme and DNA methylation in breast cancer patients undergoing tamoxifen therapy *Br. J. Nutr.* **100** 1179–82

Pu Y, Zhu G, Xu Y, Zheng S, Tang B, Huang H, Wu I X, Huang D, Liu Y and Zhang X 2021 Association between vitamin D exposure and head and neck cancer: a systematic review with meta-analysis *Front. Immunol.* **12** 627226

Ribeiro M P, Santos A E and Custódio J B 2014 Interplay between estrogen and retinoid signaling in breast cancer–current and future perspectives *Cancer Lett.* **353** 17–24

Rizvi S, Raza S T, Ahmed F, Ahmad A, Abbas S and Mahdi F 2014 The role of vitamin E in human health and some diseases *Sultan Qaboos Univ. Med.* J **14** e157

Russo I, Francesca C and Mauro A 2015 Vitamins and melanoma *Cancers* **7** 1371–87

Samykutty A, Shetty A V, Dakshinamoorthy G, Kalyanasundaram R, Zheng G, Chen A, Bosland M C, Kajdacsy-Balla A and Gnanasekar M 2013 Vitamin K2, a naturally occurring menaquinone, exerts therapeutic effects on both hormone-dependent and hormone-independent prostate cancer cells *Evid.-Based Complement. Altern. Med.* **2013** 287358

Takata Y *et al* 2012 Dietary B vitamin and methionine intakes and lung cancer risk among female never smokers in China *Cancer Causes Control* **23** 1965–75

Tokita H, Tsuchida A, Miyazawa K, Ohyashiki K, Katayanagi S, Sudo H, Enomoto M, Takagi Y and Aoki T 2006 Vitamin K2-induced antitumor effects via cell-cycle arrest and apoptosis in gastric cancer cell lines *Int. J. Mol. Med.* **17** 235–43

Tratnjek L, Jeruc J, Romih R and Zupančič D 2021 Vitamin A and retinoids in bladder cancer chemoprevention and treatment: a narrative review of current evidence, challenges and future prospects *Int. J. Mol. Sci.* **22** 3510

Tripodo G, Mandracchia D, Collina S, Rui M and Rossi D 2014 New perspectives in cancer therapy: the biotin-antitumor molecule conjugates *Med. Chem.* **8** 1–4

Van Poppel G and Van den Berg H 1997 Vitamins and cancer *Cancer Lett.* **114** 195–202

Varghese J E, Balasubramanian B, Velayuthaprabhu S, Thirunavukkarasu V, Rengarajan R L, Murugesh E, Manikandan P, Arun M and Anand A V 2021 Therapeutic effects of vitamin D and cancer: an overview *Food Front.* **2** 417–25

Wada A 2021 Chemical biology studies using vitamin a analogs *Yakugaku Zasshi: J. Pharm. Soc. Japan* **141** 557–77

Wang W, Hu W, Xue S, Chen Q, Jiang Y, Zhang H and Zuo W 2021 Vitamin D and lung cancer; association, prevention, and treatment *Nutr. Cancer* **73** 2188–200

Wei D H and Mao Q Q 2020 Vitamin B6, vitamin B12 and methionine and risk of pancreatic cancer: a meta-analysis *Nutrition J.* **19** 1–2

Wellington K W, Hlatshwayo V, Kolesnikova N I, Saha S T, Kaur M and Motadi L R 2020 Anticancer activities of vitamin K3 analogues *Invest. New Drugs* **38** 378–91

Welsh J, Bak M J and Narvaez C J 2022 New insights into vitamin K biology with relevance to cancer *Trends Mol. Med.* **28** P864–81

Welsh J 2021 Vitamin D and breast cancer: mechanistic update *JBMR Plus* **5** e10582

WHO 2022 https://who.int/news-room/fact-sheets/detail/cancer

Wu X Y and Lu L 2012 Vitamin B6 deficiency, genome instability and cancer *Asian Pac. J. Cancer Prev.* **13** 5333–8

Xin J, Jiang X, Ben S, Yuan Q, Su L, Zhang Z, Christiani D C, Du M and Wang M 2022 Association between circulating vitamin E and ten common cancers: evidence from large-scale Mendelian randomization analysis and a longitudinal cohort study *BMC Med.* **20** 168

Xv F, Chen J, Duan L and Li S 2018 Research progress on the anticancer effects of vitamin K2 *Oncol. Lett.* **15** 8926–34

Yadav D, Kwak M, Chauhan P S, Puranik N, Lee P C and Jin J O 2022 Cancer immunotherapy by immune checkpoint blockade and its advanced application using bio-nanomaterials *Seminars in Cancer Biology* (New York: Academic)vol 86 pp 909–22

Yang C S, Luo P, Zeng Z, Wang H, Malafa M and Suh N 2020 Vitamin E and cancer prevention: studies with different forms of tocopherols and tocotrienols *Mol. Carcinog* **59** 365–89

Yang C S, Suh N and Kong A N 2012 Does vitamin E prevent or promote cancer? *Cancer Prev. Res. (Phila)* **5** 701–5

Yang W, Cheng Y, Xu T, Wang X and Wen L P 2009 Targeting cancer cells with biotin–dendrimer conjugates *Eur. J. Med. Chem.* **44** 862–8

Yi Z, Wang L and Tu X 2021 Effect of Vitamin D deficiency on liver cancer risk: a systematic review and meta-analysis *Asian Pac. J. Cancer Prev: APJCP* **22** 991

Zasowska-Nowak A, Nowak P J and Ciałkowska-Rysz A 2021 High-dose vitamin C in advanced-stage cancer patients *Nutrients* **13** 735

Zastre J A, Sweet R L, Hanberry B S and Ye S 2013 Linking vitamin B1 with cancer cell metabolism *Cancer Metabol.* **1** 1–4

Zeng J, Gu Y, Fu H, Liu C, Zou Y and Chang H 2020 Association between one-carbon metabolism-related vitamins and risk of breast cancer: a systematic review and meta-analysis of prospective studies *Clin. Breast Cancer* **20** e469–80

Zhang Y F, Shi W W, Gao H F, Zhou L, Hou A J and Zhou Y H 2014 Folate intake and the risk of breast cancer: a dose-response meta-analysis of prospective studies *PLoS One* **9** e100044

Zhao Y, Guo C, Hu H, Zheng L, Ma J, Jiang L, Zhao E and Li H 2017 Folate intake, serum folate levels and esophageal cancer risk: an overall and dose–response meta-analysis *Oncotarget* **8** 10458–69

Zhao Z, Zhang Z P, Soprano D R and Soprano K J 1995 Effect of 9-cis-retinoic acid on growth and RXR expression in human breast cancer cells *Exp. Cell. Res.* **219** 555–61

Chapter 3

Phytochemicals as an epigenetic modifier to prevent cancer

Nidhi Puranik and Minseok Song

Cancer is a disease that develops as a result of a series of genetic and epigenetic changes. Despite extensive research, there are still many unsolved concerns regarding how epigenetic modifications relate to the development of cancer. Epigenetics is the modifications to the genome that affect gene expression by silencing some genes and altering the expression of other genes. These changes are frequently inherited. DNA methylation, histone modification, and non-coding RNA (ncRNA)-associated gene silencing are the three main pathways for epigenetic modifications. Even though cell differentiation and adaptability are two processes that epigenetics are crucial for maintaining on a daily basis, abnormal epigenetic modifications can impair or modify gene activity, which may eventually result in cancer. As a result, the relationship between epigenetics and cancer has been extensively researched over the past two decades, and this research has led to the production of a large amount of clinical data attesting to the effectiveness of epigenetics as a practical method for comprehending the progression of cancer or treating it. The anti-cancer benefits of natural compounds, particularly phytochemicals derived from medicinal plants, have been linked to their mechanisms of action. This chapter's goal is to examine the role of major phytochemical classes, such as polyphenols, alkaloids, terpenoids, and organosulfur compounds, as epigenetic regulators in the prevention and treatment of cancer. The relationships between cancer metabolism and epigenetic gene regulation, as well as how these processes are impacted by phytochemicals, are compiled in this chapter.

Abbreviations

DAS	Diallyl sulfide
DADS	Diallyl disulfide
DTS	Diallyl trisulfide

doi:10.1088/978-0-7503-5252-9ch3

DNMT	DNA methyltransferases
HDACs	Histone deacetylase
HAT	Hypoxanthine
KEAP1	Kelch-like ECH-associated protein 1
lncRNA	Long ncRNA
mRNA	Messenger RNA
miRNA	Micro RNA
ncRNA	Non-coding RNA
Nrf2	Nuclear factor erythroid 2–related factor 2
piRNA	Piwi interacting RNA
PTMs	Posttranslational modifications
RO/NS	Reactive oxygen/nitrogen species
SAM	S-adenosylmethionine
siRNA	Small interfering RNA

3.1 Introduction

The disruption of crucial biological processes involved in the control of the cell cycle, proliferation, differentiation, DNA repair, and cell death characterize cancer as a group of disorders. A complex web of connections includes abnormal genetic and epigenetic changes that cause cancer and coordinates cellular transformation, tumor development, tumor progression, and metastasis. Anomalies in the genome have long been thought to be the cause of cancer. But it became more obvious that epigenetics and cancer are inextricably linked as it became recognized that the genome is regulated by epigenetic mechanisms. Different facets of cancer biology, including aberrant transcription, cancer initiation, cancer progression, treatment resistance, and metastasis, can be impacted by a dysregulated epigenetic change. But because changed epigenetic systems are dynamic and reversible in nature, they make better targets for therapy than genetic mutations, which are harder to correct. Epigenetics has enormous promise for cancer treatments and gene reprogramming, which enables the altered genes to resume their normal function. Due to these benefits, epigenetic research in the field of oncology has increased exponentially, making them particularly promising and therapeutically useful targets for the fight against cancer (Pathak *et al* 2023).

Since ancient times, people have understood the effects of environment and diet on health. Cancer is a genetic and epigenetic illness with a multi-stage, complex interplay of genetic and environmental variables in which synchronized gene expression, protein synthesis, and metabolite function occur. Cancer in particular is brought on by the disruption of epigenetic mechanisms. By regulating the genome through processes including DNA methylation, histone modifications, and non-coding RNAs, epigenetics affect gene expression without affecting nucleotide sequences. Current research suggests that, in some situations, eating the right kinds of foods or getting a balanced diet can help avoid cancer. Dietary elements are a key determinant in the development and prevention of cancer, and nutrient consumption is a key environmental factor. In reaction to food components, bioactive substances, and phytochemicals acting as effective antioxidants and cancer-preventative agents, epigenetic events cause changes in DNA that affect all gene expressions. By affecting important routes and stages in carcinogenesis, such as signaling, apoptosis, differentiation, or inflammation, a number of dietary components can change the behavior of cancer cells and cancer risk. To date, a number of physiologically active food ingredients, such as methyl-group donors, fatty acids, phytochemicals, flavonoids, isothiocyanates, etc, have been strongly proposed to have preventive potential against the development of cancer. The diet has protective agents such as vitamins, antioxidants, detoxifying agents, chelating agents, etc. Therefore, the role of dietary phytochemicals as epigenetic modifiers in cancer as well as their effects on gene expression and signaling pathways have been extensively explored. A diet high in phytochemicals may influence the result of treatment as well as lowering the chance of acquiring cancer, according to recent studies on epigenetic modulations. Studies in epigenetics and cancer research showed that genetic and epigenetic mechanisms do not occur independently during the development of cancer; rather, they interact with one another. These studies also highlighted plant-derived anticancer compounds with epigenetic mechanisms of action and their potential application in epigenetic therapy (Pehlivan 2021).

Mammals' normal development and maintenance of tissue-specific gene expression patterns depend heavily on epigenetic processes. Alterations in gene activity and cancerous cellular transformation can result from epigenetic process disruption. Cancer is characterized by broad changes in the epigenetic landscape (Sharma *et al* 2010). The field of 'epigenetics' studies changes in gene expression brought on by heritable, but theoretically reversible, variations in DNA methylation and chromatin structure. Due to their early occurrence during carcinogenesis and probable role as cancer formation beginning events, epigenetic changes have been highlighted as prospective novel targets for cancer prevention techniques. Nutrigenetics, or the impact of dietary elements on factors affecting the epigenome, has arisen in recent years as an interesting new area of epigenetic study. Major cellular processes and pathways, such as drug metabolism, cell cycle control, the ability to repair DNA damage or to trigger apoptosis, the response to inflammatory stimuli, cell signaling, and control over cell proliferation and differentiation become dysregulated during carcinogenesis. Recent research suggests that epigenetic changes are responsible for these cellular defects. For instance, acetylation or methylation of histones and nonhistone proteins, such as p53, NF-kB, and the chaperone HSP90, epigenetically silences detoxifying enzymes, tumor suppressor genes, cell cycle regulators, apoptosis-inducing and DNA repair genes, nuclear receptors, signal transducers, and transcription factors (Gerhauser 2013). Growing evidence indicates that intermediary metabolites drive chromatin dynamics through chemical post-translational modifications (PTMs) that change the structures and functions of chromatin. Metabolism has recently been recognized as a key player and context-dependent regulator of epigenetic modifications (Sun *et al* 2022) (figure 3.1).

Numerous difficulties have been presented by conventional cancer therapy, such as toxicity, medication resistance, and cost. However, due to their capacity to control a variety of molecular pathways with a less harmful effect, phytochemicals used in complementary alternative medicine have recently attracted more attention.

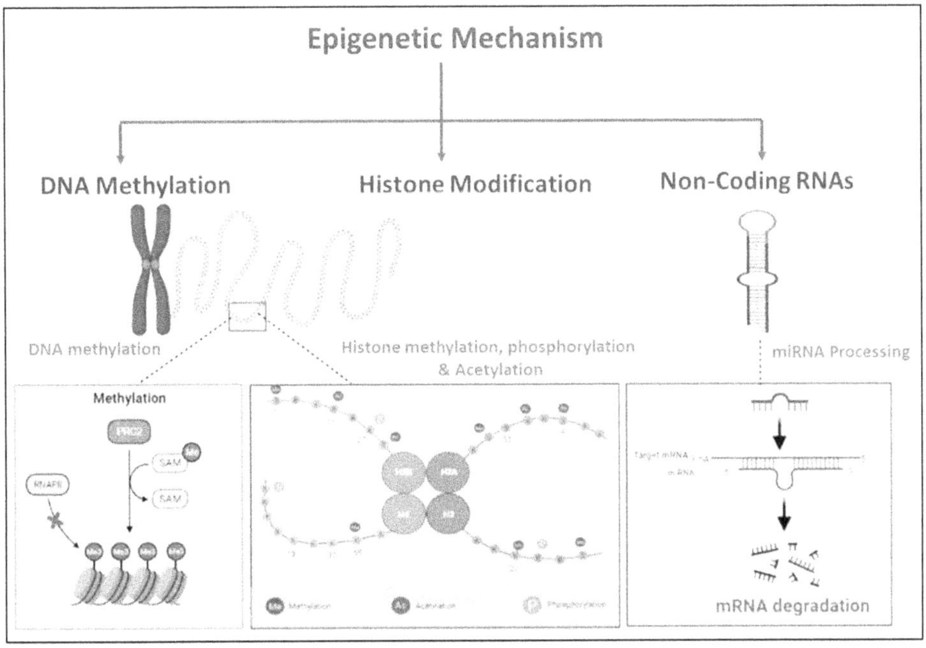

Figure 3.1. Epigenetic mechanisms involved in gene expression: DNA methylation, histone modifications, and non-coding RNAs constitute the three mechanisms involved in the epigenetic regulation of gene expression (created with BioRender.com).

Preclinical and clinical research is accumulating evidence that phytochemicals can influence the genesis and progression of cancer by favorably modulating a number of signaling pathways. Combinations of phytochemicals act as powerful alternatives to chemotherapy because they increase immune function, limit cancer cell invasion and proliferation, and promote cell death (Rizeq *et al* 2020).

Recent years have seen the emergence of 'nutri-epigenetics,' a fascinating new field in epigenetic research that focuses on the impact of dietary components on the epigenetic mechanism(s). Cancer chemoprevention research has focused a lot of attention on targeting abnormal epigenetic modifications because, unlike genetic changes, epigenetic alterations happen early in the development of cancer and can be reversed (Thakur *et al* 2014). In cell culture experiments and some animal models of cancer, there is growing evidence that dietary chemopreventive medicines can stop or undo these epigenetic alterations. All cancer types have aberrant gene expression caused by epigenetic alterations, therefore a logical and comprehensive strategy for cancer therapy would be to use these bioactive food substances to both treat and prevent cancer by neutralizing epigenomic abnormalities (Lewis and Tollefsbol 2017).

Plant-derived compounds known as phytochemicals have been used to prevent chronic and degenerative diseases because they have the potential to influence disease development. A class of low molecular weight polyphenolic phytochemicals called flavonoids is present in all types of plants. They are classified as flavonols,

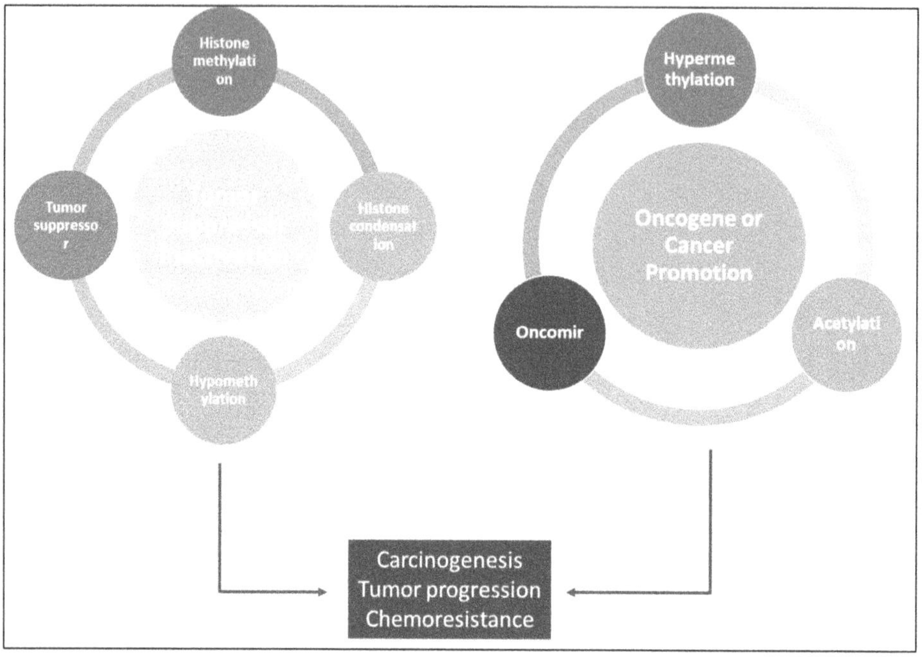

Figure 3.2. A schematic representation of tumor progression by inhibition of tumor suppressor factors and activation of oncogenes.

flavones, flavanones, isoflavones, catechins, anthocyanidins, and chalcones based on their chemical makeup (Mukherjee *et al* 2015) (figure 3.2).

3.2 Epigenetics

The term 'epigenetics' refers to heritable modifications that are not directly encoded in the DNA sequence but yet have a significant impact on how genes are expressed. It involves alterations to histones, RNA interference, and DNA methylation changes. Typically, epigenetics refer to heritable modifications of gene expression that do not affect the DNA sequence itself. The three most significant epigenetic processes are listed below. These comprise RNA interference, histone modification, and DNA methylation. The role of individual alterations as well as the synergistic impact of those modifications in the onset and development of cancer are now being studied by epigenetic research. The recruitment of different transcriptional regulatory proteins that bind to certain, modified histone structures is one way in which this mix of histone modifications has a noticeable impact on gene expression. A variety of enzymes that catalyze the addition of different chemical groups, such as acetyl-, methyl-, phosphate-, and ubiquitin-, from one substrate to another are responsible for the PTM of histones. The lysine and arginine residues found in the histone peptides are the main targets for acetylation and methylation. The residues serine, threonine, and tyrosine are phosphorylated. The presence of certain lysine and arginine methylation sites near acetylation and phosphorylation sites on the

N-terminal tails of histones shows that the various post-translational histone modifications may work together to modulate chromatin structure. The interactions of the histone tails with DNA and other proteins may be disrupted or enhanced by particular combinations of covalent modifications (Zam and Khadour 2017). The accumulating body of research strongly suggests that genomic instability plays a key role in epigenetic dysregulation in breast cancer pathogenesis and is a key feature of breast cancer hallmarks. Compared to the more unidirectional genetic changes, epigenetic processes are more accessible to therapeutic intervention since they are reversible and changeable. In this study, we describe the epigenetic reprogramming linked to breast cancer, including changes in the expression profiles of miRNAs, histone acetylation, and DNA methylation (Rahman *et al* 2019).

3.2.1 DNA methylation

DNA methylation is one epigenetic process that enables the exact gene expression cascade required for cellular development. However, as people age and develop tumors, these systems go out of control, which compromises cellular identity and function (Köhler and Rodríguez-Paredes 2020). DNA methylation is the action of DNA methyltransferases to transfer a methyl group from S-adenosylmethionine (SAM) to the C5 position of the pyrimidine ring of cytosine residues in genomic CpG dinucleotides. CpG islands, which are clusters found at gene promoters, are one location in the genome where CpG dinucleotides are preferentially found. CpG islands are short segments of the genome that are typically found every 100 kb and range in size from 0.5 to 5 kb. They are distinguished by the fact that they are unmethylated. Housekeeping and tissue-specific genes are among the CpG island-containing genes that make up about half of all human genes. DNA methyltransferases (DNMT) are enzymes that facilitate DNA methylation. DNMT1b, DNMT1o, DNMT1p, DNMT2, DNMT3A, DNMT3b along with its subtype, and DNMT3L are the DNMTs that have been identified thus far (Jin and Chen 2016).

In the future, tumor DNA methylation profiling, which has already helped to identify new entities and combine tumors with different morphologies into one biologically coherent entity, will likely become more widely used. Additionally, the DNA methylation patterns in circulating tumor DNA show significant potential for the diagnosis and categorization of cancer with minimally invasive methods (Papanicolau-Sengos *et al* 2022).

3.2.2 Histone modification

Histones, which create an octameric cylinder scaffold and are highly conserved DNA-packaging proteins, make it easier to wrap 147 bp DNA stretched around the cylindrical spool. Two sets of the core histone proteins H2A, H2B, H3, and H4 make up the octamer core. A central globular histone fold, which makes up around 75% of the mass of core histone proteins, is formed when core histone proteins come together in a certain way. The remaining histone mass primarily takes the shape of amorphous, flexible histone tails. For reversible and covalent PTMs like acetylation, methylation, ubiquitination, phosphorylation, sumoylation, poly-ADP-ribosylation, neddylation, and glycosylation, the tails (H3/H4 N-terminal tail and H2A/H2B C-terminal tail) as well as the histone fold provide sites. In the context of cancer, extensive research has been done on the histone changes that occur during carcinogenesis and metastasis in order to identify biomarkers, diagnostic tools, and therapies (Rahman *et al* 2019).

The expression and activity of histone deacetylase (HDACs) are connected to the alteration of the acetylation signature, which functions as a master epigenetic change in malignancies. In this setting, class I HDACs are important regulators of cancer and cell proliferation. Cancer stem cells (CSCs) are a minority population of tumor cells that have just lately been identified as being responsible for the invasiveness, medication resistance, and recurrence of malignancies. The acetylation pattern of chromatin may now be regulated by modulating CSCs through epigenetic reprogramming, such as by targeting HDACs. Several researches have recently identified some phytochemicals as HDAC inhibitors. The usage of phytochemicals with HDAC inhibitory properties may be effective in resolving the aforementioned issues with CSCs (Bayat *et al* 2018).

3.2.3 Non-coding RNAs

Non-coding RNA (ncRNA) transcripts have been linked to a number of epigenetic mechanisms, including DNA imprinting, paramutation, transposon silencing, X-chromosome inactivation, and transposon silencing, according to recent research. Approximately 98% of all human transcriptional output is made up of non-coding RNAs (ncRNAs), which in humans comprise the microRNA (miRNA), small interfering RNA (siRNA), and piwi interacting RNA (piRNA). Small ncRNA, which is typically less than 200 nucleotides in length, and long ncRNA (lncRNA), which are transcripts longer than 200 nucleotides, can be divided into two categories based on size. Key epigenetic pathways are regulated by small ncRNAs, especially miRNAs. MiRNAs are well known for controlling different polycomb complexes and other elements of the cellular epigenetic machinery, which has a variety of downstream effects (Shankar *et al* 2016). It was established more than ten years ago that lncRNAs produced from the rDNA promoter control the transcription of rDNA and DNA methylation. Later research showed that this type of lncRNA interacts with the rDNA promoter to produce a DNA: RNA triplex that is recognized by DNMT3B to epigenetically control the production of rDNA (Huang *et al* 2022).

The majority of ncRNAs are now recognized as important regulators in a variety of networks where they may influence particular cellular responses and destinies. The discovery of ncRNAs as both tumor suppressors and oncogenic drivers in various malignancies points to a complex regulatory network including these ncRNAs (Saw *et al* 2021) (figure 3.3).

Similar outcomes are emerging for the treatment of solid tumors, and reversal of these epigenetic modifications has been demonstrably shown to have therapeutic effects in a variety of lymphoma and preleukemia types (Ilango *et al* 2020).

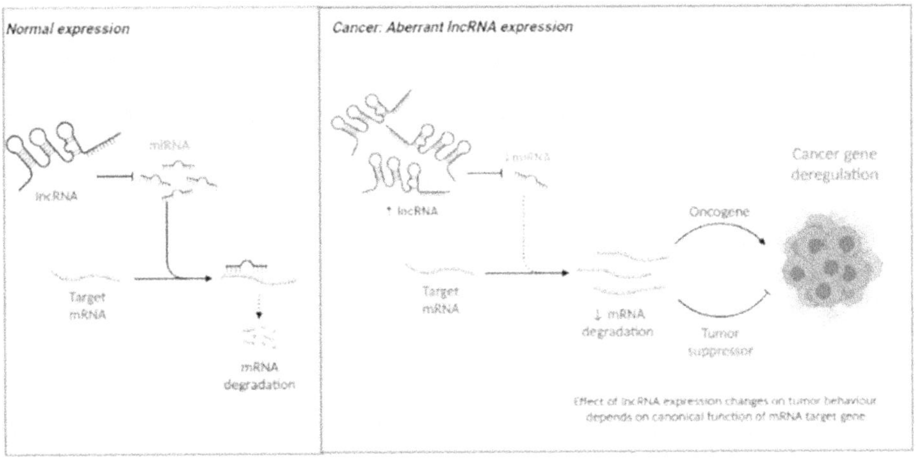

Figure 3.3. A schematic diagram shows the lncRNA-mRNA gene expression regulation in cancer (created with BioRender.com).

3.3 Oxidative stress and epigenetics

Biological redox signaling is crucial in the development of many illnesses. Reductive and oxidative pathways are used in redox signaling. When oxidative challenges outweigh the reductive mechanism, oxidative stress results. Reactive oxygen/nitrogen species (RO/NS) that are more than what the cellular reductive/antioxidant capability can handle cause cellular oxidative stress. Cellular signaling events are triggered by endogenously produced RO/NS from the mitochondrial metabolic citric-acid cycle combined with the electron transport chain or foreign stimuli, which can result in pathological damage or a homeostatic response. When the reductive system is overpowered by the oxidative challenge, oxidative stress results. Reactive oxygen/nitrogen species (RO/NS), such as superoxide, hydroxyl, hydrogen peroxide, phenoxyl, nitric oxide, nitrogen dioxide, dinitrogen trioxide, and nitrous acid radicals, among others, can accumulate to levels that are greater than the body's ability to reduce them or combat them with antioxidants such as glutathione, catalase, superoxide dismutase, and glutathione peroxidase. It is significant to note that RO/NS are secondary messengers that activate cellular signaling pathways in order to maintain the equilibrium of the intracellular redox state, which results in typical physiological homeostatic responses. Recent data suggest that RO/NS also affects the mechanisms controlling gene expression at the epigenetic level. Histone acetylation/deacetylation, DNA methylation/demethylation, or histone methylation/demethylation are all impacted by RO/NS. Numerous phytochemicals with health benefits have redox properties that neutralize RO/NS either directly by scavenging free radicals or indirectly through the induction of antioxidant/reductive enzymes in cellular defense. Surprisingly, these phytochemicals can affect epigenetic processes. Numerous dietary phytochemicals with positive health effects that are plentiful in fruit and vegetables are redox-active and have epigenetic effects. These redox-active phytochemicals interact with the citric acid cycle, cellular metabolism,

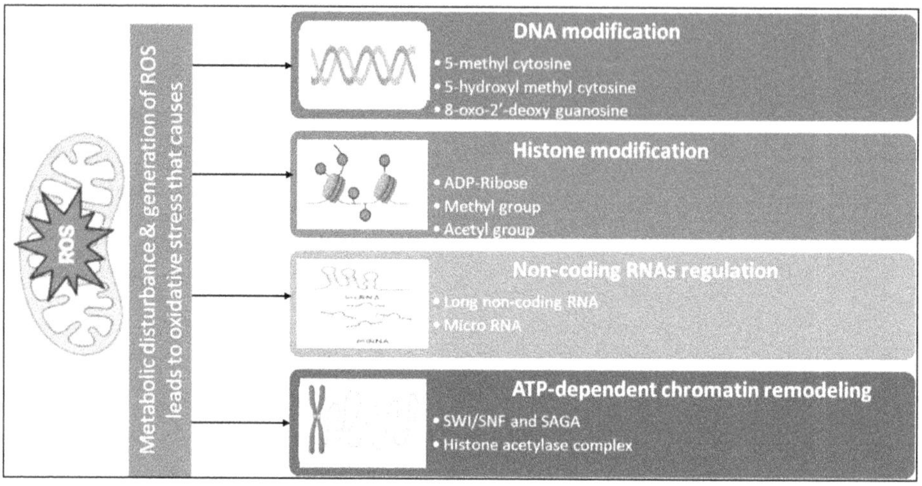

Figure 3.4. Oxidative stress leads to epigenetic modification.

and the epigenetic apparatus, and they change the cellular redox status. We will briefly review the most prevalent types of these redox-active phytochemicals with the ability to influence epigenetic processes (Wu *et al* 2022) (figure 3.4).

3.4 Phytochemicals

Epigenetic markers, which refer to a group of alterations influencing gene expression without changing the actual sequence of DNA, ensure the persistence of cellular memory. DNA methylation, histone modification, chromatin remodeling, and mRNA and ncRNA activity are a few examples of epigenetic alterations. Enzymes that catalyze these events in particular ways, such as DNMT, HDAC, and HAT, are responsible for all of these alterations. Recently, a strong correlation and demonstration of the relationship between the disruption of epigenetic modifications, loss of cellular memory, and tumor transformation have been made. The word 'epidrugs' refers to a class of chemicals that act on epigenetic processes and are used as anti-cancer medications (El Omari *et al* 2021).

Phytochemicals are secondary metabolites derived from plants that have a variety of biological effects on people, including anti-cancer qualities. This topic is still debatable despite current research that seems to support their involvement in both preventing and treating cancer. The primary mechanism by which phytochemicals fight cancer is a multi-targeted action that includes antimutagenic, antioxidant, and anti-proliferative properties (Catalano 2016).

Through research using *in vitro* and *in vivo* animal models, as well as results from various epidemiologic studies, many kinds of dietary phytochemicals have been demonstrated to have cancer-preventive characteristics (Dave *et al* 2020). Unexpectedly, it has been discovered that these dietary cancer-preventative substances also control epigenetic activity (Kong *et al* 2013).

It has been demonstrated that a number of active food components with anti-cancer potential might affect epigenetic activities. These dietary molecules, which include folate, polyphenols, selenium, retinoids, fatty acids, isothiocyanates, and allyl compounds, are components of various chemical classes. These bioactive food components may have an impact on cancer prevention mechanisms such as signal transduction pathways, cell growth, differentiation, and apoptosis by interfering with epigenetic processes deregulated during carcinogenesis, such as global DNA hypomethylation, tumor suppressor gene promoter hypermethylation, and histone onco-modification (Ong *et al* 2012).

Epigenetics, transcriptomics, and nutrigenomics are all included in nutrigenomics, along with other 'omic disciplines like metabolomics and proteomics that clearly illustrate the wide variation in tumor risk across people with similar dietary preferences. Numerous research on a variety of food components, such as phytochemicals, important nutrients, and chemicals derived from bacteria, and fungal chemicals, had produced varying outcomes in terms of how well they reduced the risk of cancer and tumor development. In nutrigenetics and nutrigenomics, foods interact with cancer-related genes, while their effects on epigenetic processes such as DNA methylation and histone modifications are the focus of nutrigenetics (Nasir *et al* 2022). Figure 3.5 is showing the phytochemicals-based regulation of DNA methylation and demethylation.

The context of cancer research is the greatest place to understand how epigenetic processes might silence genes. During the development of cancer, epigenetic modification silences a large number of tumor suppressor genes. DNA seems to be hypomethylated globally and certain genes appear to be hypermethylated (Gilbert *et al* 2010).

Numerous anti-cancer medications have been created that target epigenetic machinery, including HDAC and DNMT inhibitors. Although these medications

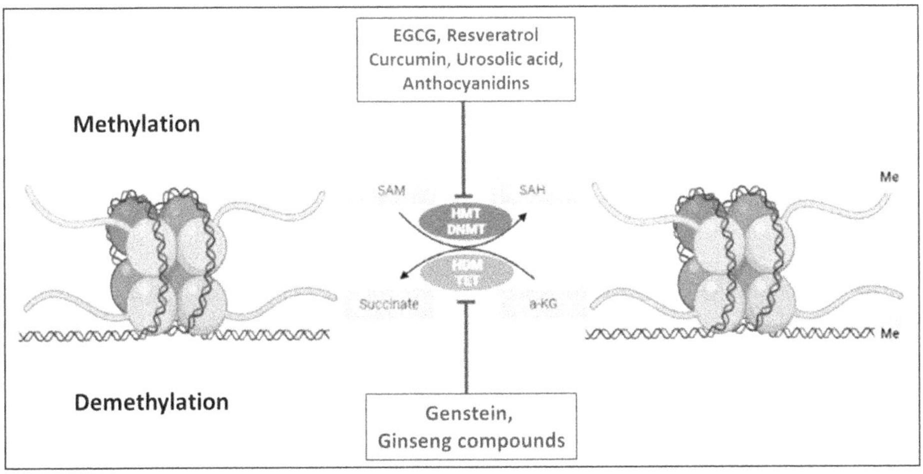

Figure 3.5. Phytochemicals-based regulation of methylation and demethylation (created with BioRender.com).

had some effect on various forms of cancer, modest to severe negative side effects have been noted (Unoki 2011).

Histone deacetylase/acetyltransferase activator can increase HDAC/hypoxanthine (HAT) activity, which in turn can either increase or decrease gene expression. In addition to HAT and HDAC inhibitors, HAT and HDAC activators also have the potential to be used as breast cancer therapy. The activators of HAT or HDAC may also turn into medications for treating breast cancer since histone acetylation or deacetylation can stop the growth of breast cancer (Guo *et al* 2018). A basic schematic diagram of role of phytochemicals in histone modification is shown in figure 3.6.

Our understanding of nuclear factor erythroid 2-related factor 2 (Nrf2)/Kelch-like ECH-associated protein 1 (Keapl) signaling has been expanded by the study of epigenetics. The reversible nature of epigenetic alterations, in contrast to hereditary changes in an acting DNA sequence, offers an alluring method of cancer prevention (Bhattacharjee and Dashwood 2020).

3.4.1 Polyphenols

The most significant class of phytochemicals found in plants are polyphenols. They are byproducts of plants that can be found in natural foods such as fruit, vegetables, cereals, and beverages. These substances play biological functions in human cells, including those of antioxidants, antimicrobials, detoxifiers, immune system stimulators, platelet-aggregation inhibitors, hormone metabolism regulators, and antitumor agents (Carlos-Reyes *et al* 2019). Based on their chemical makeup, purpose, bioavailability, and stability, polyphenols can be categorized. Today, flavonoids make up half of the more than 8000 polyphenols that have been found. Despite this, several studies have produced results that are difficult to put into practice since they were conducted using excessively high concentrations of polyphenols without taking

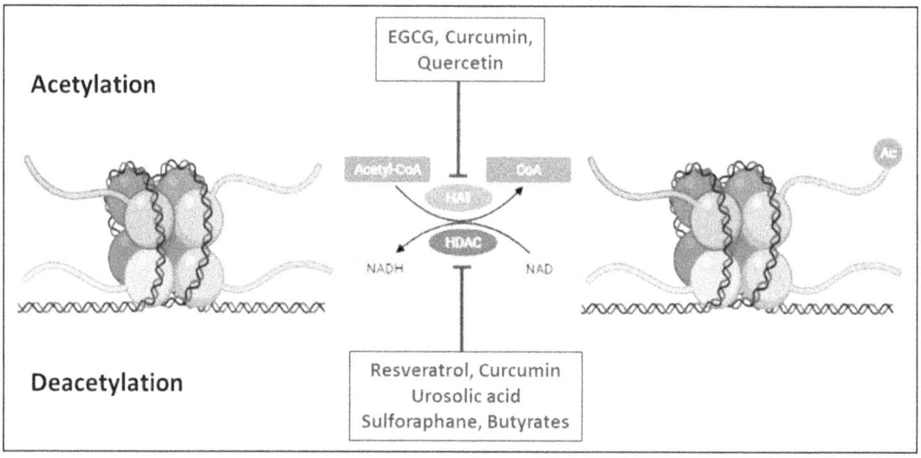

Figure 3.6. Phytochemicals-based regulation of acetylation and deacetylation (created with BioRender.com).

daily intake or bioavailability into account (Khan *et al* 2021). Various research studies support the potential of flavonoids as epigenetic regulators including flavonols, flavanones, anthocyanidins, isoflavones, and flavones.

A large class of chemicals known as phenolic compounds have anti-cancer, anti-inflammatory, and antioxidant properties. These traits appear to be connected to inhibiting the formation, microenvironment, and metabolism of CSCs through epigenetic pathways (Ghasemi *et al* 2021). These phytochemicals and polyphenols can have an improved impact on epigenetic alterations, which are critical for the treatment and prevention of cancer when administered in a dose-dependent and combinatorial manner (Arora *et al* 2019).

According to recent findings, natural substances and dietary supplements may be able to restore the normal epigenetic markers that are changed during carcinogenesis. The phytochemicals that have been examined the most in relation to cancer are epigallocatechin gallate (EGCG), quercetin, resveratrol, curcumin, and sulforaphane. These organic substances are known to suppress a number of cellular processes linked to cancer, according to numerous researches. These substances specifically prevented the growth and spread of tumors by focusing on important signaling transducers, which led to the restoration of tumor suppressor genes and the inhibition of oncogene expression. These effects are partly mediated by altering the epigenetic apparatus, which controls the activity of DNMTs and HDACs (Carlos-Reyes *et al* 2019). For instance, it has been demonstrated that the enzymes DNMTs and HDACs are inhibited by EGCG. Regular use of EGCG, a polyphenolic catechin mostly found in green tea, may greatly lower the risk of breast and prostate cancer. By using epigenetic pathways, this natural substance may cause apoptosis and prevent cell proliferation (Aggarwal *et al* 2015).

Numerous researches suggest that curcumin possesses anti-inflammatory, anti-proliferative, anti-cancer, and anti-anti-inflammatory activities. In brain cancer cells, it causes apoptosis and histone hypoacetylation in conjunction with PARP activity. Additionally, curcumin enhanced neuronal differentiation linked to the hypoacetylation of H3 and H4 and inhibited astrocyte differentiation (Hewlings and Kalman 2017). In accordance with additional research, curcumin boosted RANK protein levels in human glioblastoma cells via a demethylation process. Neurogenesis of neural progenitor cells and caspase-3-dependent glioma cell death were both increased by curcumin-induced histone hypoacetylation. Additionally, low STAT3 levels resulted in RANK promoter demethylation, which led to the gene's reactivation (Wu *et al* 2013).

Substantial evidence from both preclinical and clinical investigations supports the idea that bioactive natural substances have substantial anti-cancer activities. Some of these effects are synchronized by altering the epigenetic machinery of the altered cells. Only a very small amount of data, however, is known on the clinical application of phytochemicals that modulate epigenetic processes in the treatment of human breast cancer. To get these epigenetic modulators from the laboratory to the bedside and validate the preclinical information, additional clinical trials are necessary (Shukla *et al* 2019).

Through the control of epigenetic mechanisms such as DNA methylation, histone modification, or miRNA expression, phenolic substances have the capacity to modify gene expression. Generally speaking, a number of phenolic substances can activate HDACs (e.g., fisetin), genistein, or inhibit HATs (e.g., EGCG, curcumin), sirtuins (e.g., resveratrol), and DNMTs (e.g., EGCG). Some phenolic substances, such as genistein and curcumin, are connected to the control of miRNA expression. Numerous phenolic substances have the capacity to influence NF-B activity and chromatin remodeling via the control of HDACs and HATs (Číž *et al* 2020). An isoflavone called genistein can stop unchecked cell proliferation in colon cancer by blocking the Wnt signaling pathway through epigenetic alteration (Wang *et al* 2012). Effects of trichostatin A and EGCG on p16INK4a gene expression and tumor progression in human malignant lymphoma (Wu *et al* 2013). Through altering the epigenome, curcumin and trichostatin A can reduce cell viability and cause apoptosis. Effects of trichostatin A and curcumin on hepatocellular carcinoma (HCC) Hepa 1–6 cell line DNMT1 gene expression, cell growth suppression, and induction of apoptosis (Kavoosi 2018). Effect of curcumin versus trichostatin A on the reactivation of estrogen receptor alpha gene expression by epigenetic alteration that results in cell growth suppression and induction of death in the HCC cell line (Sanaei *et al* 2020). However, some investigations have demonstrated that the amount of demethylation or the reactivation of methylation-silenced genes does not significantly vary when EGCG is administered. Additionally, the findings from various studies looking at how EGCG affects the reactivation of silenced genes seem to be still up for debate. More research is necessary to demonstrate the effectiveness of EGCG in preventing cancer by altering the epigenome (Shirakami *et al* 2015).

3.4.2 Alkaloids

Early epigenetic evidence for the prevention and treatment of colorectal cancer is provided by the effect of evodiamine and berberine on the interaction between DNMTs and target microRNAs during the malignant transformation of the colon by TGF-1. They also increased the expression of DNMT1, DNMT3A, and DNMT3B as well as miR-152, miR-429, and miR-29a genes (Huang *et al* 2017). Via suppressing the production of DNMT1 and DNMT3B, which leads to hypomethylation of TP53 via altering the DNA methylation level and the p53-dependent signal pathway, berberine causes death in the human multiple myeloma cell line U266 (Qing *et al* 2014). In acute myelocytic leukemia, berberine affects the histone code by suppressing the expression of EZH2 and DNMT1 in HL-60/ADR and KG1-cells, both in terms of protein and mRNA. In terms of DNA methylation, BBR caused the SFRPs' level of methylation to drop, which in turn suppressed the Wnt/-catenin pathway. The findings of this investigation point to the possibility that berberine may modify the expression of epigenetic regulators crucial for some downstream pathways, resulting in the manifestation of its diverse biological actions in acute myeloid leukaemia (AML) cells (Wang *et al* 2017). Berberine affects the expression of the histone code by reducing the levels of the proteins H3K4me3,

H3K27me3, and H3K36me3 in a potential epigenetic modulator (Wang *et al* 2016). The impact of harmalin on DNMT1 expression reduction, P15 promoter hypomethylation, and P15 reactivation in this cell line shows that it might be recommended as a treatment approach, suited for monotherapy or as an addition to medication that is frequently used to treat acute promyeloid leukemia (Nikkhoo *et al* 2017). In the HL-60 leukemia cell line, harmine alkaloid affects the expression of P16 and DAPK and causes DAPK to be up-regulated (Aghide *et al* 2016). Mahanine stimulates the proteasomal degradation of DNMT1 and DNMT3B via the inhibition of Akt, which allows the demethylation of the RASSF1A promoter and restores its expression in prostate cancer cells, making it a promising therapeutic agent for the treatment of advanced prostate cancer (Agarwal, *et al* 2013). By inhibiting the tumor suppressor miR-203, butyric acid, nicotinamide, and calcium glucarate, which are all naturally occurring substances, were found to have chemopreventive effects on mouse skin tumors caused by 7,12-dimethylbenz [a] anthracene (Tiwari and Gupta 2014). Vincristine's role in the therapy of colorectal cancer cells was investigated by Moon and their group. They discovered that vincristine demethylates the RUNX3 gene in these cells and restores its expression (Moon *et al* 2014). The well-known anti-cancer drug trichostatin A inhibits histone deacetylase and efficiently and specifically triggers tumor growth arrest and apoptosis. A recent study found that CTCF is recruited into the demethylated core promoter region of human telomerase reverse transcriptase (hTERT) in HCT-116, which in turn causes TSA-induced DNMT1 down-regulation to suppress hTERT expression (Choi *et al* 2010).

3.4.3 Terpenoids

Triterpenoids' biological effects on health and the prevention of cancer work through a variety of pathways, including their anti-inflammatory and antioxidant qualities, their ability to regulate the cell cycle, and their control of epigenetic/epigenomic processes. Triterpenoids may be able to prevent colon cancer via altering the epigenome, according to growing research. Triterpenoids play a key role in the epigenetic regulation of genes, which includes gene-specific methylation via DNMT and miRNA alterations, in the prevention of cancer (Li *et al* 2020).

Triterpenoid corosolic acid modulates the global CpG methylation and transcriptome of tumor-promoting TPA-induced mouse epidermal JB6 P+ cells, revealing that CA may be able to reverse these changes, elucidating novel molecular targets for future prevention of early stages of skin cancer studies in humans (Hudlikar *et al* 2020). By altering the DNA methylation status of a number of tumor suppressor genes in colorectal cancer cells, boswellic acid causes epigenetic changes (Shen *et al* 2012). c-Myc, cyclin D1, and survivin are among the oncogenes whose promoters are hypermethylated by cucurbitacin B in breast cancer cells, suggesting that it may be used as a cancer treatment for the disease (Dittharot *et al* 2019). Another study on cucurbitacin B found that it could inhibit DNMTs and HDACs in H1299 cells, leading to the reactivation of important tumor suppressor genes like CDKN1A and CDKN2A as well as down-regulation of important tumor promoter genes, including hTERT and oncogenes c-MYC and K-RAS. This implies that it can prevent NNK-induced lung carcinogenesis and alter the expression of genes associated with tumors in non-small cell lung cancer (NSCLC) through epigenetic alterations (Shukla *et al* 2015). Grifolin's anti-tumor effects come from the epigenetic reactivation of genes related to metastasis inhibitory factors via ERK1/2-Elk1-DNMT1 signaling (Ye *et al* 2007). Grifolin may be an effective ERK1/2 kinase inhibitor as well as an epigenetic agent to improve our understanding of DNMT1 activity. It may also be a viable therapeutic lead chemical for the prevention of cancer metastasis (Luo *et al* 2015). By preventing the expression of DNMT1 and UHRF1 in colon cancer cells, hinokitiol might affect DNA methylation. expression of DNMT1, UHRF1, and the ubiquitin-like plant homeodomain in HCT-116 cells. In addition, treatment with hinokitiol boosted the expression of TET1, a recognized DNA demethylation initiator. Hinokitiol enhanced the 5-hydroxymethylcytosine level in both colon cancer cells, but the 5-methylcytosine level was unaffected. Hinokitiol also considerably improved the methylation status of HCT-116 cells while also significantly restoring the mRNA expression of B-cell translocation gene 4, carbohydrate sulfotransferase 10, and O6-methylguanine DNA methyltransferase (Seo *et al* 2017). In our test leukemia cells, parthenolide, an epigenetic modulator, produces global DNA hypomethylation and increases histone acetylation in a dose- and time-dependent manner. With an EC50 of 5.0 M, parthenolide inhibits M. SssI activity, depletes DNMT1 protein at a concentration of 10 M, and downregulates DNMT1 transcription in a time- and dose-dependent manner. The docking model shows that parthenolide inhibits DNMT activity presumably by covalently interacting with the catalytic active site through the Michael addition of the cysteine of DNMT1 to the parthenolide's -methylene lactone. In addition, we discovered that parthenolide markedly ups histone acetylation without changing the quantity of the enzyme, indicating that parthenolide may inhibit HDAC. P21 transcription was upregulated in correlation with enhanced histone acetylation and DNA demethylation (Liu *et al* 2007). Another study confirmed parthenolide's promise as a chemopreventive medication by demonstrating that it suppresses tumor promotion and epigenetically modifies p21 expression (Ghantous *et al* 2012). The function of parthenolide as a therapeutic molecule in the treatment of AML was investigated by Yun Dai and his team. The study found that parthenolide interacts with inhibitors of histone deacetylase to cause MKK7/JNK1-dependent apoptosis in human acute myeloid leukemia cells. Parthenolide increases the lethality of HDACI in human AML cells by inhibiting NF-B and then activating the SAPK/JNK pathway under the control of MKK7 (Dai *et al* 2010). Through the inhibition of Sp1 by AMPK, which in turn causes the inhibition of DNMT1, ursolic acid reduces the growth of HCC. This result implies that DNMT1 may be a novel target for HCC chemoprevention and treatment and uncovers a possibly novel mechanism by which UA regulates the development of HCC cells (Yie *et al* 2015). Leukocytes expressing iNos and the epigenetic markers DNA methyltransferases and HDACs in response to LPS were suppressed by UA (Zhang *et al* 2017).

3.4.4 Organosulfur compounds

Allium vegetables like garlic and onions contain organosulfur chemicals that are known to be anti-carcinogenic. Garlic oil contains a significant amount of diallyl sulfide (DAS), which inhibits the growth of tumors caused by different metabolically active carcinogens. Through the inhibition of N-nitroso methyl benzylamine carcinogen-promoted DNA methylation in rats, the anti-carcinogenic effect of DAS was reported, although not enough chemopreventive efficacy. In SiHa cervical cancer cells, allyl sulfide (AS), another organosulfur component present in garlic, led to the reversal of hypermethylation of the RAR2 promoter. Several investigations found that diverse rat and mouse cells, human cancer cells, xenografts, and HDAC inhibition-mediated hyperacetylation of histone H3 and H4 were present (Kumar *et al* 2016). The sulfur-containing organic molecules known as organosulfur compounds are responsible for the strong aromas of allium vegetables like garlic and onions. Additionally, cruciferous veggies like broccoli and cabbage are widely available in them. One of the main components of the allyl derivatives found in garlic oils is DAS. This chemical has pharmacological and biological properties such as anti-inflammatory, anti-carcinogenic, and antiangiogenic effects, along with other allyl derivatives such as diallyl disulfide (DADS) and diallyl trisulfide (DTS). Cancer cells have been demonstrated to experience cytotoxic and apoptotic effects from AS. However, it is currently unclear how cancer prevention in CRCs works mechanistically. Inhibiting invasion and metastasis in colon cancer cells has been demonstrated for all three of these allyl sulfides, with DTS being more effective than DADS and DAS at doses of 10 and 25 M. These modifications were discovered to be mediated by the down-regulation of the cell proliferation-related pathways COX-2 and NF-B. Also suppressed were participants in the cell invasion and migration pathway (PI3K, Ras, MEKK3, MKK7, ERK1/2, JNK1/2, p38, and MMPs 2, 7, and 9) (Lai *et al* 2012). At doses of 200 m in Caco-2 and HT-29 cells, it has been demonstrated that DADS and its metabolite, allyl mercaptan (AM), promote the production of p21 through a decrease in HDACs and an increase in H3 and H4 hyperacetylation. Lysine residues at positions 12 and 16 were more frequently found to be acetylated. When compared to DADS, AM was found to be a more effective HDAC inhibitor (92%) (Druesne *et al* 2004). Additionally, DADS have been demonstrated to cause cell cycle arrest in the G2/M phase in HCT-116 cells due to an increase in cyclin B1 expression in a p53-independent way (Jo *et al* 2008). Similar to this, DAS therapy caused G2/M arrest in Colo 320 DM colon cancer cells, which was accompanied by enhanced caspase-3 expression and ERK2 inhibition (Sriram *et al* 2008). Collectively, these and numerous other studies demonstrate DAS's capacity to stop colon cancer cells from proliferating, inducing apoptosis, and migrating. However, additional *in vivo* and clinical research is necessary to confirm the chemopreventive properties of this allylic molecule (Arya and Saldanha 2019). Another investigation found that AM reduces HDAC activity and increases the binding of Sp3 to the P21WAF1 promoter, repressing epigenetically repressed genes in cancer cells (Nian *et al* 2008).

Bioactive dietary substances known as organosulfur compounds are mostly found in cruciferous vegetables like broccoli, cabbage, cauliflower, watercress, and Brussels sprouts. Notably, the naturally occurring tiny chemical compounds known as organosulfur compounds including sulforaphane, phenethyl isothiocyanate, allicin, benzyl isothiocyanate, and DADS are produced from the glucosinolate precursors present in cruciferous plants. According to epidemiological research, eating cruciferous veggies may lower one's overall chance of contracting a number of diseases, including several cancers. Organosulfur compounds have previously been demonstrated to influence epigenetic regulation to have chemopreventive effects on a number of malignancies. Organosulfur compounds target DNA methylation, histone changes, and microRNA control specifically, which may significantly aid in the epigenetic regulation of cancer prevention. The synergistic potential of organosulfur compounds in combination with another molecule or a common cancer medication has also been demonstrated in a number of preclinical investigations. It is critical to note that there is a dearth of clinical research on the epigenetic modifications caused by organo-sulfur compounds in cancer cells (Shoaib *et al* 2023).

Although it has been assumed that DNA methylation in cancer cells is primarily responsible for the effects of EGCG on epigenetic change, a prior study found that EGCG also acts as a histone modifier. When human esophageal cancer cells are treated with EGCG, DNA methyltransferase activity is inhibited, which causes cytosine-phosphate guanine demethylation and the reactivation of suppressed tumor-suppressor genes like p16INK4a, retinoic acid receptor (RAR), and O6-methylguanine-DNA methyltransferase. In breast cancer cell lines, EGCG is also said to partially stimulate the demethylation of hypermethylated RAR. The ability of sulforaphane and indole-3-carbinol derivatives to influence the activity of enzymes governing the epigenetic status of prostate cancer cells has been established by recent studies (Watson *et al* 2013) and in colon cancer, sulforaphane induces NRF2 and inhibits HDAC activity and protein expression (Rajendran *et al* 2015) (tables 3.1 and 3.2).

3.5 Concluding remark and future prospective

Cancer continues to be the leading cause of death in both industrialized and developing countries, despite breakthroughs in modern medicine. To improve patient care, it is necessary to look for safer and more efficient chemoprevention and treatment methods (Pratheeshkumar *et al* 2015). Natural remedies have long been utilized to cure a variety of illnesses. Plant-based foods are linked to advantageous health effects brought on by bioactive substances. Phytochemicals are bioactive, non-nutritive substances that are present in fruit, vegetables, and other plant sources and have health-promoting properties including antioxidants and anti-inflammatories. Importantly, because of their cumulative or synergistic effects, a mixture of phytochemicals found in whole foods may be more protective against carcinogenesis. Natural compounds have recently attracted a lot of attention due to their potential to fight cancer by altering different cancer-associated signaling

Table 3.1. A table summarizes the effect of phytochemicals as an epigenetic modifier to suppress cancer development and progression.

Phytochemical	Cancer	Epigenetic activity	Gene	Outcome	References
Curcumin	Prostate cancer	DNA hypomethylation	Nrf2 regulation	Induction of the Nrf2-mediated anti-oxidative stress cellular defense pathway	Khor *et al* (2011)
EGCG	Breast cancer	Hypomethylation	SCUBE2	Inhibition of breast cancer progression	Sheng *et al* (2019)
Anthocyanin delphinidin	Skin cancer	DNA demethylation	Nrf2 promoter	Prevents neoplastic transformation	Kuo *et al* (2019)
Resveratrol	Breast cancer	Histone methylation and acetylation	BRCA1, p53, and p21	Restored expression of tumor suppressor genes	Chatterjee *et al* (2019)
Fucoxanthin	Skin cancer	DNA demethylation	Nrf2 promoter	Blocks the TPA-induced transformation	Yang *et al* (2018)
Curcumin	Colorectal cancer	DNA methylation	CDX2 promoter	Inhibit epithelial-mesenchymal transition	Chen *et al* (2020)
Flavone luteolin	Colorectal cancer	DNA demethylation	Nrf2 gene	Inhibit cell transformation	Zuo *et al* (2018)
Fisetin	Pancreatic adenocarcinoma	Histone H3K36 demethylation	KDM4A promoter	DNA damage & inhibition of cell proliferation	Ding *et al* (2020)
Cinnamaldehyde	Gastric cancer	Histone–lysine N-methyltransferase (G9a)	LC3B promoter	Autophagy-mediated cell death	Kim (2022)
Luteolin	Colon cancer	DNA demethylation	Nrf2 promoter	Apoptotic cell death	Kang *et al* (2019)
Pelargonidin	Skin cancer	DNA demethylation	Nrf2 promoter	Blocks TPA-induced cell transformation	Li *et al* (2019)
Pterostilbene	Hepatocellular carcinoma	Acetylation	PTEN	Anti-cancer and antimetastatic	Qian *et al* (2018)
Pelargonidin	Colon adenocarcinoma	DNA methylation	Regulate DNA methyltransferase enzyme activity	Cell cycle arrest	Karthi *et al* (2017)

Triterpenoid corosolic acid	Skin cancer	CpG methylation	CDK1 and RASSF2	Inhibit tumor formation	Hudlikar *et al* (2020)
sulforaphane derivatives	Breast cancer	Histone deacetylases	Nrf2 chromatin	Inhibits cell proliferation, causes apoptosis	Kaboli *et al* (2020)
EGCG	Breast cancer	Histone modification (prevent deacetylation)	Estrogen receptor-α	Can restore ERα expression	Li *et al* (2010)

Table 3.2. A summary of the effect of phytochemicals on miRNA regulation to suppress cancer development and progression.

Phytochemical	miR	Regulation	Cancer type	Outcome	References
Epigallocatechin gallate (EGCG)	miR-16	Up-regulation	Human cancer cells	Apoptosis	Tsang and Kwok (2010)
EGCG	mir-485-5p	Down-regulation	NSCLC	Induced cell apoptosis	Jiang *et al* (2018)
EGCG	miR-204	Up-regulation	Oral squamous cell carcinomas OSCC	Suppression of cancer stemness	Yu *et al* (2016)
EGCG	miR-1	Up-regulation	Osteosarcoma	Suppresses osteosarcoma cell growth	Zhu *et al* (2016)
EGCG	miR-7–1	Up-regulation	Malignant neuroblastoma	Apoptosis	Chakrabarti *et al* (2013)
Curcumin	miR-21	Up-regulation	NSCLC	Suppresses the anti-cancer activities	Zhang *et al* (2014)
Curcumin	miR-9	Up-regulation	OSCC	Inhibit cell proliferation	Xiao *et al* (2014)
Quercetin	miR-200b-3p	Up-regulation	Pancreatic Ductal Adenocarcinoma (PDA)	Regulating the division mode of cancer stem cells	Nwaeburu *et al* (2017)
Diindolylmethane	miR-21	Up-regulation	Breast cancer	Inhibit cell growth	Jin (2011)
Sulforaphane	miR-124	Knockdown	Gastric carcinoma	Inhibit cell proliferation	Wang *et al* (2016)
Genistein	miR-1260b	Down-regulation	Prostate cancer	Demethylation and histone modification	Hirata *et al* (2014)
Genistein	miR-27a	Down-regulation	Pancreatic cancer	Inhibits cell growth and invasion	Xia *et al* (2014)
Genistein	miR A-27a	Down-regulation	Ovarian cancer	Cancer cell growth and metastasis	Xu *et al* (2013)
Genistein	mir-23b	Breast cancer	Inhibits the growth	Up-regulated	Avci *et al* (20150
Genistein	miR-27a	Up-regulation	Lung cancer	Inhibit cell proliferation	Yang *et al* (2016)
β-Sitosterol-D-glucoside	miR-10a	Up-regulation	Breast cancer	Suppresses tumor growth	Xu *et al* (2018)
Curcumin with emodin	miR-34a	Up-regulation	Breast cancer	Inhibit cell proliferation	Guo *et al* (2013)
Curcumin	miR-181b	Up-regulation	Breast cancer	Inhibits metastasis	Kronski *et al* (2014)
Curcumin	miR-19	Down-regulation	Breast cancer	Inhibit cell proliferation	Li *et al* (2014)
Curcumin	miR-33b	Up-regulation	Melanoma	Suppresses the epithelial-to-mesenchymal transition	Zhang *et al* (2015)
EGCG	miR-126	Up-regulation	Osteosarcoma	Induce apoptosis	Jiang *et al* (2014)
EGCG	miR-98–5p	Down-regulation	Enhanced efficacy of cisplatin	NSCLC	Zhou *et al* (2014)

pathways at various stages of carcinogenesis. Natural substances primarily have geno-protective, proapoptotic, antiangiogenic, antimutagenic, and anti-proliferative properties. Furthermore, DNA damage or repair mechanisms, as well as epigenome modulatory mechanisms that maintain gene expression, can mediate the anti-neoplastic activity of plant natural substances. Post-translational histone modifications may be regulated by plant natural chemicals in addition to miRNA expression or DNA methylation (Samec *et al* 2019). Epidrugs are chemicals that specifically target the epigenome program and can thus help treat cancer by regaining cell memory. Flavonoids and phenolic acids, which are naturally occurring substances derived from medicinal plants, have demonstrated their capacity to exert a variety of effects on epigenetic modifiers, including the inhibition of DNMT, HMT, and HAT. The use of these chemicals as anti-cancer epidrugs is currently a noteworthy strategy in the fight against human tumors. The mechanisms of these substances are specific, pleiotropic, and occasionally stochastic (Bouyahya *et al* 2022).

Acknowledgments

Authors thank their respective organizations for providing infrastructure facilities for book chapter writing.

References

Agarwal S, Amin K S, Jagadeesh S, Baishay G, Rao P G, Barua N C, Bhattacharya S and Banerjee P P 2013 Mahanine restores RASSF1A expression by down-regulating DNMT1 and DNMT3B in prostate cancer cells *Mol. Cancer* **12** 1–2

Aggarwal R, Jha M, Shrivastava A and Jha A K 2015 Natural compounds: role in reversal of epigenetic changes *Biochemistry (Moscow)* **80** 972–89

Aghide A N, Samarkhazan H S and Ahmadnezhad M 2016 Effect of harmine alkaloid on the expression of P16 and DAPK in HL60 leukemia cell line *Paramed. Sci. Mil. Health* **11** 28–33

Arora I, Sharma M and Tollefsbol T O 2019 Combinatorial epigenetics impact of polyphenols and phytochemicals in cancer prevention and therapy *Int. J. Mol. Sci.* **20** 4567

Arya R and Saldanha S N 2019 Dietary phytochemicals, epigenetics, and colon cancer chemo-prevention *Epigenetics of Cancer Prevention* (New York: Academic) pp 205–29

Avci C B, Susluer S Y, Caglar H O, Balci T, Aygunes D, Dodurga Y and Gunduz C 2015 Genistein-induced mir-23b expression inhibits the growth of breast cancer cells *Contemp. Oncol./Współczesna Onkol.* **19** 32–5

Bayat S, Khaniani M S, Choupani J, Alivand M R and Derakhshan S M 2018 HDACis (class I), cancer stem cell, and phytochemicals: cancer therapy and prevention implications *Biomed. Pharmacother.* **97** 1445–53

Bhattacharjee S and Dashwood R H 2020 Epigenetic regulation of NRF2/KEAP1 by phyto-chemicals *Antioxidants* **9** 865

Bouyahya A *et al* 2022 The role of epigenetic modifications in human cancers and the use of natural compounds as epidrugs: mechanistic pathways and pharmacodynamic actions *Biomolecules* **12** 367

Carlos-Reyes Á, López-González J S, Meneses-Flores M, Gallardo-Rincón D, Ruíz-García E, Marchat L A, Astudillo-De La Vega H, Hernández de la Cruz O N and López-Camarillo C 2019 Dietary compounds as epigenetic modulating agents in cancer *Front. Genet.* **10** 79

Catalano E 2016 Role of phytochemicals in the chemoprevention of tumors *arXiv preprint* arXiv:1605.04519

Chakrabarti M, Ai W, Banik N L and Ray S K 2013 Overexpression of miR-7-1 increases efficacy of green tea polyphenols for induction of apoptosis in human malignant neuroblastoma SH-SY5Y and SK-N-DZ cells *Neurochem. Res.* **38** 420–32

Chatterjee B, Ghosh K and Kanade S R 2019 Resveratrol modulates epigenetic regulators of promoter histone methylation and acetylation that restores BRCA1, p53, p21CIP1 in human breast cancer cell lines *BioFactors* **45** 818–29

Chen T, Yang C, Xi Z, Chen F and Li H 2020 Reduced caudal type homeobox 2 (CDX2) promoter methylation is associated with curcumin's suppressive effects on epithelial-mesenchymal transition in colorectal cancer cells *Med. Sci. Monit: Int. Med. J. Experimen. Clin. Res.* **26** e926443–1

Choi J H *et al* 2010 TSA-induced DNMT1 down-regulation represses hTERT expression via recruiting CTCF into demethylated core promoter region of hTERT in HCT116 *Biochem. Biophys. Res. Commun.* **391** 449–54

Číž M, Dvořáková A, Skočková V and Kubala L 2020 The role of dietary phenolic compounds in epigenetic modulation involved in inflammatory processes *Antioxidants* **9** 691

Dai Y, Guzman M L, Chen S, Wang L, Yeung S K, Pei X Y, Dent P, Jordan C T and Grant S 2010 The NF (nuclear factor)-κB inhibitor parthenolide interacts with histone deacetylase inhibitors to induce MKK7/JNK1-dependent apoptosis in human acute myeloid leukaemia cells *Br. J. Haematol.* **151** 70–83

Dave A, Parande F, Park E J and Pezzuto J M 2020 Phytochemicals and cancer chemoprevention *J. Cancer Metastasis Treat.* **6** 46

Ding G, Xu X, Li D, Chen Y, Wang W, Ping D, Jia S and Cao L 2020 Fisetin inhibits proliferation of pancreatic adenocarcinoma by inducing DNA damage via RFXAP/KDM4A-dependent histone H3K36 demethylation *Cell Death Dis.* **11** 893

Dittharot K, Dakeng S, Suebsakwong P, Suksamrarn A, Patmasiriwat P and Promkan M 2019 Cucurbitacin B induces hypermethylation of oncogenes in breast cancer cells *Planta Med.* **85** 370–8

Druesne N, Pagniez A, Mayeur C, Thomas M, Cherbuy C, Duée P H, Martel P and Chaumontet C 2004 Diallyl disulfide (DADS) increases histone acetylation and p21 waf1/cip1 expression in human colon tumor cell lines *Carcinogenesis* **25** 1227–36

El Omari N, Bakrim S, Bakha M, Lorenzo J M, Rebezov M, Shariati M A, Aboulaghras S, Balahbib A, Khayrullin M and Bouyahya A 2021 Natural bioactive compounds targeting epigenetic pathways in cancer: a review on alkaloids, terpenoids, quinones, and isothiocyanates *Nutrients* **13** 3714

Gerhauser C 2013 Cancer chemoprevention and nutri-epigenetics: state of the art and future challenges *Natural Products in Cancer Prevention and Therapy* (Berlin, Heidelberg: Springer) pp 73–132

Ghantous A, Saikali M, Rau T, Gali-Muhtasib H, Schneider-Stock R and Darwiche N 2012 Inhibition of tumor promotion by parthenolide: epigenetic modulation of p21parthenolide inhibits tumor promotion *Cancer Prev. Res.* **5** 1298–309

Ghasemi S, Xu S, Nabavi S M, Amirkhani M A, Sureda A, Tejada S and Lorigooini Z 2021 Epigenetic targeting of cancer stem cells by polyphenols (cancer stem cells targeting) *Phytother. Res.* **35** 3649–64

Gilbert E R and Liu D 2010 Flavonoids influence epigenetic-modifying enzyme activity: structure-function relationships and the therapeutic potential for cancer *Curr. Med. Chem.* **17** 1756–68

Guo J *et al* 2013 Synergistic effects of curcumin with emodin against the proliferation and invasion of breast cancer cells through upregulation of miR-34a *Mol. Cell. Biochem.* **382** 103–11

Guo P, Chen W, Li H, Li M and Li L 2018 The histone acetylation modifications of breast cancer and their therapeutic implications *Pathol. Oncol. Res.* **24** 807–13

Hewlings S J and Kalman D S 2017 Curcumin: a review of its effects on human health *Foods* **6** 92

Hirata H, Hinoda Y, Shahryari V, Deng G, Tanaka Y, Tabatabai Z L and Dahiya R 2014 Genistein downregulates onco-miR-1260b and upregulates sFRP1 and Smad4 via demethylation and histone modification in prostate cancer cells *Br. J. Cancer* **110** 1645–54

Huang C, Liu H, Gong X L, Wu L Y and Wen B 2017 Effect of evodiamine and berberine on the interaction between DNMTs and target microRNAs during malignant transformation of the colon by TGF-β1 *Oncol. Rep.* **37** 1637–45

Huang W, Li H, Yu Q, Xiao W and Wang D O 2022 DNA LncRNA-mediated methylation: an emerging mechanism in cancer and beyond *J. Exp. Clin. Cancer Res.* **41** 100

Hudlikar R R, Sargsyan D, Wu R, Su S, Zheng M and Kong A N 2020 Triterpenoid corosolic acid modulates global CpG methylation and transcriptome of tumor promotor TPA induced mouse epidermal JB6 P+ cells *Chem. Biol. Interact.* **321** 109025

Ilango S, Paital B, Jayachandran P, Padma P R and Nirmaladevi R 2020 Epigenetic alterations in cancer *Front. Biosci.-Landmark* **25** 1058–109

Jiang L, Tao C, He A and He X 2014 Overexpression of miR-126 sensitizes osteosarcoma cells to apoptosis induced by epigallocatechin-3-gallate *World J. Surg. Oncol.* **12** 1–7

Jiang P, Xu C, Chen L, Chen A, Wu X, Zhou M, Haq I U, Mariyam Z and Feng Q 2018 Epigallocatechin-3-gallate inhibited cancer stem cell–like properties by targeting hsa-mir-485-5p/RXRα in lung cancer *J. Cell. Biochem.* **119** 8623–35

Jin P and Chen X 2016 Current status of epigenetics and anticancer drug discovery *Anti-Cancer Agents Medi. Chem. (Formerly Curr. Med. Chem.-Anti-Cancer Agents)* **16** 699–712

Jin Y 2011 3, 3′-Diindolylmethane inhibits breast cancer cell growth via miR-21-mediated Cdc25A degradation *Mol. Cell. Biochem.* **358** 345–54

Jo H J, Song J D, Kim K M, Cho Y H, Kim K H and Park Y C 2008 Diallyl disulfide induces reversible G2/M phase arrest on a p53-independent mechanism in human colon cancer HCT-116 cells *Oncol. Rep.* **19** 275–80

Kaboli P J *et al* 2020 Targets and mechanisms of sulforaphane derivatives obtained from cruciferous plants with special focus on breast cancer–contradictory effects and future perspectives *Biomed. Pharmacother.* **121** 109635

Kang K A, Piao M J, Hyun Y J, Zhen A X, Cho S J, Ahn M J, Yi J M and Hyun J W 2019 Luteolin promotes apoptotic cell death via upregulation of Nrf2 expression by DNA demethylase and the interaction of Nrf2 with p53 in human colon cancer cells *Exp. Mol. Med.* **51** 1–4

Karthi N, Karthiga A, Kalaiyarasu T, Stalin A, Manju V, Singh S K, Cyril R and Lee S M 2017 Exploration of cell cycle regulation and modulation of the DNA methylation mechanism of pelargonidin: insights from the molecular modeling approach *Comput. Biol. Chem.* **70** 175–85

Kavoosi F 2018 Effect of curcumin and trichostatin a on the expression of DNA methyltransfrase 1 in hepatocellular carcinoma cell line hepa 1–6 *Iran. J. Pediatr. Hematol. Oncol.* **8** 193–201

Khan H *et al* 2021 Targeting epigenetics in cancer: therapeutic potential of flavonoids *Crit. Rev. Food Sci. Nutr.* **61** 1616–39

Khor T O, Huang Y, Wu T Y, Shu L, Lee J and Kong A N 2011 Pharmacodynamics of curcumin as DNA hypomethylation agent in restoring the expression of Nrf2 via promoter CpGs demethylation *Biochem. Pharmacol.* **82** 1073–8

Kim T W 2022 Cinnamaldehyde induces autophagy-mediated cell death through ER stress and epigenetic modification in gastric cancer cells *Acta Pharmacol. Sin.* **43** 712–23

Köhler F and Rodríguez-Paredes M 2020 DNA methylation in epidermal differentiation, aging, and cancer *J. Investig. Dermatol.* **140** 38–47

Kong A N, Zhang C and Su Z Y 2013 Targeting epigenetics for cancer prevention by dietary cancer preventive compounds—the case of miRNAEpigenetic miRNA regulation by cancer preventive phytochemicals *Cancer Prev. Res.* **6** 622–4

Kronski E *et al* 2014 miR181b is induced by the chemopreventive polyphenol curcumin and inhibits breast cancer metastasis via down-regulation of the inflammatory cytokines CXCL1 and-2 *Mol. Oncol.* **8** 581–95

Kumar A, Butt N A and Levenson A S 2016 Natural epigenetic-modifying molecules in medical therapy *Medical Epigenetics* (New York: Academic) pp 747–98

Kuo H C, Wu R, Li S, Yang A Y and Kong A N 2019 Anthocyanin delphinidin prevents neoplastic transformation of mouse skin JB6 P+ cells: epigenetic re-activation of Nrf2-ARE pathway *AAPS* J **21** 1–0

Lai K C, Kuo C L, Ho H C, Yang J S, Ma C Y, Lu H F, Huang H Y, Chueh F S, Yu C C and Chung J G 2012 Diallyl sulfide, diallyl disulfide and diallyl trisulfide affect drug resistant gene expression in colo 205 human colon cancer cells *in vitro* and *in vivo Phytomedicine* **19** 625–30

Lewis K A and Tollefsbol T O 2017 The influence of an epigenetics diet on the cancer epigenome *Epigenomics* **9** 1153–5

Li S, Kuo H C, Yin R, Wu R, Liu X, Wang L, Hudlikar R, Peter R M and Kong A N 2020 Epigenetics/epigenomics of triterpenoids in cancer prevention and in health *Biochem. Pharmacol.* **175** 113890

Li S, Li W, Wang C, Wu R, Yin R, Kuo H C, Wang L and Kong A N 2019 Pelargonidin reduces the TPA induced transformation of mouse epidermal cells–potential involvement of Nrf2 promoter demethylation *Chem. Biol. Interact.* **309** 108701

Li X *et al* 2014 Curcumin modulates miR-19/PTEN/AKT/p53 axis to suppress bisphenol A-induced MCF-7 breast cancer cell proliferation *Phytother. Res.* **28** 1553–60

Li Y, Yuan Y Y, Meeran S M and Tollefsbol T O 2010 Synergistic epigenetic reactivation of estrogen receptor-α (ERα) by combined green tea polyphenol and histone deacetylase inhibitor in ERα-negative breast cancer cells *Mol. Cancer* **9** 1–2

Liu Z, Liu S, Xie Z, Li C, Aimiuwu J, Chen P, Pang J, Marcucci G and Chan K 2007 NF-kappaB inhibitor Parthenolide mediates DNA demethylation and histone acetylation in leukemia cells *Cancer Res.* **67** 1466

Luo X *et al* 2015 Grifolin directly targets ERK1/2 to epigenetically suppress cancer cell metastasis *Oncotarget.* **6** 42704

Moon J W, Lee S K, Lee J O, Kim J H, Kim N, Kim J, Kim H S and Park S H 2014 Demethylation of RUNX3 by vincristine in colorectal adenocarcinoma cells *Anticancer Res.* **34** 133–40

Mukherjee N, Kumar A P and Ghosh R 2015 DNA methylation and flavonoids in genitourinary cancers *Curr.Pharmacol. Rep.* **1** 112–20

Nasir A, Bullo M M, Ahmed Z, Imtiaz A, Yaqoob E, Safdar M, Ahmed H, Afreen A and Yaqoob S 2022 Nutrigenomics: epigenetics and cancer prevention: a comprehensive review *Crit. Rev. Food Sci. Nutr.* **60** 1375–87

Nian H, Delage B, Pinto J T and Dashwood R H 2008 Allyl mercaptan, a garlic-derived organosulfur compound, inhibits histone deacetylase and enhances Sp3 binding on the P21WAF1 promoter *Carcinogenesis* **29** 1816–24

Nikkhoo P, Oodi A and Sotoodehnejadnematalahi F 2017 Effect of harmalin on Dnmt1 expression and hypomethylation of P15 gene promoter in NB4 leukemic cell *Sci. J. Iran Blood Transfus Organ.* **14** 314–24

Nwaeburu C C, Abukiwan A, Zhao Z and Herr I 2017 Quercetin-induced miR-200b-3p regulates the mode of self-renewing divisions in pancreatic cancer *Mol. Cancer* **16** 1–0

Ong T P, Moreno F S and Ross S A 2012 Targeting the epigenome with bioactive food components for cancer prevention *Lifestyle Genom.* **4** 275–92

Papanicolau-Sengos A and Aldape K 2022 DNA methylation profiling: an emerging paradigm for cancer diagnosis *Annu. Rev. Pathol: Mech. Dis.* **17** 295–321

Pathak A, Tomar S and Pathak S 2023 Epigenetics and cancer: a comprehensive review *Asian Pac. J. Cancer Biol.* **8** 75–89

Pehlivan F E 2021 Diet-epigenome interactions: epi-drugs modulating the epigenetic machinery during cancer prevention *Epigenetics to Optogenetics: A New Paradigm in the Study of Biology* (London: IntechOpen)

Pratheeshkumar P, Son Y O, Korangath P, Manu K A and Siveen K S 2015 Phytochemicals in cancer prevention and therapy *BioMed Res. Int.* **2015** 324021

Qian Y Y, Liu Z S, Yan H J, Yuan Y F, Levenson A S and Li K 2018 Pterostilbene inhibits MTA1/HDAC1 complex leading to PTEN acetylation in hepatocellular carcinoma *Biomed. Pharmacother.* **101** 852–9

Qing Y, Hu H, Liu Y, Feng T, Meng W, Jiang L, Sun Y and Yao Y 2014 Berberine induces apoptosis in human multiple myeloma cell line U266 through hypomethylation of p53 promoter *Cell Biol. Int.* **38** 563–70

Rahman M M, Brane A C and Tollefsbol T O 2019 MicroRNAs and epigenetics strategies to reverse breast cancer *Cells* **8** 1214

Rajendran P *et al* 2015 Nrf2 status affects tumor growth, HDAC3 gene promoter associations, and the response to sulforaphane in the colon *Clin. Epigenetics* **7** 1–2

Rizeq B, Gupta I, Ilesanmi J, AlSafran M, Rahman M M and Ouhtit A 2020 The power of phytochemicals combination in cancer chemoprevention *J. Cancer* **11** 4521

Samec M *et al* 2019 Fluctuations of histone chemical modifications in breast, prostate, and colorectal cancer: an implication of phytochemicals as defenders of chromatin equilibrium *Biomolecules* **9** 829

Sanaei M, Kavoosi F and Arabloo M 2020 Effect of curcumin in comparison with trichostatin A on the reactivation of estrogen receptor alpha gene expression, cell growth inhibition and apoptosis induction in hepatocellular carcinoma Hepa 1–6 cell lline *Asian Pac. J. Cancer Prev: APJCP* **21** 1045

Saw P E, Xu X, Chen J and Song E W 2021 Non-coding RNAs: the new central dogma of cancer biology *Sci. China Life Sci.* **64** 22–50

Seo J S, Choi Y H, Moon J W, Kim H S and Park S H 2017 Hinokitiol induces DNA demethylation via DNMT1 and UHRF1 inhibition in colon cancer cells *BMC Cell Biol.* **18** 1

Shankar E, Kanwal R, Candamo M and Gupta S 2016 Dietary phytochemicals as epigenetic modifiers in cancer: promise and challenges *Seminars in Cancer Biology* (New York: Academic)40 pp 82–99

Sharma S, Kelly T K and Jones P A 2010 Epigenetics in cancer *Carcinogenesis* **31** 27–36

Shen Y, Takahashi M, Byun H M, Link A, Sharma N, Balaguer F, Leung H C, Boland C R and Goel A 2012 Boswellic acid induces epigenetic alterations by modulating DNA methylation in colorectal cancer cells *Cancer Biol. Ther.* **13** 542–52

Sheng J, Shi W, Guo H, Long W, Wang Y, Qi J, Liu J and Xu Y 2019 The inhibitory effect of (−)-epigallocatechin-3-gallate on breast cancer progression via reducing SCUBE2 methylation and DNMT activity *Molecules* **24** 2899

Shirakami Y, Sakai H, Kubota M, Kochi T and Shimizu M 2015 Dietary phytochemicals as cancer preventive agents: efficacy and mechanisms *J. Bioanal. Biomed.* **7** 2

Shoaib S *et al* 2023 Prospective epigenetic actions of organo-sulfur compounds against cancer: perspectives and molecular mechanisms *Cancers* **15** 697

Shukla S, Khan S, Kumar S, Sinha S, Farhan M, Bora H K, Maurya R and Meeran S M 2015 Cucurbitacin B alters the expression of tumor-related genes by epigenetic modifications in NSCLC and inhibits NNK-induced lung tumorigenesis *Cancer Prev. Res.* **8** 552–62

Shukla S, Penta D, Mondal P and Meeran S M 2019 Epigenetics of breast cancer: clinical status of epi-drugs and phytochemicals *Adv. Exp. Med. Biol.* **1152** 293–310

Sriram N, Kalayarasan S, Ashokkumar P, Sureshkumar A and Sudhandiran G 2008 Diallyl sulfide induces apoptosis in Colo 320 DM human colon cancer cells: involvement of caspase-3, NF-κB, and ERK-2 *Mol. Cell. Biochem.* **311** 157–65

Sun L, Zhang H and Gao P 2022 Metabolic reprogramming and epigenetic modifications on the path to cancer *Protein Cell* **13** 877–919

Thakur V S, Deb G, Babcook M A and Gupta S 2014 Plant phytochemicals as epigenetic modulators: role in cancer chemoprevention *AAPS* J **16** 151–63

Tiwari P and Gupta K P 2014 Modulation of miR-203 and its regulators as a function of time during the development of 7, 12 dimethylbenz [a] anthracene induced mouse skin tumors in presence or absence of the antitumor agents *Toxicol. Appl. Pharmacol.* **278** 148–58

Tsang W P and Kwok T T 2010 Epigallocatechin gallate up-regulation of miR-16 and induction of apoptosis in human cancer cells *J. Nutr. Biochem.* **21** 140–6

Unoki M 2011 Current and potential anticancer drugs targeting members of the UHRF1 complex including epigenetic modifiers *Recent Pat. Anti-Cancer Drug Discov.* **6** 116–30

Watson G W, Beaver L M, Williams D E, Dashwood R H and Ho E 2013 Phytochemicals from cruciferous vegetables, epigenetics, and prostate cancer prevention *AAPS* J. **15** 951–61

Wang H, Li Q and Chen H 2012 Genistein affects histone modifications on Dickkopf-related protein 1 (DKK1) gene in SW480 human colon cancer cell line *PLoS One* **7** e40955

Wang X *et al* 2016 Sulforaphane improves chemotherapy efficacy by targeting cancer stem cell-like properties via the miR-124/IL-6R/STAT3 axis *Sci. Rep.* **6** 1

Wang Z, Liu Q, Jiang X, Zhang Y, Jiang L and Meng F 2017 Berberine acts as a putative epigenetic modulator by affecting histone code in acute myelocytic leukemia cells *Blood.* **130** 4989

Wang Z, Liu Y, Xue Y, Hu H, Ye J, Li X, Lu Z, Meng F and Liang S 2016 Berberine acts as a putative epigenetic modulator by affecting the histone code *Toxicol. In Vitro* **36** 10–7

Wu B, Yao X, Nie X and Xu R 2013 Epigenetic reactivation of RANK in glioblastoma cells by curcumin: involvement of STAT3 inhibition *DNA Cell Biol.* **32** 292–7

Wu D S, Shen J Z, Yu A F, Fu H Y, Zhou H R and Shen S F 2013 Epigallocatechin-3-gallate and trichostatin A synergistically inhibit human lymphoma cell proliferation through epigenetic modification of p16INK4a *Oncol. Rep.* **30** 2969–75

Wu R, Li S, Hudlikar R, Wang L, Shannar A, Peter R, Chou P J, Kuo H C, Liu Z and Kong A N 2022 Redox signaling, mitochondrial metabolism, epigenetics and redox active phytochemicals *Free Radical Biol. Med.* **179** 328–36

Xia J, Cheng L, Mei C, Ma J, Shi Y, Zeng F, Wang Z and Wang Z 2014 Genistein inhibits cell growth and invasion through regulation of miR-27a in pancreatic cancer cells *Curr. Pharm. Des.* **20** 5348–53

Xiao C, Wang L, Zhu L, Zhang C and Zhou J 2014 Curcumin inhibits oral squamous cell carcinoma SCC-9 cells proliferation by regulating miR-9 expression *Biochem. Biophys. Res. Commun.* **454** 576–80

Xu H *et al* 2018 Anti-breast-cancer activity exerted by β-sitosterol-D-glucoside from sweet potato via upregulation of microRNA-10a and via the PI3K–Akt signaling pathway *J. Agric. Food Chem.* **66** 9704–18

Xu L, Xiang J, Shen J, Zou X, Zhai S, Yin Y, Li P, Wang X and Sun Q 2013 Oncogenic MicroRNA-27a is a target for genistein in ovarian cancer cells *Anticancer Agents Med. Chem. (Formerly Curr. Med. Chem.-Anti-Cancer Agents)* **13** 1126–32

Yang Y, Yang I, Cao M, Su Z Y, Wu R, Guo Y, Fang M and Kong A N 2018 Fucoxanthin elicits epigenetic modifications, Nrf2 activation and blocking transformation in mouse skin JB6 P+ cells *AAPS* J. **20** 1

Yang Y, Zang A, Jia Y, Shang Y, Zhang Z, Ge K, Zhang J, Fan W and Wang B 2016 Genistein inhibits A549 human lung cancer cell proliferation via miR-27a and MET signaling *Oncol. Lett.* **12** 2189–93

Ye M, Luo X, Li L, Shi Y, Tan M, Weng X, Li W, Liu J and Cao Y 2007 Grifolin, a potential antitumor natural product from the mushroom Albatrellus confluens, induces cell-cycle arrest in G1 phase via the ERK1/2 pathway *Cancer Lett.* **258** 199–207

Yie Y, Zhao S, Tang Q, Zheng F, Wu J, Yang L, Deng S and Hann S S 2015 Ursolic acid inhibited growth of hepatocellular carcinoma HepG2 cells through AMPKα-mediated reduction of DNA methyltransferase 1 *Mol. Cell. Biochem.* **402** 63–74

Yu C C, Chen P N, Peng C Y, Yu C H and Chou M Y 2016 Suppression of miR-204 enables oral squamous cell carcinomas to promote cancer stemness, EMT traits, and lymph node metastasis *Oncotarget.* **7** 20180

Zam W and Khadour A 2017 Impact of phytochemicals and dietary patterns on epigenome and cancer *Nutri. Cancer* **69** 184–200

Zhang C, Wang C, Li W, Wu R, Guo Y, Cheng D, Yang Y, Androulakis I P and Kong A N 2017 Pharmacokinetics and pharmacodynamics of the triterpenoid ursolic acid in regulating the antioxidant, anti-inflammatory, and epigenetic gene responses in rat leukocytes *Mol. Pharmaceut.* **14** 3709–17

Zhang P *et al* 2015 MicroRNA-33b, upregulated by EF24, a curcumin analog, suppresses the epithelial-to-mesenchymal transition (EMT) and migratory potential of melanoma cells by targeting HMGA2 *Toxicol. Lett.* **234** 151–61

Zhang W, Bai W and Zhang W 2014 MiR-21 suppresses the anticancer activities of curcumin by targeting PTEN gene in human non-small cell lung cancer A549 cells *Clin. Transl. Oncol.* **16** 708–13

Zhou D H, Wang X and Feng Q 2014 EGCG enhances the efficacy of cisplatin by downregulating hsa-miR-98-5p in NSCLC A549 cells *Nutr. Cancer* **66** 636–44

Zhu K and Wang W 2016 Green tea polyphenol EGCG suppresses osteosarcoma cell growth through upregulating miR-1 *Tumor Biol.* **37** 4373–82

Zuo Q, Wu R, Xiao X, Yang C, Yang Y, Wang C, Lin L and Kong A N 2018 The dietary flavone luteolin epigenetically activates the Nrf2 pathway and blocks cell transformation in human colorectal cancer HCT116 cells *J. Cell. Biochem.* **119** 9573–82

Chapter 4

Role of dietary natural food as a therapeutic drug to prevent lung cancer

Sagarkumar Joshi and Nidhi Saxena

Smoking and tobacco use are the main causes of lung cancer-related death. Because it cannot be cured with surgery or radiation therapy, lung cancer spreads rapidly and has a higher fatality rate. In this chapter, we discuss the role of dietary habits and nutrition on lung cancer. Lung cancer has been found to be prevented by diets rich in fruit, vegetables, fish, nuts, soy, and foods containing vitamins A, B, D, E, C, calcium, magnesium, selenium, and zinc. They can also aid in the treatment of the disease using chemotherapeutic drugs.

4.1 Introduction

Lung cancer is frequently diagnosed and leads to cancer-related deaths globally. Lung cancer accounts for 8.1% of all cancer-related fatalities in India and 5.9% of all cancer cases [1]. According to Mohan *et al* [2], smoking is responsible for roughly 80% of lung cancer cases [2]. Lung cancer is also greatly influenced by genetic, familial, demographic, environmental, and behavioral factors [3–5]. According to [6], tobacco use and burning produce about 60 different carcinogens that cause oxidative stress, free radical production, DNA damage, such as breaks in DNA strands or changes in genomic processing, and are particularly harmful to the lungs.

According to numerous studies [7–9], eating a lot of fruit, vegetables, and fish lowers the risk of developing lung cancer, but consuming red meat and processed food raises that risk. Consequently, in addition to quitting smoking, food adjustment may also be a desirable strategy for the prevention and management of lung cancer.

In this chapter, we discuss the use of specific dietary components, such as fisetin, β-carotene, lycopene, lutein, β-cryptoxanthin, astaxanthin, canthaxanthin, and fucoxanthin, probiotics, carvone, alliin, shogaol, carnosic acid, and rosamarinic

doi:10.1088/978-0-7503-5252-9ch4

acid, as preventive or therapeutic agents for the prevention and cure of lung cancer. The reported effects of these dietary agents against lung cancer are summarized in table 4.1 and figure 4.1.

4.2 Epigallocatechin gallate

4.2.1 Structure

EGCG, or epigallocatechin-3-gallate, is another name for epigallocatechin gallate. It is created through the esterification of gallic acid and epigallocatechin (figure 4.2). It is a phenolic antioxidant substance that is present in many plants, including green tea and black tea. It protects the cells from free radical and oxidative damage.

4.2.2 Function

Epigallocatechin gallate has a number of anti-cancer properties, including the modulation of enzymes that break down carcinogens, the induction of apoptosis and cell cycle arrest, the modulation of cell signaling pathways, and the suppression of the transcription factors activation, which all work together to slow the growth of cancer ([39, 67, 68]).

Inhibiting MDM2-mediated p53 ubiquitination and anchorage-independent proliferation of human lung cancer cells, epigallocatechin gallate promotes the phosphorylation of p53 at Ser^{15} and Ser^{20} and improves its transcriptional activity [10]. It inhibits transforming growth factor (TGF)-β via downregulation of phosphorylated Smad2 and ERK1/2 [12], inhibits the HIF and miR-210 proteins that are responsible for tumor suppression, and so enhances the death of tumor cells.

4.3 Isothiocyanates

4.3.1 Structure

Isothiocyanates are a class of sulfur-containing phytochemicals that are found as conjugated glucosinolates (figure 4.3). This compound is converted into glucosinolates like glucoraphanin and isothiocyanate sulforaphane by the enzyme myrosinase which is present in plant tissues or intestinal flora [69]. Cruciferous vegetables like cabbage, cauliflower, kale, broccoli, brussels sprouts and others contain isothiocyanates.

4.3.2 Function

According to [70, 71], isothiocyanates and their metabolites help to lower the chance of developing a variety of cancers, including lung, breast, liver, esophagus, gastrointestinal tract, and others. According to [72, 73], isothiocyanates exhibit a variety of mechanisms, including modulation of cytoprotective enzymes, inhibition of nuclear factor kappa B (NFκB), prevention of proliferation through induction of cell cycle arrest and apoptosis, induction of expression of hormone receptors, antiangiogenic and anti-metastasis potential, and autophagy induction.

Table 4.1. Food and its components work as therapeutic agents for lung cancer [165].

S. No.	Compound	Food	Effect	References
1.	Epigallocatechin	Green tea (*Camellia sinensis*)	The transcriptional activity of p53 is enhanced by phosphorylation	Jin *et al* [10]
			Expression of miR-210 increases	Wang *et al* [11]
			Vimentin expression is reduced and E-cadherin expression is increased, which prevents NSCLC cells from migrating and invading in response to TGF-β	Liu *et al* [12]
			Reduces DNA fragmentation, decreased caspases-3 and −9, decreased telomerase activity, and S-phase cell cycle arrest	Sadava *et al* [166]
			Lowers tumor growth, enhances tumor cell apoptosis, and reduces oxidative DNA damage in athymic nude mice	Li *et al* [13]
			A rise in apoptotic cells and a decrease in hyperplasia, dysplasia, and cancer *in situ*	Banerjee *et al* [14]
			In NNK-induced lung adenomas, green tea solution reduced lung tumor multiplicity, inhibited angiogenesis, and triggered apoptosis in A/J mice	Liao *et al* [15]
2.	Isothiocyanates	Cruciferous vegetables such as cauliflower, cabbage, broccoli, and others	Caspase-3 activation, cell cycle arrest in the G2/M phase, production of reactive oxygen species, and glutathione depletion causes apoptosis	Liu *et al* [16]
			Actin fiber deconstruction, tubulin degradation, and cell cycle arrest in the G2/M phase are all induced	Pawlik *et al* [17]
			Reduces cell proliferation, causes apoptosis induction, mitotic arrest, and disrupted microtubule polymerization	Mi *et al* [18]

(*Continued*)

Table 4.1. *(Continued)*

S. No.	Compound	Food	Effect	References
			DNA fragmentation, chromatin condensation, p38 activation, caspase-3 activity, sub-G(1) phase DNA content, and downregulation of ERK1/2 and Akt are all induced	Jin *et al* [19]
			Sulforaphane reduces H_2O_2, increases cytochrome C release from mitochondria, decreases Bcl-2 and increases Bax and caspase-3 in Swiss albino mice	Kalpana Deepa Priya *et al* [20]
			In neonatal mice exposed to cigarette smoke, there was less pulmonary carcinogenicity	Balansky *et al* [21]
			Reduced lung tumor multiplicity brought on by toxins in cigarette smoke in A/J mice	Hecht *et al* [22]
3.	Indole-3-carbinol	Brassica plants include broccoli, brussels sprouts, cabbage, cauliflower, kale, and others	Less instances of all tumor size classes at all levels of efficacy, as well as fewer instances of hyperplastic foci, adenomas, and adenocarcinomas	Qian *et al* [23]
			Inhibit the multiplication of tumors, and pulmonary adenocarcinoma	Qian *et al* [23]
			Decrease in the multiplicities of tumors on the surface of the lung and adenocarcinoma. Modification of p-Akt, p-ERK, cyclin D1 and PARP cleavage in NNK-treated mice	Dagne *et al* [24]
			In A/J mice, decreases the levels of miR-21, mir-31, miR-130a, miR-146b and miR-377	Melkamu *et al* [25]
			Decrease in tumor multiplicities, cancer incidence, and inhibition NF-κB activation, COX-2, p-Akt, caspase-3 and PARP cleavage	Kassie *et al* [26]
			Reduces the expression of Ki-67, PCNA, p-Akt, p-BAD and induction of apoptosis in the lung tissues	Kassie *et al* [27]
			Inhibited production of Nitrous Oxide, IL-6 and IL-1β	Jiang *et al* [28]

4.	Genistein	Soybean (*Glycine max*)	Blockage of the G2/M phase of the cell cycle, activation of apoptosis, inhibition of cell migration	Tian *et al* [29]
			Erlotinib and gefitinib together led to a decrease in EGFR, p-Akt, COX-2, PGE2, and NF-κB	Gadgeel *et al* [30]
			Decreases the NF-κB activity	Li *et al* [31]
			In a xenograft model, the combination of gefitinib and genistein significantly reduced tumor growth	Zhu *et al* [32]
			C57BL/6 mice treated with genistein and diadzein had decreased lung tumor nodule formation, increased lung collagen hydroxyproline content, lower serum sialic acid levels, and longer lifespans	Menon *et al* [33]
5.	Curcumin	Turmeric (*Curcuma longa*)	Decrease in the weight of intra-lung tumors, a drop in COX-2 expression in subcutaneous tumors, and an improvement in survival rate. Orthotopic human NSCLC xenograft tumor growth was inhibited, and athymic nude mice survived longer	Lev-Ari *et al* [34]
			Liposomal curcumin decreased lung fibrosis and made LL/2 cells more sensitive to radiation	Shi *et al* [35]
			Inhibition of Cdc42 results in decreased tumor growth and invasion in BALB/c mice	Chen *et al* [36]
			Lewis lung carcinoma primary tumor growth inhibition in C57BL/6 mice. Neutrophil elastase decreased and α1-antitrypsin increased in tumor tissues	Xu *et al* [37]
			Increased survival, slowed tumor progression, and boosted the T cell-mediated adaptive immune response	Luo *et al* [38]

(Continued)

Table 4.1. (*Continued*)

S. No.	Compound	Food	Effect	References
6.	Polyphenol	Pomegranate (*Punica granatum*)	Reduces the tumor growth and enhances the survival of athymic nude mice	Khan *et al* [39]
			Inhibiting NF-κB, MAPK, PI3K, phosphorylation of Akt, mTOR, c-met, indicators of cell proliferation, and angiogenesis led to a reduction in the number of lung tumors in A/J mice	Khan *et al* [40]
			Fruit extract decreased cell viability, G0-G1 phase arrest, decreased cyclin D1, D2, E, cdk-2, -4, and -6 levels, increased cell cycle regulatory molecules, and inhibited MAPK, PI3K, Akt, NF-κB, Ki-67, and PCNA phosphorylation	Khan *et al* [41]
7.	Fisetin	Strawberry (*Fragaria ananassa*), persimmon (*Diospyros kaki*), grape (*Vitis vinifera*), apple (*Malus domestica*), cucumber (*Cucumis sativus*) and onion (*Allium cepa*)	Cell growth inhibition, tumorigenesis inhibition, reduction in PI3K protein expression, inhibition of Akt, mTOR, p70S6K1, eIF-4E, 4E-BP1, members of the mTOR signaling complex, phosphorylation of TSC2, phosphorylation of mTOR and its target proteins, and augmentation of AMPKα phosphorylation	Khan *et al* [42]
			Reduced STAT-3 tyrosine phosphorylation and inhibition of hypoxia-induced VEGF production	Anso *et al* [43]
			Reduces the adhesion, migration, and invasion by downregulation of the ERK1/2, MMP-2, uPA NF-κB, c-Fos, c-Jun, and NF-κB binding	Liao *et al* [44]
			Decrease in mitochondrial dysfunction	Ravichandran *et al* [45]
			Decrease in PCNA, lipid peroxidation, a decrease in histological lesions, and a modification of enzymatic and non-enzymatic antioxidants	Ravichandran *et al* [46]
			Angiogenesis is prevented, and tumor growth is decreased	Touil *et al* [47]

8.	α-Carotene	Orange yellow and green vegetables	Antioxidant, enhance gap junctional intercellular communication	Rutovskikh *et al* [48]
9.	β-Carotene	Orange and yellow fruits and vegetables, as well as green leafy veggies	Antioxidant, enhance gap junctional intercellular communication	Rutovskikh *et al* [48]
10.	Lycopene	Tomatoes (*Solanum lycopersicum*), watermelon (*Citrullus lanatus*), apricot (*Prunus armeniaca*), peaches (*Prunus persica*)	Antioxidant, various human cancer cell lines are inhibited from growing	Levy *et al* [49]
11.	Lutein	Dark-green vegetables with leaves	Antioxidant, effective at advancing the cell cycle, and effective at preventing the growth of several cancer cell types	Hyang-Sook *et al* [50]
12.	β-Cryptoxanthin	Orange fruits (*Citrus sinensis*)	Antioxidant, anti-inflammatory, and reduces certain cancer risk	Tanaka *et al* [51]
13.	Astaxanthin	Green algae (*Chlorophyta*), salmon (Salmo salar), trout (*Oncorhynchus* and *Salvelinus*)	Antioxidant, modify gap junction communications	Kurihara *et al* [52]
14.	Canthaxanthin	Salmon (*Salmo salar*), crustaceans (*Crustacea*)	Antioxidant, powerful reactive oxygen species quenchers, and free radical scavengers	Tanaka *et al* [51]
15.	Fucoxanthin	Brown algae (*Phaeophyceae*), heterokonts (*Heterokonta*)	Anti-inflammatory, antioxidant, and anti-cancer	Tanaka *et al* [51]
16.	Probiotics	*Lactobacillus casei* YIT 9018	Long survival time and pulmonary metastasis inhibition in Lewis lung carcinoma	Matsuzaki *et al* [53]
		Enterococcus faecium K-50 and *Saccharomyces cerevisiae* 14K	Prevented metastatic Lewis's lung cancer and solid sarcoma from spreading	Tanasienko *et al* [167]
		Recombin-ant *Bifidobacterium infantis* with sFlt-1 gene	Tumor growth inhibition in lung cancer	Zhu *et al* [54]
		B. infantis with soluble kinase domain receptor (sKDR)	Tumor growth suppression by increase the necrosis rate of the tumor, and prolonged survival time of mice	Li *et al* [55]

(*Continued*)

Table 4.1. (*Continued*)

S. No.	Compound	Food	Effect	References
		Lactobacillus acidophil-lus	Cisplatin's anti-tumor effects were boosted when combined with *L. acidophilus*	Gui *et al* [56]
		Lactococcus lactis NK34	Shows more than 77% of cytotoxic activity in lung cancer and breast cancer	Han *et al* [57]
		L. lactis KC24	Increase cytotoxic effects in cells of lung and breast cancer	Lee *et al* [58]
		Mixture of *Bifidobacterium bifidum*, *Bifidobacterium longum*, *Bifidobacterium lactis*, and *Bifidobacterium breve*	Tumor controlled by checkpoint blockade	Sivan *et al* [59]
		Bacteroides fragilis	Effects of immunostimulation in non-small cell lung cancer (NSCLC) or metastatic melanoma	Vetizou *et al* [168]
		Lactobacillus casei CRL 431	Reduced tumor vascularity, extravasation of tumor cells, and lung metastasis; decreased tumor growth	Aragon *et al* [60]
		Kefir	Increases cytotoxic T cells and helper T cells, and reduces metastases to the lungs and bone marrow	Zamberi *et al* [61]
		Enterococcus hirae and *Barnesiella intestinihominis*	Increased cyclophosphamide-anti-cancer effects is observed in lung and ovarian cancer patients during advanced stage	Daillere *et al* [62]
17.	Carvone	Caraway (*Carum carvi*)	Increased glutathione level	Zhang *et al* [63]
18.	Alliin	Garlic (*Allium sativum*)	Anti-proliferative, depression of CYP1A1, 2B1, and 3A1 protein products	Sakamoto *et al* [64]
19.	Shogaol	Ginger (*Zingiber officinale*)	Antitumorigenic, causes apoptosis by increasing the expression of GADD153	Chen *et al* [65]
20.	Carnosic acid and rosmarinic acid	Rosemary (*Salvia rosmarinus*)	By reducing TNF-α -induced reactive oxygen species formation and NF-κB activation, you can inhibit proliferation and trigger apoptosis	Moon *et al* [66]

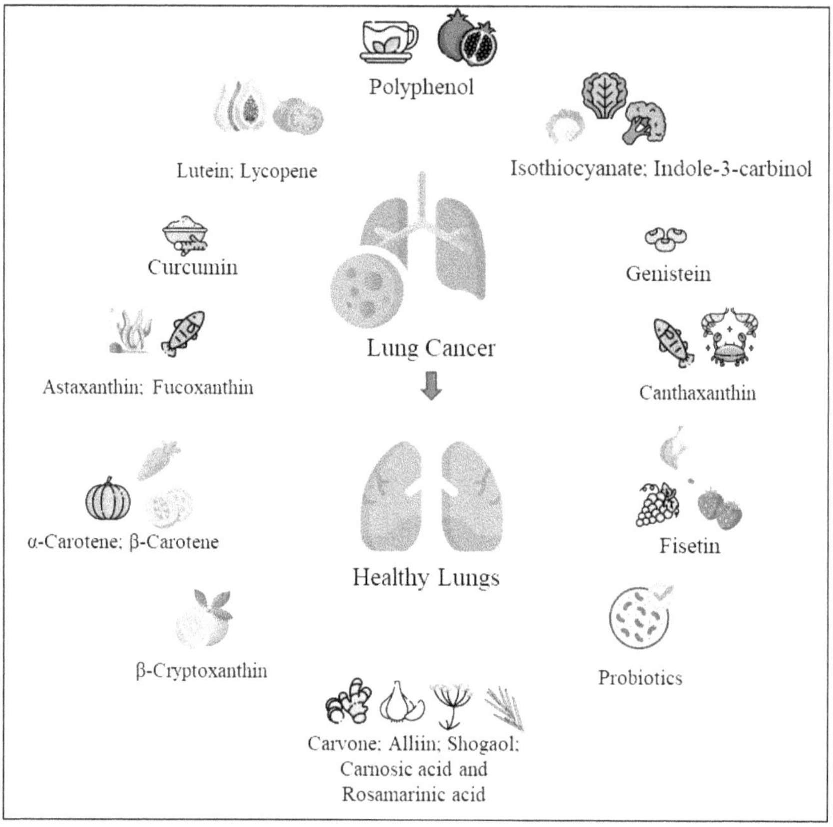

Figure 4.1. Dietary ingredients used to prevent lung cancer.

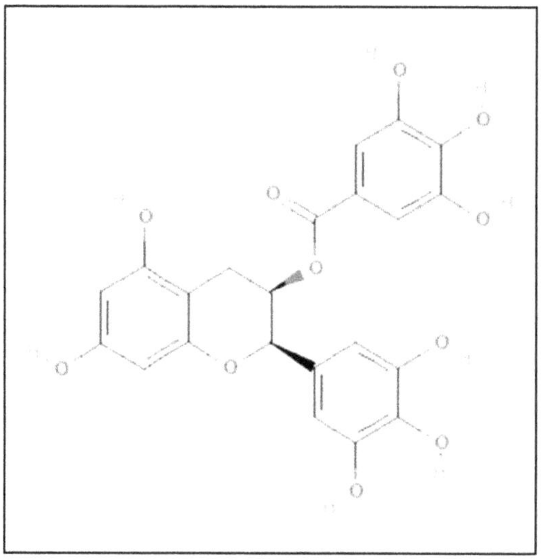

Figure 4.2. Structure of epigallocatechin gallate [165].

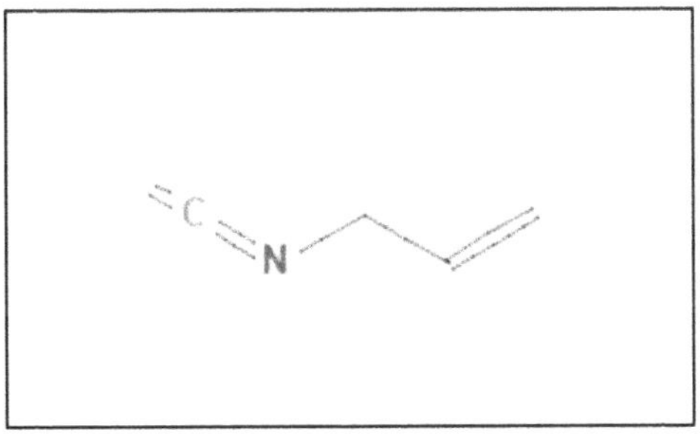

Figure 4.3. Structure of allyl isothiocyanate [165].

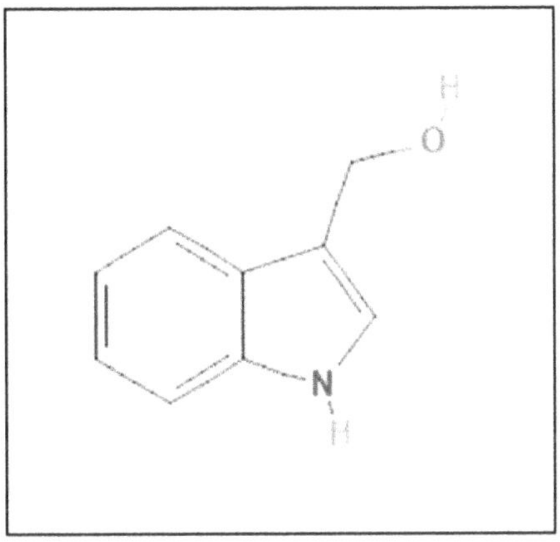

Figure 4.4. Structure of indole-3-carbinol [165].

According to a study [18], isothiocyanates bind with tubulin and induce apoptosis and mitotic arrest. When isothiocyanates are administered orally, less hydrogen peroxide is produced, more cytochrome C is released from mitochondria, less Bcl-2 is expressed, and more Bax and caspase-3 are expressed [18]. By reducing cell proliferation and inducing apoptosis in tobacco carcinogen-treated A/J mice, isothiocyanates and their conjugates also have an impact on the development of lung adenomas into adenocarcinomas [74].

4.4 Indole-3-carbinol

4.4.1 Structure

With antioxidant and possible chemo-preventive characteristics, indole-3-carbinol (I3C) is found in brassica plants such as cabbage, cauliflower, kale, broccoli, and Brussels sprouts [75], and is an autolysis product of glucosinolate (figure 4.4).

4.4.2 Function

By activating the Fas and caspase-8 pathways, indole-3-carbinol is utilized for treating lung cancer cells by inducing an arrest of the cell cycle at the phase of G0/G1

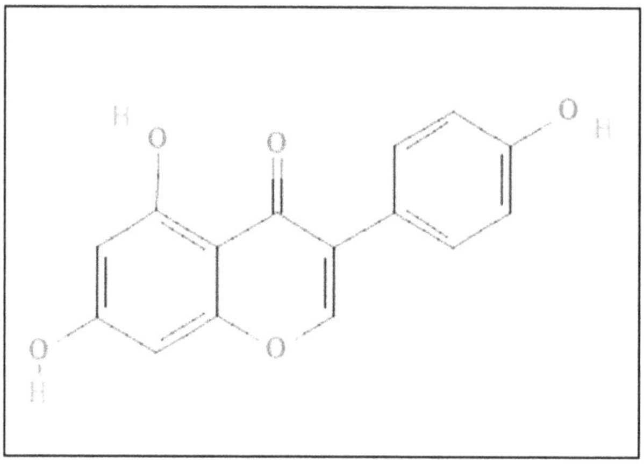

Figure 4.5. Structure of genistein [165].

and apoptosis [76]. Indole-3-Carbinol can reduce tumor multiplication, hyperplastic foci, adenoma, adenoma with malformations, and adenocarcinoma by resulting in the inhibition of IκBα deterioration, activation of NF-B, COX-2, p-Akt and stimulating caspase-3 and PARP cleavage [26], modulation of phosphatidylinositol-3-kinase (PI3K)/Akt signaling process [23], impacts the level of miRNA and regulates its abnormal expression during lung cancer [25].

4.5 Genistein

4.5.1 Structure

Genistein belongs to the family flavonoid and subgroup isoflavones. It is a phytoestrogen that shows a similar chemical structure to mammalian estrogens and is mainly derived from legumes (figure 4.5).

4.5.2 Function

According to [30], genistein attaches and inhibits protein-tyrosine kinase, altering signal transduction and causing cell differentiation. Additionally, it causes G2/M cell cycle arrest and inhibits topoisomerase-II, which results in DNA fragmentation and apoptosis [77]. According to studies, genistein affects tumor necrosis factor (TNFR)-1 signaling. It increases caspase-3 activity to accelerate trichostatin-A-induced apoptosis in human lung carcinoma cells, while it does not affect normal human lung fibroblasts. According to [33], genistein also suppresses lung tumor nodule formation, lung collagen hydroxyproline content, and serum sialic acid level.

4.6 Curcumin

4.6.1 Structure

For its antiseptic, antioxidant, analgesic, antiangiogenic, and anti-inflammatory characteristics, the compound curcumin (diferuloylmethane) (figure 4.6), which is derived from the turmeric plant (*Curcuma longa*), has been extensively researched [78].

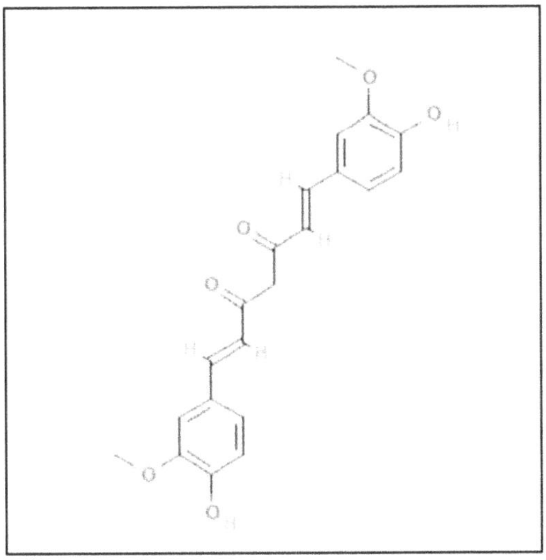

Figure 4.6. Structure of curcumin [165].

4.6.2 Function

Curcumin inhibits cell proliferation and invasion, and induces cell cycle arrest in G0/G1 phase in non-small cell lung cancer cells through inactivation of Wnt/β-catenin pathway by inhibiting the metastasis-associated protein 1 (MTA1) [79], enhances erlotinib-induced apoptosis, decreases the expressions of growth factor receptor of epidermal cells, survivin and inhibited NF-κB activation [80], increases phosphorylation of acetyl Co-A carboxylase and AMP-activated protein kinase (AMPKα), and induces autophagy in the human lung adenocarcinoma cells [81].

Curcumin is useful to treat metastatic lung cancer by inhibiting the migration, and invasion of cells by downregulating Cdc42 gene [36]. Curcumin also upregulates the Bax expression, downregulates the Bcl-2 and Bcl-xl expression, responsible for release of cytochrome *c* into the cytosol, activates the caspase-9, -3, and increases the intracellular reactive oxygen species (ROS) level in SCLC NCI-H446 cells that causes apoptosis [82]. It inhibits the expression of Cdc42 [36], upregulates the α1-antitrypsin expression and decreases the neutrophil elastase protein level, and this modulates the lung tumor proliferation [37]. Curcumin treatment decreases the Bcl-2 expression during anoikis and causes detachment-induced cell apoptosis [83].

4.7 Polyphenol from pomegranate

4.7.1 Structure

Pomegranate (*Punica granatum*) is an edible fruit that has 80% juice and 20% seeds, and is commonly farmed in India, China, Japan, Afghanistan, Russia, and the United States. Polyphenols contain repeating phenolic moieties of pyrocatechol, resorcinol, pyrogallol, and phloroglucinol connected by esters (hydrolyzable tannins) or more stable C-C bonds (nonhydrolyzable condensed tannins) (figure 4.7).

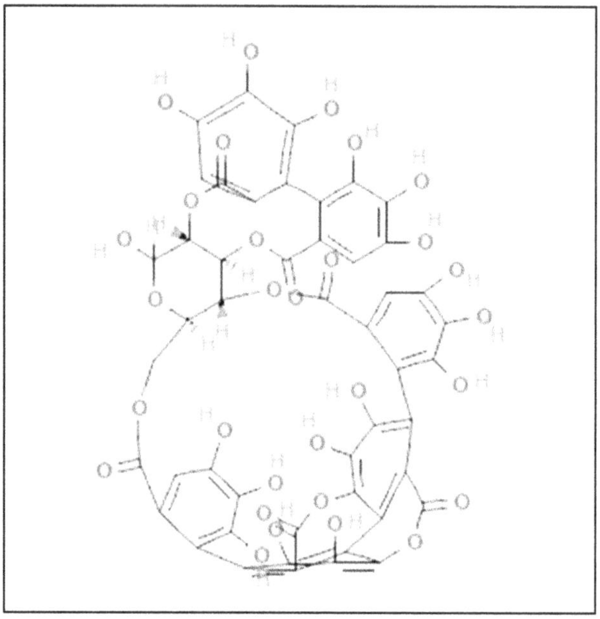

Figure 4.7. Structure of polyphenol from pomegranate [165].

Punicalagin and ellagitannins discovered in pomegranate fruit peel inhibit the formation of DNA adducts when incubated with B(a)P, rat liver microsomes, suitable cofactors, and DNA [84].

4.7.2 Function

Peel extract of pomegranate inhibits myeloperoxidase activity *in vitro* [169], arrests cell cycle in the G0/G1 phase, decreases the expression of cyclin and cyclin-dependent kinase protein, increases the rxpression of regulatory molecules of cell cycle, inhibits the expression of MAPK and PI3K, inhibits the phosphorylation of Akt, NF-κB, and is an indicator of cell proliferation [39]. Pomegranate blossom ingestion reduces development and progression [39] of lung tumor multiplicities by inhibiting the NFκ-B, MAPK, PI3K, phosphorylation of Akt, mTOR, c-met, cell proliferation and angiogenesis indicators [39].

4.8 Fisetin

4.8.1 Structure

Fisetin comes under flavonoid group, known as 3,3′,4′,7-tetrahydroxyflavone (figure 4.8) and is present in grapes, apples, strawberries, cucumber and onion. It is a plant metabolite and works as a geroprotector, antioxidatant, and anti-inflammatory agent by inhibiting the DNA topoisomerase (ATP hydrolyzing), proliferation, angiogenesis and apoptosis in cancer cells [85].

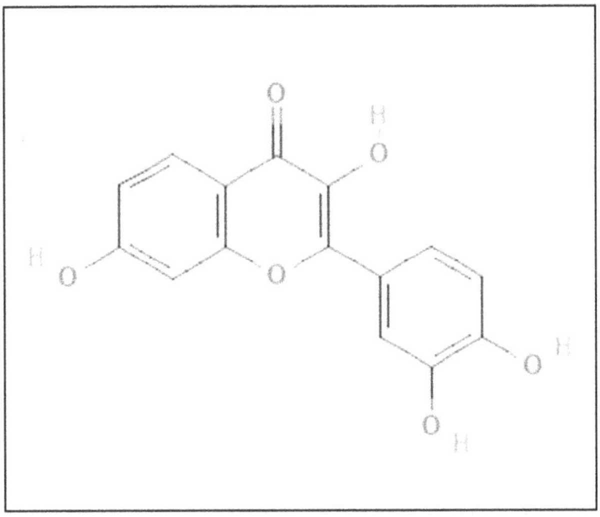

Figure 4.8. Structure of fisetin [165].

4.8.2 Function

Fisetin controls the tumor metastasis by downregulating of PI3K gene expression, Akt phosphorylation, hindering the mTOR signaling [42], inducing HIF-1 alpha expression, and reducing VEGF expression [43]. It also obstructs the adhesion, migration, and invasion by downregulating the expression of MMP-2, ERK1/2, uPA, c-Jun, c-Fos and inhibits the NF-κB binding, therefore controling the tumor metastasis and is useful in cancer treatment [44].

4.9 α-Carotene

4.9.1 Structure

α-Carotene is a carotene with a α-ionone ring at one end and a β-ionone ring at the other (figure 4.9). α-carotene is found in carrots, pumpkin, tangerines, tomatoes, collards, tangerines, winter squash, and peas.

4.9.2 Function

α-carotene has been found to be more effective at inhibiting cancer of the lungs, skin, colorectum, and liver in animal experiments [86, 87].

4.10 β-Carotene

4.10.1 Structure

β-Carotene is a pro-vitamin A present in yellow foods, orange, and colored vegetables. The presence of beta-rings at both ends of the molecule distinguishes β-carotene [88] and it is produced through the biosynthesis of geranylgeranyl pyrophosphate [89]. Figure 4.10 depicts the molecular structure of β-carotene.

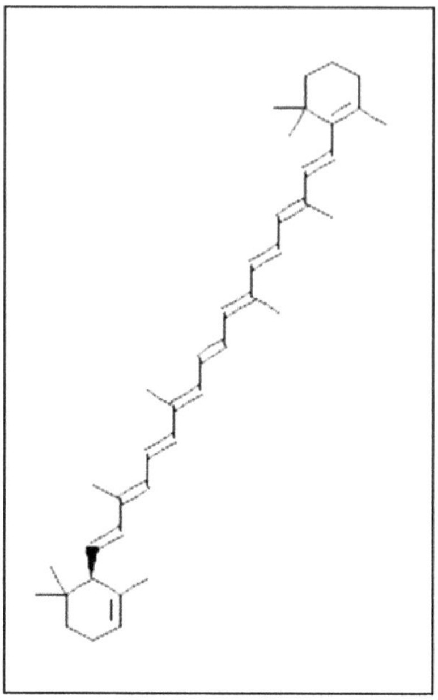

Figure 4.9. Structure of α-carotene [165].

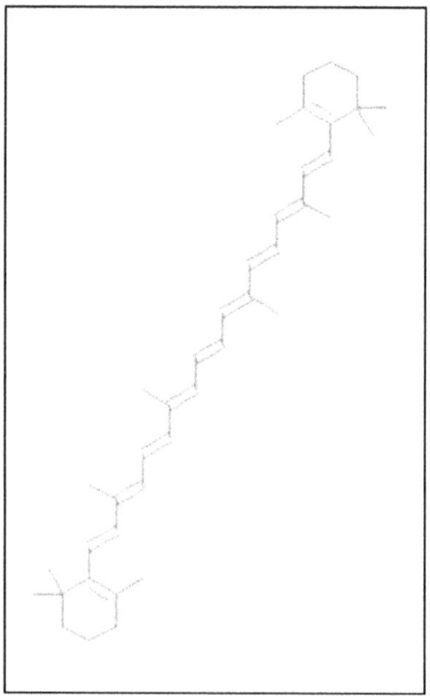

Figure 4.10. Structure of β-carotene [165].

4.10.2 Function

Through transcriptional activation of the RARβ gene, β-carotene acts as pro-apoptotic, anti-proliferative, and antioxidative agent [90–92]. *In vitro*, β-carotene and lutein quench per-oxy radicals and exhibit antioxidant properties against oxidative damage [93, 94], and they decrease lung cancer by 13% when combined with vitamin E and selenium [95].

4.11 Lycopene

4.11.1 Structure

Lycopene is a 40-carbon molecule with a hydrocarbon chain that has linearly arranged two non-conjugated and 11 conjugated double bonds (figure 4.11) [170]. Watermelon, grapes, pawpaw, pink guava, apricots, tomatoes, and tomato-based products contain lycopene [96]. Lycopene's conjugated double bonds are responsible for its many protective actions, including peroxyl radical trapping and singlet oxygen quenching [97].

4.11.2 Function

Lycopene shows various biological properties so that it is used in the therapy of different diseases [35]. Lycopene inhibits the development of human cancer cells by interfering with growth factor receptor signaling and cell cycle progression in the G1 and S phases [98].

4.12 Lutein

4.12.1 Structure

Lutein is a xanthophyll with two hydroxyl groups, one on each side of the molecule (figure 4.12). Lutein is an oxygenated carotenoid present in fruit and vegetables. Lutein exhibits antioxidant properties, protecting cells from the detrimental effects of free radicals.

4.12.2 Function

Lutein is found in spinach, sweet corn, sweet peppers, peas, zucchini, kiwi, grapes, orange, and egg yolk [99]. Lutein is a very good antioxidant and therefore protects the cells from free radical damage and inhibits the development of certain cancers [100].

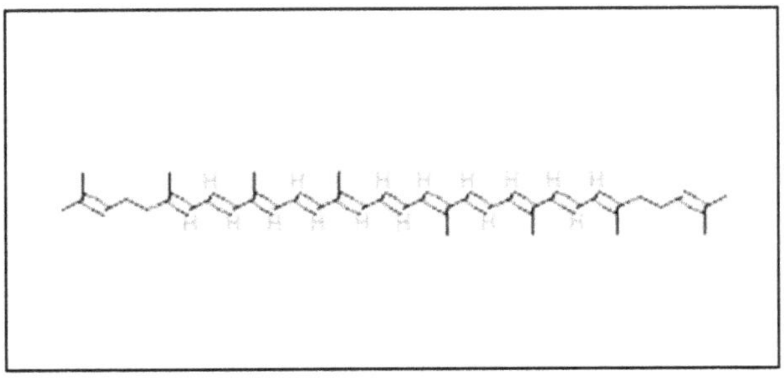

Figure 4.11. Structure of lycopene [165].

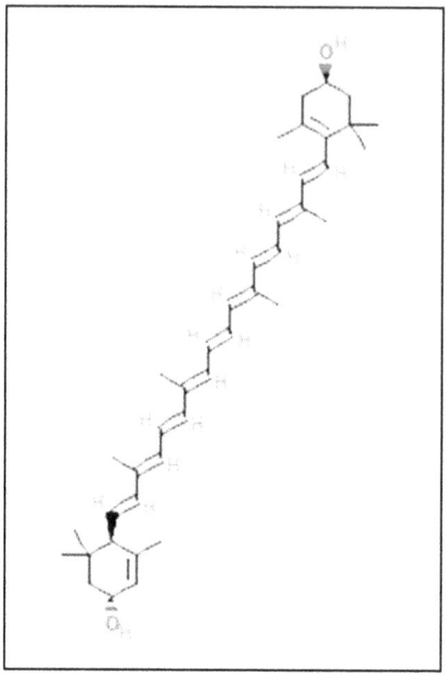

Figure 4.12. Structure of lutein [165].

4.13 β-Cryptoxanthin

4.13.1 Structure

Red bell peppers, black olives, plums, grapefruit, watermelon, mango, papaya, peach, orange, human milk, whole wheat flour, and bran/germ fraction, and other foods contain β-cryptoxanthin which is an oxygenated carotenoid (figure 4.13) [101, 102]. It is a vitamin A precursor that is converted to retinol in the body [103].

4.13.2 Function

β-Cryptoxanthin are immunomodulators, can scavenge free radicals, increase gap junctions, and control carcinogenesis by regulating enzyme activity [104]. β-cryptoxanthin decreases the risk of lung cancer [105].

4.14 Astaxanthin

4.14.1 Structure

Astaxanthin is a type of oxygenated carotenoid that is an alpha-hydroxyl-keto-carotenoid (figure 4.14). Astaxanthin is an effective antioxidant, anti-inflammatory, and anti-cancer agent. It is contained in most red-colored aquatic animals, including Pacific krill (*Euphausia pacifica*), Antarctic krill (*Euphausia superba*), algae (*Haematococcus pluvialis*), Arctic shrimp (*Pandalus borealis*) and yeast (*Xanthophyllomyces dendrorhous*).

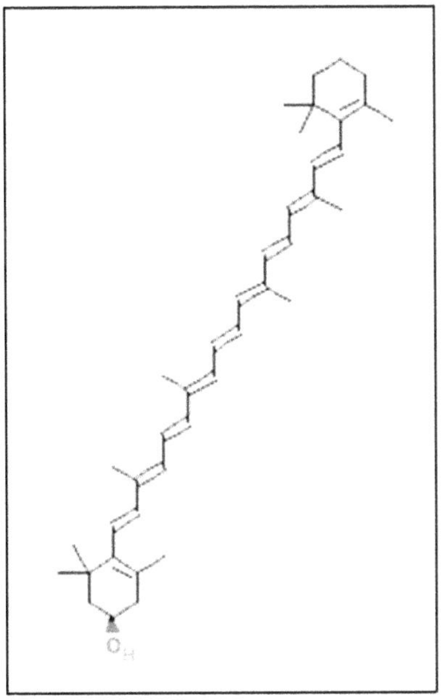

Figure 4.13. Structure of β-cryptoxanthin [165].

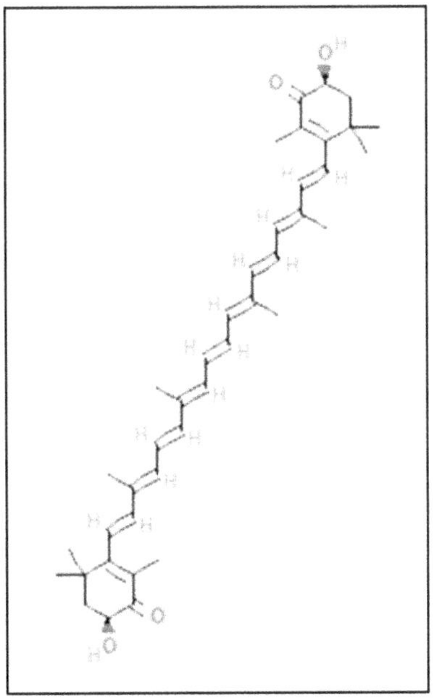

Figure 4.14. Structure of astaxanthin [165].

4.14.2 Function

Astaxanthin can protect against oxidation, scavenge and limit free radical production [51, 106], change the phosphorylation pattern of gap junction protein, connexion [52, 107], modulate nuclear factor kappa B (NFκ-B), COX-2, matrix metalloproteinases (MMP) 2/9, protein kinase B (Akt) and extracellular signal-regulated kinase (ERK)-2 [108] and therefore causes the apoptosis of lung cancer cells.

4.15 Canthaxanthin

4.15.1 Structure

Canthaxanthin belongs to the class terpenoids and is a keto-carotenoid (figure 4.15), found in the edible mushroom, *Cantharellus cinnabarinus*, green algae, blue-green algae, various species of fish such as carp (*Cyprinus carpio*), annular seabream (*Diplodus annularis*), golden mullet (*Mugil auratus*), and trush wrasse (*Crenilabrus tinca*), bacteria, and crustacea [51].

4.15.2 Function

Canthaxanthin are antioxidants, free radical quenchers, and potent quenchers of ROS and nitrogen oxygen species [109], that increase gap junctional cell–cell communication by upregulating the gene expression [110, 111], inducing xenobiotic metabolizing enzymes in the liver, lungs, and kidneys [112, 113].

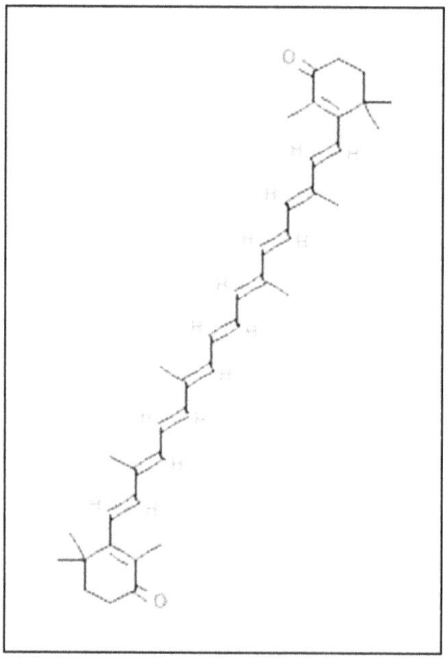

Figure 4.15. Structure of canthaxanthin [165].

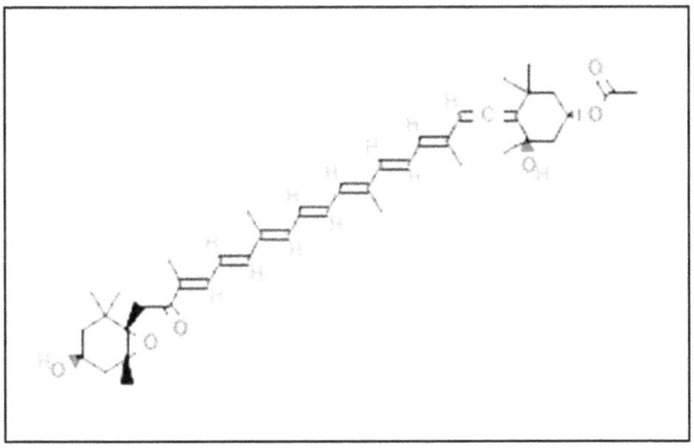

Figure 4.16. Structure of fucoxanthin [165].

4.16 Fucoxanthin

4.16.1 Structure

Fucoxanthin is a hydrocarbon carotenoid with an epoxide bond and hydroxyl groups in the polyene chain, as well as an allenic bond (two contiguous carbon–carbon double bonds) and a conjugated carbonyl group (carbon–oxygen double bond) (figure 4.16). It is found in brown seaweeds and diatoms and has antioxidative, anti-cancer, anti-diabetic, and neuroprotective activities [114].

4.16.2 Function

Fucoxanthin, which acts as an antioxidant in anoxic conditions [51], inhibits the induction of apoptosis [115, 116] and the prevention of cyclin D levels [117], both of which are required for cancer cell proliferation. Fucoxanthin can selectively inhibit mammalian DNA polymerase activities, particularly replicative DNA polymerases implying an anti-neoplastic impact [118] and the ability to alter cell cycle progression [119].

4.17 Probiotics

4.17.1 Structure

According to WHO, probiotics are defined as 'living microorganisms which when ingested in certain amounts, show positive effects on human health, by improvement of the balance of the intestinal microflora' [120]. A few strains such as *Enterococcus faecium*, *Lactobacillus acidophilus*, *Bifidobacterium breve*, *Lactobacillus casei*, *Lactococcus lactis*, *Saccharomyces cerevisiae*, *Bifidobacterium bifidum*, *Bifidobacterium infantis*, *Bifidobacterium longum*, *Bifidobacterium lactis*, and *Bacteroides fragilis* show anti-cancer activity.

4.17.2 Function

Probiotic microorganisms affect lung cancer cell metastasis and homeostasis, inhibit checkpoints, decrease the rate of intestinal dyspepsia [171], downregulate gastro-intestinal complaints, prevent depletion of the gut microflora, reduce Vegfa and Ras expression levels, and enhance Cdkn1b and Bax genes expression, as well as upregulating the Gzmb, interferon (IFN)-γ, and Prf1 mRNA expression [56].

L. casei YIT 9018 (LC 9018) has anti-tumor action in mice and guinea pigs by reducing pulmonary and regional lymph node metastases [53]. *L. lactis* KC24 and NK34 have a substantial cytotoxic effect on the SK-MES-1 lung cancer cell line [57]. Tanasienko *et al* [121] found that *E. faecium* K-50 and *S. cerevisiae* 14-K combination have 2 to 2.5 times more efficacy against metastatic Lewis's lung cancer and solid sarcoma 37 (S37). *L. casei* CRL 431 reduces or inhibits tumor growth by decreasing macrophage infiltration in tumor and lungs and increasing $CD4^+$ lymphocytes and anti-tumor response associated with $CD8^+$ immune cells [60].

Kefir has cytotoxic effects on 4T1 breast cancer cells and inhibits metastases to the lung and bone marrow [61]. T cells and IL17 produced by commensal bacteria help the host immune response against cancer [122].

Oral administration of *B. bifidum*, *B. longum*, *B. lactis*, and *B. breve* improved tumor control via $CD8^+$ T cell activation and co-stimulation, as well as cytokine-cytokine receptor interaction [59]. *B. infantis*-mediated soluble kinase insert domain receptor (sKDR) [55] and soluble fms-like tyrosine kinase receptor (sFlt-1) [54] improve tumor growth suppression efficacy by increasing tumor necrosis rate and extending survival time in lung cancer.

4.18 Carvone

4.18.1 Structure

Caraway (*Carum carvi*), also known as cumin or meridian fennel, grows primarily in northern Africa, western Asia, and Europe. Caraway oil is mostly made of carvone, and limonene, which are also known as *p*-mentha-1,8-dien-2-one, and p-mentha-1,8-diene, respectively (figure 4.17). They are precursors to carvone and anethofuran [123].

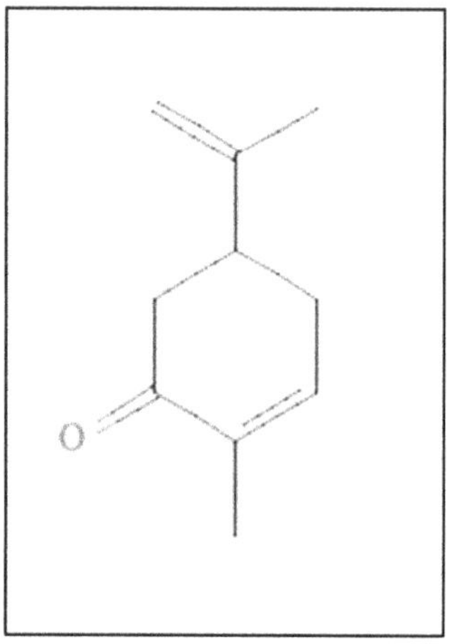

Figure 4.17. Structure of carvone [165].

4.18.2 Function

Caraway essential oil and oleoresins are powerful antioxidants that improve carcinogen elimination [123] and hence reduce cancer risk [124]. Carvone also raises glutathione (GSH) in the lung and regulates carcinogen activation by modifying carcinogen bioactivation [125].

4.19 Alliin

4.19.1 Structure

Garlic (*Allium sativum*) has been utilized for centuries for both medicinal and culinary purposes. Garlic gets its characteristic flavor from sulfur, which accounts for around 1% of its dry weight. Alliin is a sulfoxide formed from cysteine amino acid (figure 4.18) that is found naturally in fresh garlic. Allicin and other thiosulfinates in garlic are unstable and can be converted into a variety of different chemicals, including ajoene, dithiins, diallyl trisulfide (DAT), diallyl disulfide (DADS), and diallyl sulfide (DAS).

4.19.2 Function

Garlic and its constituents reduce the risk of lung, esophagus, skin, breast, uterine, and colon cancers [126–128] via altering the CYP1A1, 1A2, 2B1, or 3A4 genes [129]. Alliin and its sulfur compounds inhibit neoplastic cells [64], increase cell cycle blockage between the G2/M phase [130], act as an antioxidant [131], and affect histone homeostasis [132], resulting in cell cycle arrest and apoptosis.

4.20 Shogaol

4.20.1 Structure

Shogaol is a monomethoxybenzene, a member of phenols and an enone (figure 4.19), isolated from ginger (*Zingiber officinale*), which relates to the family Zingiberaceae and is consumed as a spice and as medicine. Shogaols are pungent constituents of ginger and are produced when ginger is dried or cooked.

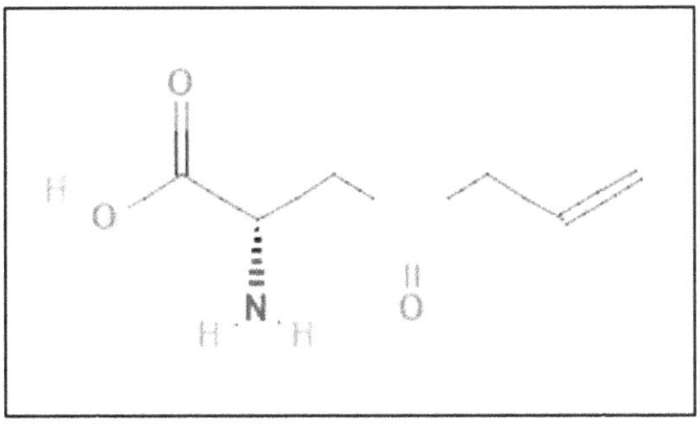

Figure 4.18. Structure of alliin [165].

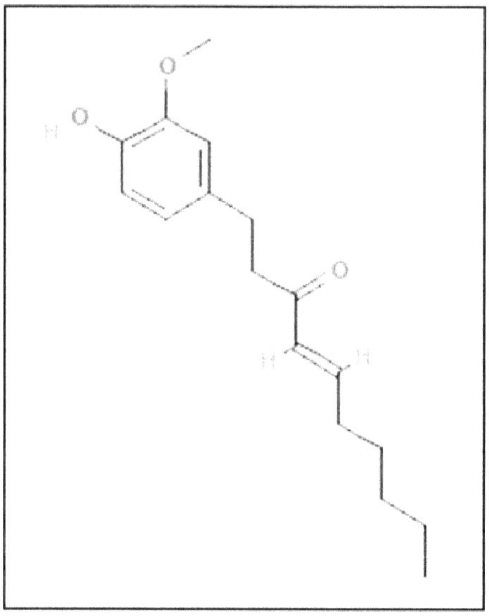

Figure 4.19. Structure of shogaol [165].

4.20.2 Function

Gingerol, paradol, shogaol (dehydrated gingerols), and zingerone are the primary ingredients of ginger. Several investigations on ginger's antioxidant capabilities have been conducted [133]. Shogaol enhances GADD153 gene expression, which accelerates apoptosis and causes DNA damage via an oxidative stress-mediated caspase-dependent mechanism [65].

4.21 Carnosic acid and rosmarinic acid

4.21.1 Structure

Rosemary (*Rosmarinus officinalis*) is a woody herb with fragrant needle-like leaves that has a bitter, astringent flavor and is highly scented. It is a member of the Lamiaceae family and includes a variety of biologically active chemicals such as rosmanol, rosmaridiphenol, rosmarinic acid, betulinic acid, ursolic acid, camphor, caffeic acid, and carnosic acid. Carnosic acid is an abietane diterpenoid substituted by hydroxy groups at positions 11 and 12 and a carboxy group at position 20; rosamarinic acid is ester of caffeic acid with 3,4-dihydroxyphenyllactic acid (figure 4.20).

4.21.2 Function

Several studies have shown that rosemary extract protects human against oxidative stress [134], inhibits the human small cell lung carcinoma cell lines NCI-H82 [172] proliferation by reducing ROS generation and increases TNF-α-induced apoptosis [66].

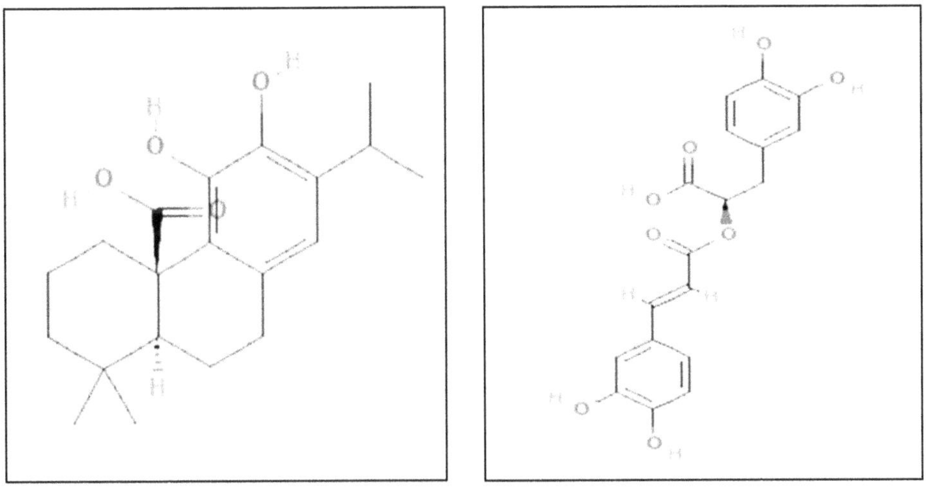

A. B.

Figure 4.20. Structure of (A) carnosic acid and (B) rosmarinic acid [165].

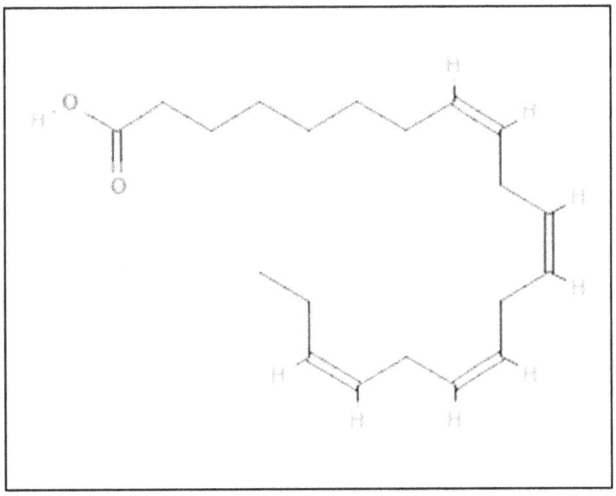

Figure 4.21. Structure of omega-3 [165].

4.22 Omega-3

4.22.1 Structure

Linolenic acid is the source of omega-3 fatty acids. Omega-3 fatty acids are a type of polyunsaturated fatty acid with double bond at the third carbon atom from methyl end (figure 4.21). Alpha-linolenic acid (ALA), the basic omega-3 fatty acid, eicosapentaenoic acid (EPA), and docosahexaenoic acid (DHA) are the three principal forms of omega-3 fatty acids. Omega-3 fatty acids are present in high-oil-content fatty fish, some green vegetables, nuts, and oils.

4.22.2 Function

Various research has indicated that omega-3 fatty acid supplementation in the diet has a negative link with psoriasis, rheumatoid arthritis, inflammatory bowel disease, and cancer [135–137].

4.23 Vitamin A

4.23.1 Structure

Vitamin A is soluble in fats and binds to and activates retinoid receptors (RARs), causes cancer cell differentiation and apoptosis, and suppresses carcinogenesis. Vitamin A and its derivatives are natural retinoids (figure 4.22) found in eggs, butter, cereals, and dark-colored vegetables like squash and carrots. Vitamin A is required for several physiological functions, including appropriate retinal function, target tissue growth and differentiation, reproductive organ function, and immune function modulation.

4.23.2 Function

Retinoid molecules have anti-proliferative properties, such as cell growth inhibition and cell differentiation, and are utilized to treat lung illnesses [138, 139]. Vitamin A has been shown to significantly reduce the incidence of lung cancer [140, 141].

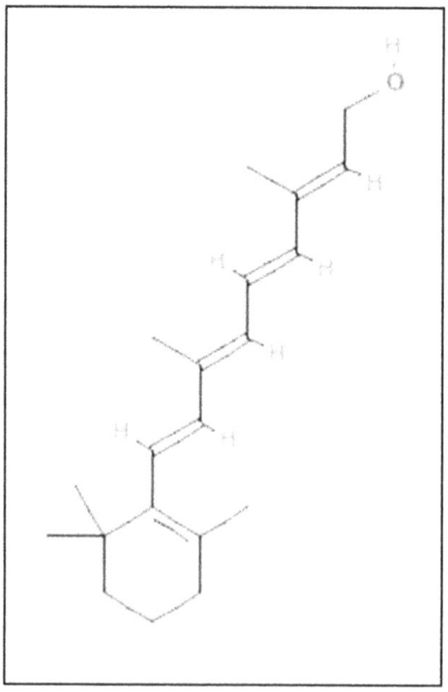

Figure 4.22. Structure of vitamin A [165].

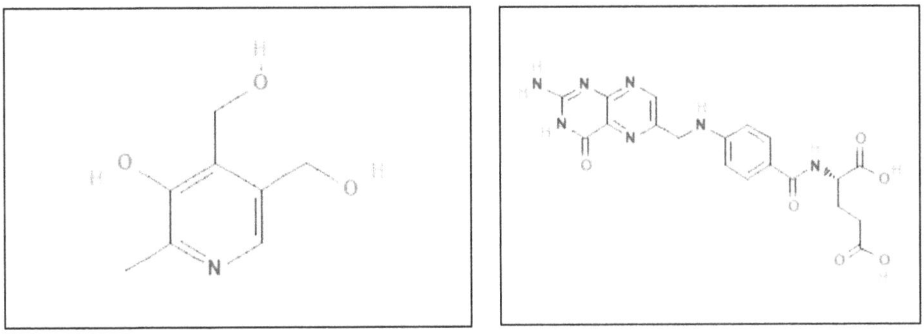

A B

Figure 4.23. Structure of (A) pyridoxin and (B) folic acid [165].

4.24 Vitamin B

4.24.1 Structure

Vitamins of B group are soluble in water, and are essential for cell metabolism. They are present in vegetables, banana, legumes and meat [142]. Cobalamin (vitamin B12), folate (vitamin B9), biotin (vitamin B7), pyridoxine (vitamin B6), pantothenic acid (vitamin B5), niacin (vitamin B3), riboflavin (vitamin B2), and thiamin (vitamin B1) are all included in vitamin B complex (figure 4.23).

4.24.2 Function

Various studies show that smokers have lower levels of circulating folate and vitamin B6, and that B vitamin intake could reverse metaplasia. Various studies show that increased levels of vitamin B6 and folate lower the risk of lung cancer [143], and also show a protective effect on lung cancer development [144, 145].

4.25 Vitamin D

4.25.1 Structure

Vitamin D is a steroid hormone obtained from dietary sources, and human skin can produce it from ultraviolet light. The active form of vitamin D is 1,25-dihydroxycholecalciferol (calcitriol) (figure 4.24), which is responsible for maintaining phosphorus and calcium levels in the blood.

4.25.2 Function

Vitamin D is a fat-soluble steroid that is important in several biological processes, including bone metabolism, immune system modulation, angiogenesis, and cell proliferation regulation [146, 147]. As a result, increasing serum vitamin D levels reduced lung cancer mortality [148–152].

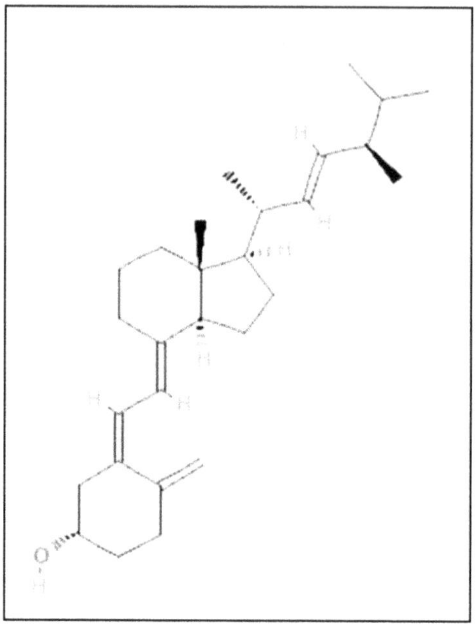

Figure 4.24. Structure of vitamin D [165].

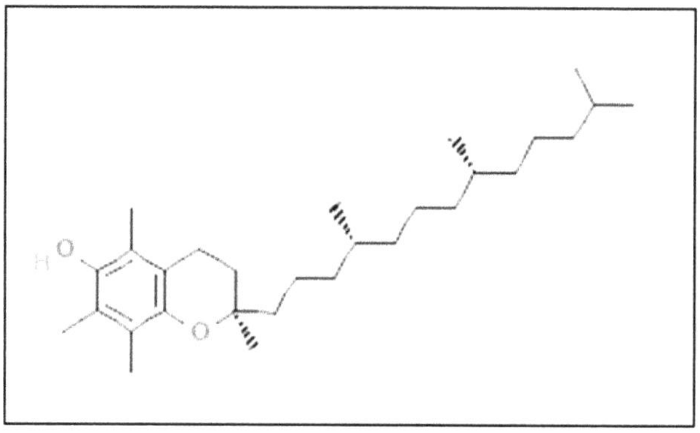

Figure 4.25. Structure of vitamin E [165].

4.26 Vitamin E

4.26.1 Structure

The naturally occurring fat-soluble vitamin E, alpha-tocopherol (figure 4.25), is orally accessible. It is abundant in the flesh of oily fish and fish liver oils, but it is also found in smaller levels in egg yolks, cheese, and beef liver.

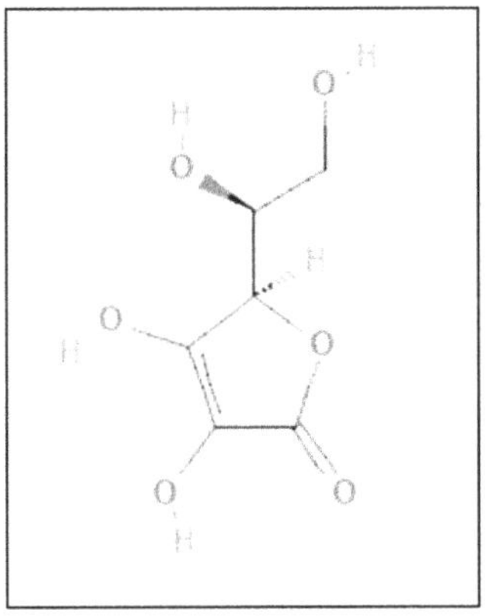

Figure 4.26. Structure of ascorbic acid [165].

4.26.2 Function

Free radicals are neutralized by alpha-tocopherol, which is absorbed into biological membranes, prevents protein oxidation, and inhibits lipid peroxidation, hence maintaining cell membrane integrity and protecting cells and organs from oxidative damage [153].

4.27 Vitamin C

4.27.1 Structure

Vitamin C is a water-soluble vitamin which cannot be stored or produced by humans. Ascorbic acid or vitamin C is a furan-based lactone of 2-ketogluconic acid (figure 4.26). It is a potent reducing and antioxidant agent found in citrus and other fruit and vegetables.

4.27.2 Function

Vitamin C is one of the most important antioxidant vitamins found in fruit and vegetables, capable of influencing immunity and preventing DNA damage [154–156].

4.28 Micronutrients

Calcium is primarily found in dairy products. It protects against lung cancer in both smokers and non-smokers [157–160]. Magnesium was found to be protective by boosting the DNA repair pathway after damage [160, 161]. Zinc deficiency raises the risk of lung cancer because it is a cofactor for key enzymes such as superoxide dismutase, which protects against free radicals [160]. Selenium is a trace element that is needed for numerous enzymes, including glutathione peroxidase, which is responsible for eliminating hydrogen peroxides produced by free radicals [162].

4.29 Summary

In summary, adequate diets that include probiotics, vitamins, minerals, flavonoids, polyphenols, carotenes, and xanthophyll in sufficient levels can minimize the high risk of lung cancer in both smokers and non-smokers.

Acknowledgments

The authors are thankful to their organization for providing infrastructure facilities to write a book chapter. All the images of compounds (figures 4.2–4.26) are retrieved from PubChem (https://pubchem.ncbi.nlm.nih.gov/) [165].

References

[1] Bray F, Ferlay J, Soerjomataram I, Siegel R L, Torre L A and Jemal A 2018 Global cancer statistics 2018: GLOBOCAN estimates of incidence and mortality worldwide for 36 cancers in 185 countries *CA Cancer J. Clin.* **68** 394–424

[2] Mohan A *et al* 2020 Clinical profile of lung cancer in North India: a 10-year analysis of 1862 patients from a tertiary care center *Lung. India.* **37** 190–7

[3] Amos C I, Xu W and Spitz M R 1999 Is there a genetic basis for lung cancer susceptibility? *Recent Res. Cancer Res.* **151** 3–12

[4] de Groot P M, Wu C C, Carter B W and Munden R F 2018 The epidemiology of lung cancer *Transl. Lung Cancer Res.* **7** 220–33

[5] Ferlay J, Soerjomataram I, Dikshit R, Eser S, Mathers C, Rebelo M, Parkin D M, Forman D and Bray F 2015 Cancer incidence and mortality worldwide: sources, methods and major patterns in GLOBOCAN 2012 *Int. J. Cancer.* **136** E359–86

[6] Costa F and Soares R 2009 Nicotine: a pro-angiogenic factor *Life Sci.* **84** 785–90

[7] Song J, Su H, Wang B L, Zhou Y Y and Guo L L 2014 Fish consumption and lung cancer risk: systematic review and meta-analysis *Nutr. Cancer.* **66** 539–49

[8] Sun Y, Li Z, Li J, Li Z and Han J 2016 A healthy dietary pattern reduces lung cancer risk: a systematic review and meta-analysis *Nutrients* **8** 134

[9] Wang Y, Li F, Wang Z, Qiu T, Shen Y and Wang M 2015 Fruit and vegetable consumption and risk of lung cancer: a dose-response meta-analysis of prospective cohort studies *Lung Cancer* **88** 124–30

[10] Jin L *et al* 2013 Epigallocatechin gallate promotes p53 accumulation and activity via the inhibition of MDM2-mediated p53 ubiquitination in human lung cancer cells *Oncol. Rep.* **29** 1983–90

[11] Wang H, Bian S and Yang C S 2011 Green tea polyphenol EGCG suppresses lung cancer cell growth through upregulating miR-210 expression caused by stabilizing HIF-1alpha *Carcinogenesis* **32** 1881–9

[12] Liu L C, Tsao T C, Hsu S R, Wang H C, Tsai T C, Kao J Y and Way T D 2012 EGCG inhibits transforming growth factor-beta-mediated epithelial-to-mesenchymal transition via the inhibition of Smad2 and Erk1/2 signaling pathways in non-small cell lung cancer cells *J. Agric. Food Chem.* **60** 9863–73

[13] Li G X *et al* 2010 Pro-oxidative activities and dose-response relationship of (–)-epigallocatechin-3-gallate in the inhibition of lung cancer cell growth: a comparative study *in vivo* and *in vitro* *Carcinogenesis* **31** 902–10

[14] Banerjee S, Manna S, Saha P, Panda C K and Das S 2005 Black tea polyphenols suppress cell proliferation and induce apoptosis during benzo(a)pyrene-induced lung carcinogenesis *Eur. J. Cancer Prev.* **14** 215–21

[15] Liao J, Yang G Y, Park E S, Meng X, Sun Y, Jia D, Seril D N and Yang C S 2004 Inhibition of lung carcinogenesis and effects on angiogenesis and apoptosis in A/J mice by oral administration of green tea *Nutr. Cancer* **48** 44–53

[16] Liu B N, Yan H Q, Wu X, Pan Z H, Zhu Y, Meng Z W, Zhou Q H and Xu K 2013 Apoptosis induced by benzyl isothiocyanate in gefitinib-resistant lung cancer cells is associated with Akt/MAPK pathways and generation of reactive oxygen species *Cell Biochem. Biophys.* **66** 81–92

[17] Pawlik A, Szczepanski M A, Klimaszewska A, Gackowska L, Zuryn A and Grzanka A 2012 Phenethyl isothiocyanate-induced cytoskeletal changes and cell death in lung cancer cells *Food Chem. Toxicol.* **50** 3577–94

[18] Mi L, Xiao Z, Hood B L, Dakshanamurthy S, Wang X, Govind S, Conrads T P, Veenstra T D and Chung F L 2008 Covalent binding to tubulin by isothiocyanates: a mechanism of cell growth arrest and apoptosis *J. Biol. Chem.* **283** 22136–46

[19] Jin C Y, Moon D O, Lee J D, Heo M S, Choi Y H, Lee C M, Park Y M and Kim G Y 2007 Sulforaphane sensitizes tumor necrosis factor-related apoptosis-inducing ligand-mediated apoptosis through downregulation of ERK and Akt in lung adenocarcinoma A549 cells *Carcinogenesis* **28** 1058–66

[20] Kalpana Deepa Priya D, Gayathri R, Gunassekaran G R, Murugan S and Sakthisekaran D 2013 Apoptotic role of natural isothiocyanate from broccoli (*Brassica oleracea italica*) in experimental chemical lung carcinogenesis *Pharm. Biol.* **51** 621–8

[21] Balansky R, Ganchev G, Iltcheva M, Steele V E and De Flora S 2010 Prevention of cigarette smoke-induced lung tumors in mice by budesonide, phenethyl isothiocyanate, and N-acetylcysteine *Int. J. Cancer* **126** 1047–54

[22] Hecht S S, Kenney P M, Wang M and Upadhyaya P 2002 Benzyl isothiocyanate: an effective inhibitor of polycyclic aromatic hydrocarbon tumorigenesis in A/J mouse lung *Cancer Lett.* **187** 87–94

[23] Qian X, Melkamu T, Upadhyaya P and Kassie F 2011 Indole-3-carbinol inhibited tobacco smoke carcinogen-induced lung adenocarcinoma in A/J mice when administered during the post-initiation or progression phase of lung tumorigenesis *Cancer Lett.* **311** 57–65

[24] Dagne A, Melkamu T, Schutten M M, Qian X, Upadhyaya P, Luo X and Kassie F 2011 Enhanced inhibition of lung adenocarcinoma by combinatorial treatment with indole-3-carbinol and silibinin in A/J mice *Carcinogenesis* **32** 561–7

[25] Melkamu T, Zhang X, Tan J, Zeng Y and Kassie F 2010 Alteration of microRNA expression in vinyl carbamate-induced mouse lung tumors and modulation by the chemopreventive agent indole-3-carbinol *Carcinogenesis* **31** 252–8

[26] Kassie F, Kalscheuer S, Matise I, Ma L, Melkamu T, Upadhyaya P and Hecht S S 2010 Inhibition of vinyl carbamate-induced pulmonary adenocarcinoma by indole-3-carbinol and myo-inositol in A/J mice *Carcinogenesis* **31** 239–45

[27] Kassie F, Matise I, Negia M, Upadhyaya P and Hecht S S 2008 Dose-dependent inhibition of tobacco smoke carcinogen-induced lung tumorigenesis in A/J mice by indole-3-carbinol *Cancer Prev. Res. (Phila)* **1** 568–76

[28] Jiang J, Kang T B, Shim do W, Oh N H, Kim T J and Lee K H 2013 Indole-3-carbinol inhibits LPS-induced inflammatory response by blocking TRIF-dependent signaling pathway in macrophages *Food Chem. Toxicol.* **57** 256–61
[29] Tian T, Li J, Li B, Wang Y, Li M, Ma D and Wang X 2014 Genistein exhibits anti-cancer effects via down-regulating FoxM1 in H446 small-cell lung cancer cells *Tumour Biol.* **35** 4137–45
[30] Gadgeel S M, Ali S, Philip P A, Wozniak A and Sarkar F H 2009 Genistein enhances the effect of epidermal growth factor receptor tyrosine kinase inhibitors and inhibits nuclear factor kappa B in non-small cell lung cancer cell lines *Cancer* **115** 2165–76
[31] Li Y, Ahmed F, Ali S, Philip P A, Kucuk O and Sarkar F H 2005 Inactivation of nuclear factor kappa B by soy isoflavone genistein contributes to increased apoptosis induced by chemotherapeutic agents in human cancer cells *Cancer Res.* **65** 6934–42
[32] Zhu H, Cheng H, Ren Y, Liu Z G, Zhang Y F and De Luo B 2012 Synergistic inhibitory effects by the combination of gefitinib and genistein on NSCLC with acquired drug-resistance *in vitro* and *in vivo Mol. Biol. Rep.* **39** 4971–9
[33] Menon L G, Kuttan R, Nair M G, Chang Y C and Kuttan G 1998 Effect of isoflavones genistein and daidzein in the inhibition of lung metastasis in mice induced by B16F-10 melanoma cells *Nutr. Cancer* **30** 74–7
[34] Lev-Ari S, Starr A, Katzburg S, Berkovich L, Rimmon A, Ben-Yosef R, Vexler A, Ron I and Earon G 2014 Curcumin induces apoptosis and inhibits growth of orthotopic human non-small cell lung cancer xenografts *J. Nutr. Biochem.* **25** 843–50
[35] Shi H S *et al* 2012 A systemic administration of liposomal curcumin inhibits radiation pneumonitis and sensitizes lung carcinoma to radiation *Int. J. Nanomed.* **7** 2601–11
[36] Chen Q Y, Jiao D M, Yao Q H, Yan J, Song J, Chen F Y, Lu G H and Zhou J Y 2012 Expression analysis of Cdc42 in lung cancer and modulation of its expression by curcumin in lung cancer cell lines *Int. J. Oncol.* **40** 1561–8
[37] Xu Y, Zhang J, Han J, Pan X, Cao Y, Guo H, Pan Y, An Y and Li X 2012 Curcumin inhibits tumor proliferation induced by neutrophil elastase through the upregulation of alpha1-antitrypsin in lung cancer *Mol. Oncol.* **6** 405–17
[38] Luo F, Song X, Zhang Y and Chu Y 2011 Low-dose curcumin leads to the inhibition of tumor growth via enhancing CTL-mediated antitumor immunity *Int. Immunopharmacol.* **11** 1234–40
[39] Khan N, Afaq F, Kweon M H, Kim K and Mukhtar H 2007 Oral consumption of pomegranate fruit extract inhibits growth and progression of primary lung tumors in mice *Cancer Res.* **67** 3475–82
[40] Khan N, Hadi N, Afaq F, Syed D N, Kweon M H and Mukhtar H 2007 Pomegranate fruit extract inhibits prosurvival pathways in human A549 lung carcinoma cells and tumor growth in athymic nude mice *Carcinogenesis* **28** 163–73
[41] Khan N and Mukhtar H 2007 Tea polyphenols for health promotion *Life Sci.* **81** 519–33
[42] Khan N, Afaq F, Khusro F H, Mustafa Adhami V, Suh Y and Mukhtar H 2012 Dual inhibition of phosphatidylinositol 3-kinase/Akt and mammalian target of rapamycin signaling in human nonsmall cell lung cancer cells by a dietary flavonoid fisetin *Int. J. Cancer* **130** 1695–705
[43] Anso E, Zuazo A, Irigoyen M, Urdaci M C, Rouzaut A and Martinez-Irujo J J 2010 Flavonoids inhibit hypoxia-induced vascular endothelial growth factor expression by a HIF-1 independent mechanism *Biochem. Pharmacol.* **79** 1600–9

[44] Liao Y C, Shih Y W, Chao C H, Lee X Y and Chiang T A 2009 Involvement of the ERK signaling pathway in fisetin reduces invasion and migration in the human lung cancer cell line A549 *J. Agric. Food Chem.* **57** 8933–41
[45] Ravichandran N, Suresh G, Ramesh B, Manikandan R, Choi Y W and Vijaiyan Siva G 2014 Fisetin modulates mitochondrial enzymes and apoptotic signals in benzo(a)pyrene-induced lung cancer *Mol. Cell. Biochem.* **390** 225–34
[46] Ravichandran N, Suresh G, Ramesh B and Siva G V 2011 Fisetin, a novel flavonol attenuates benzo(a)pyrene-induced lung carcinogenesis in Swiss albino mice *Food Chem. Toxicol.* **49** 1141–7
[47] Touil Y S, Seguin J, Scherman D and Chabot G G 2011 Improved antiangiogenic and antitumour activity of the combination of the natural flavonoid fisetin and cyclophosphamide in Lewis lung carcinoma-bearing mice *Cancer Chemother. Pharmacol.* **68** 445–55
[48] Rutovskikh V, Asamoto M, Takasuka N, Murakoshi M, Nishino H and Tsuda H 1997 Differential dose-dependent effects of alpha-, beta-carotenes and lycopene on gap-junctional intercellular communication in rat liver *in vivo Jpn. J. Cancer Res.* **88** 1121–24
[49] Levy J, Bosin E, Feldman B, Giat Y, Miinster A, Danilenko M and Sharoni Y 1995 Lycopene is a more potent inhibitor of human cancer cell proliferation than either α or β-carotene *Nutr. Cancer* **24** 257–66
[50] Hyang-Sook K, Bowen P, Longwen C, Duncan C and Ghosh L 2003 Effects of tomato sauce consumption on apoptotic cell death in prostate benign hyperplasia and carcinoma *Nutr. Cancer* **47** 40–7
[51] Tanaka T, Shnimizu M and Moriwaki H 2012 Cancer chemoprevention by carotenoids *Molecules* **17** 3202–42
[52] Kurihara H, Koda H, Asami S, Kiso Y and Tanaka T 2002 Contribution of the antioxidative property of astaxanthin to its protective effect on the promotion of cancer metastasis in mice treated with restraint stress *Life Sci.* **70** 2509–20
[53] Matsuzaki T, Yokokura T and Azuma I 1985 Anti-tumour activity of *Lactobacillus casei* on Lewis lung carcinoma and line-10 hepatoma in syngeneic mice and guinea pigs *Cancer Immunol. Immunother.* **20** 18–22
[54] Zhu H *et al* 2011 Antitumor effect of sFlt-1 gene therapy system mediated by *Bifidobacterium Infantis* on Lewis lung cancer in mice *Cancer Gene Ther.* **18** 884–96
[55] Li Z J, Zhu H, Ma B Y, Zhao F, Mao S H, Liu T G, He J P, Deng L C, Yi C and Huang Y 2012 Inhibitory effect of *Bifidobacterium infantis* mediated sKDR prokaryotic expression system on angiogenesis and growth of Lewis lung cancer in mice *BMC Cancer* **12** 155
[56] Gui Q F, Lu H F, Zhang C X, Xu Z R and Yang Y M 2015 Well-balanced commensal microbiota contributes to anti-cancer response in a lung cancer mouse model *Genet. Mol. Res.* **14** 5642–51
[57] Han K, Lee N, Park H and Paik H 2015 Anticancer and anti-inflammatory activity of probiotic *Lactococcus lactis* NK34 *J. Microbiol. Biotechnol.* **25** 1697–701
[58] Lee N K, Han K J, Son S H, Eom S J, Lee S K and Paik H D 2015 Multifunctional effect of probiotic *Lactococcus lactis* KC24 isolated from kimchi *LWT Food Sci. Technol.* **64** 1036–41
[59] Sivan A, Corrales L and Hubert N 2015 Commensal *Bifidobacterium* promotes anti-tumor immunity and facilitates anti PD-L1 efficacy *Science* **350** 1084–9
[60] Aragon F, Carino S, Perdigon G and de-Moreno de-LeBlanc A 2015 Inhibition of growth and metastasis of breast cancer in mice by milk fermented with *Lactobacillus casei* CRL 431 *J. Immunother.* **38** 185–96

[61] Zamberi N R, Abu N, Mohamed N E, Nordin N, Keong Y S, Beh B K, Zakaria Z A B, Rahman N M A N A and Alitheen N B 2016 The antimetastatic and antiangiogenesis effects of kefir water on murine breast cancer cells *Integr. Cancer Ther.* **15** 53–66
[62] Daillere R *et al* 2016 *Enterococcus ´hirae* and *Barnesiella intestinihominis* facilitate cyclophosphamide-induced therapeutic immunomodulatory effects *Immunity* **45** 931–43
[63] Zhang Y, Blattman J N and Kennedy N J 2004 Regulation of innate and adaptive immune responses by MAP kinase phosphatase 5 *Nature* **430** 793–7
[64] Sakamoto K, Lawson L D and Milner J A 1997 Allyl sulfides from garlic suppress the *in vitro* proliferation of human A549 lung tumor cells *Nutr. Cancer* **29** 152–6
[65] Chen C Y, Liu T Z and Liu Y W 2007 6-Shogaol (alkanone from ginger) induces apoptotic cell death of human hepatoma p53 mutant Mahlavu subline via an oxidative stress-mediated caspase-dependent mechanism *J. Agric. Food Chem.* **55** 948–54
[66] Moon D O, Kim M O, Lee J D, Choi Y H and Kim G Y 2010 Rosmarinic acid sensitizes cell death through suppression of TNF-alpha-induced NF-kappaB activation and ROS generation in human leukemiaU937 cells *Cancer Lett.* **288** 183–91
[67] Khan N, Afaq F and Mukhtar H 2008 Cancer chemoprevention through dietary antioxidants: progress and promise *Antioxid. Redox Sign.* **10** 475–510
[68] Khan N and Mukhtar H 2010 Cancer and metastasis: prevention and treatment by green tea *Cancer Metastasis Rev.* **29** 435–45
[69] Shapiro T A, Fahey J W, Wade K L, Stephenson K K and Talalay P 2001 Chemoprotective glucosinolates and isothiocyanates of broccoli sprouts: metabolism and excretion in humans *Cancer Epidemiol. Biomark. Prev.* **10** 501–8
[70] Hecht S S 2004 Chemoprevention by Isothiocyanates ed G J Kelloff, E T Hawk and C C Sigman *Promising Cancer Chemopreventive Agents, Volume 1: Cancer Chemopreventive Agents* (Totowa, NJ: Humana Press)
[71] Conaway C C, Yang Y M and Chung F L 2002 Iso-thiocyanates as cancer chemo-preventive agents: their biological activities and metabolism in rodents and humans *Curr. Drug Metab.* **3** 233–55
[72] Singh S V and Singh K 2012 Cancer chemoprevention with dietary isothiocyanates mature for clinical translational research *Carcinogenesis* **33** 1833–42
[73] Navarro S L, Li F and Lampe J W 2011 Mechanisms of action of isothiocyanates in cancer chemoprevention: an update *Food Funct.* **2** 579–87
[74] Conaway C C, Wang C X, Pittman B, Yang Y M, Schwartz J E, Tian D, McIntee E J, Hecht S S and Chung F L 2005 Phenethyl isothiocyanate and sulforaphane and their N-acetylcysteine conjugates inhibit malignant progression of lung adenomas induced by tobacco carcinogens in A/J mice *Cancer Res.* **65** 8548–57
[75] Steinmetz K A and Potter J D 1996 Vegetables, fruit, and cancer prevention: a review *J. Am Diet Assoc.* **96** 1027–39
[76] Choi H S, Cho M C, Lee H G and Yoon D Y 2010 Indole-3-carbinol induces apoptosis through p53 and activation of caspase-8 pathway in lung cancer A549 cells *Food Chem. Toxicol.* **48** 883–90
[77] Zou H, Zhan S and Cao K 2008 Apoptotic activity of genistein on human lung adenocarcinoma SPC-A-1 cells and preliminary exploration of its mechanisms using microarray *Biomed. Pharmacother.* **62** 583–9
[78] Ye M X, Li Y, Yin H and Zhang J 2012 Curcumin: updated molecular mechanisms and intervention targets in human lung cancer *Int. J. Mol. Sci.* **13** 3959–78

[79] Lu Y, Wei C and Xi Z 2014 Curcumin suppresses proliferation and invasion in non-small cell lung cancer by modulation of MTA1-mediated Wnt/beta-catenin pathway *In Vitro Cell Dev. Biol. Anim.* **50** 840–50

[80] Li S, Liu Z, Zhu F, Fan X, Wu X, Zhao H and Jiang L 2014 Curcumin lowers erlotinib resistance in non-small cell lung carcinoma cells with mutated EGF receptor *Oncol. Res.* **21** 137–44

[81] Xiao K, Jiang J, Guan C, Dong C, Wang G, Bai L, Sun J, Hu C and Bai C 2013 Curcumin induces autophagy via activating the AMPK signaling pathway in lung adenocarcinoma cells *J. Pharmacol. Sci.* **123** 102–9

[82] Yang C L, Ma Y G, Xue Y X, Liu Y Y, Xie H and Qiu G R 2012 Curcumin induces small cell lung cancer NCI-H446 cell apoptosis via the reactive oxygen species-mediated mitochondrial pathway and not the cell death receptor pathway *DNA Cell Biol.* **31** 139–50

[83] Pongrakhananon V, Nimmannit U, Luanpitpong S, Rojanasakul Y and Chanvorachote P 2010 Curcumin sensitizes non-small cell lung cancer cell anoikis through reactive oxygen species-mediated Bcl-2 downregulation *Apoptosis* **15** 574–85

[84] Zahin M, Ahmad I, Gupta R C and Aqil F 2014 Punicalagin and ellagic acid demonstrate antimutagenic activity and inhibition of benzo[a]pyrene induced DNA adducts *BioMed. Res. Int.* **2014** 467465

[85] Arai Y, Watanabe S, Kimira M, Shimoi K, Mochizuki R and Kinae N 2000 Dietary intakes of flavonols, flavones and isoflavones by Japanese women and the inverse correlation between quercetin intake and plasma LDL cholesterol concentration *J. Nutr.* **130** 2243–50

[86] Narisawa T, Fukaura Y, Hasebe M, Ito M, Aizawa R, Murakoshi M, Uemura S, Khachik F and Nishino H 1996 Inhibitory effects of natural carotenoids, α-carotene, β-carotene, lycopene and lutein, on colonic aberrant crypt foci formation in rats *Cancer Lett.* **107** 137–42

[87] Murakoshi M, Nishino H, Satomi Y, Takayasu J, Hasegawa T, Tokuda H, Iwashima A, Okuzumi J, Okabe H and Kitano H 1992 Potent preventive action of α-carotene against carcinogenesis: spontaneous liver carcinogenesis and promoting stage of lung and skin carcinogenesis in mice are suppressed more effectively by α-carotene than by β-carotene *Cancer Res.* **52** 6583–87

[88] Senge M O, Hope H and Smith K M 1992 Notes: Structure and conformation of photosynthetic pigments and related compounds 3. Crystal structure of β-carotene *Z. Naturforsch. C.* **47** 474–6

[89] Van Arnum S D 2000 Niacin, nicotinamide, and nicotinic acid *Kirk-Othmer Encyclopedia of Chemical Technology. (1999–2018)* (New York: Wiley)

[90] Burton G W and Ingold K U 1984 β-Carotene: an unusual type of lipid antioxidant *Science* **224** 569–76

[91] Prakash P, Liu C, Hu K Q, Krinsky N I, Russell R M and Wang X D 2004 β-Carotene and β-apo-14′-carotenoic acid prevent the reduction of retinoic acid receptor β in benzo[a] pyrene-treated normal human bronchial epithelial cells *J. Nutr.* **134** 667–73

[92] Zhang P and Omaye S T 2000 β-Carotene and protein oxidation: effects of ascorbic acid and α-tocopherol *Toxicology* **146** 37–45

[93] Sujak A, Gabrielska J, Grudzinski W, Borc R, Mazurek P and Gruszecki W I 1999 Lutein and zeaxanthin as protectors of lipid membranes against oxidative damage: the structural aspects *Arch. Biochem. Biophys.* **371** 301–7

[94] Iannone A, Rota C, Bergamini S, Tomasi A and Canfield L M 1998 Antioxidant activity of carotenoids: an electron-spin resonance study on β-carotene and lutein interaction with free radicals generated in a chemical system *J. Biochem. Mol. Toxicol.* **12** 299–304
[95] Ziegler R G, Mayne S T and Swanson C A 1996 Nutrition and lung cancer *Cancer Causes Control* **7** 157–77
[96] Porrini M, Riso P and Testolin G 1998 Absorption of lycopene from single or daily portions of raw and processed tomato *Br. J. Nutr.* **80** 353–61
[97] Stahl W and Sies H 1996 Lycopene: a biologically important carotenoid for humans? *Arch. Biochem. Biophys.* **336** 1–9
[98] Heber D and Lu Q Y 2002 Overview of mechanisms of action of lycopene *Exp. Biol. Med.* **227** 920–23
[99] Sommerburg O, Keunen J E, Bird A C and van Kuijk F J 1998 Fruits and vegetables that are sources for lutein and zeaxanthin: the macular pigment in human eyes *Br. J. Ophthalmol.* **82** 907–10
[100] Kruger C L, Murphy M, DeFreitas Z, Pfannkuch F and Heimbach J 2002 An innovative approach to the determination of safety for a dietary ingredient derived from a new source: case study using a crystalline lutein product *Food Chem. Toxicol.* **40** 1535–49
[101] Landrum J T, Bone R A and Herrero C 2002 Astaxanthin, β-cryptoxanthin, lutein, and zeaxanthin *Phytochemicals in Nutrition and Health* ed M S Meskin (Boca Raton, FL: CRC Press)
[102] Liu R H 2007 Whole grain phytochemicals and health *J. Cereal Sci.* **46** 207–19
[103] Astorg P 1997 Food carotenoids and cancer prevention: an overview of current research *Trends Food Sci. Technol.* **8** 406–13
[104] Tanaka T, Sugiura H, Inaba R, Nishikawa A, Murakami A, Koshimizu K and Ohigashi H 1999 Immunomodulatory action of citrus auraptene on macrophage functions and cytokine production of lymphocytes in female BALB/c mice *Carcinogenesis* **20** 1471–76
[105] Nishino H, Tokuda H and Satomi Y 2000 Cancer prevention by carotenoids and curcumins *Phytochemicals as Bioactive Agents* ed W R Bidlack, H Tokuda and Y Satomi (Lancaster, PA: Technomic Publishing Company) p 9
[106] Naguib Y M 2000 Antioxidant activities of astaxanthin and related carotenoids *J. Agric. Food Chem.* **48** 1150–4
[107] Jyonouchi H, Sun S, Iijima K and Gross M 2000 Antitumor activity of astaxanthin and its mode of action *Nutr. Cancer* **36** 59–65
[108] Nagendraprabhu P and Sudhandiran G 2011 Astaxanthin inhibits tumor invasion by decreasing extracellular matrix production and induces apoptosis in experimental rat colon carcinogenesis by modulating the expressions of ERK-2, NFkB and COX-2 *Invest. N. Drug.* **29** 207–24
[109] Pashkow F J, Watumull D G and Campbell C L 2008 Astaxanthin: a novel potential treatment for oxidative stress and inflammation in cardiovascular disease *Am. J. Cardiol.* **101** 58D–68D
[110] Zhang L X, Cooney R V and Bertram J S 1992 Carotenoids up-regulate Connexin43 gene expression independent of their provitamin A or antioxidant properties *Cancer Res.* **52** 5707–15
[111] Hanusch M, Gillette C and O'Neill C 1995 Induction of gap junctional communication by 4-oxoretinoic acid generated from its precursor canthaxanthin *Arch. Biochem. Biophys.* **317** 423–35

[112] Gradelet S, Le Bon A M, Berges R, Suschetet M and Astorg P 1998 Dietary carotenoids inhibit aflatoxin B1-induced liver preneoplastic foci and DNA damage in the rat: role of the modulation of aflatoxin B1 metabolism *Carcinogenesis* **19** 403–11

[113] Jewell C and O'Brien N M 1999 Effect of dietary supplementation with carotenoids on xenobiotic metabolizing enzymes in the liver, lung, kidney and small intestine of the rat *Br. J. Nutr.* **81** 235–43

[114] Beppu F, Niwano Y, Tsukui T, Hosokawa M and Miyashita K 2009 Single and repeated oral dose toxicity study of fucoxanthin (FX), a marine carotenoid, in mice *J. Toxicol Sci.* **34** 501–10

[115] Zhang Z, Zhang P, Hamada M, Takahashi S, Xing G, Liu J and Sugiura N 2008 Potential chemoprevention effect of dietary fucoxanthin on urinary bladder cancer EJ-1 cell line *Oncol. Rep.* **20** 1099–103

[116] Hosokawa M, Kudo M, Maeda H, Kohno H, Tanaka T and Miyashita K 2004 Fucoxanthin induces apoptosis and enhances the anti-proliferative effect of the PPAR gamma ligand, troglitazone, on colon cancer cells *Biochem. Biophys. Acta* **1675** 113–19

[117] Das S K, Hashimoto T and Kanazawa K 2008 Growth inhibition of human hepatic carcinoma HepG2 cells by fucoxanthin is associated with down-regulation of cyclin D *Biochem. Biophys. Acta* **1780** 743–49

[118] Murakami C, Takemura M, Sugiyama Y, Kamisuki S, Asahara H, Kawasaki M, Ishidoh T, Linn S, Yoshida S and Sugawara F 2012 Vitamin A-related compounds, all-trans retinal and retinoic acids, selectively inhibit activities of mammalian replicative DNA polymerases *Biochem. Biophys. Acta* **1574** 85–92

[119] Yoshiko S and Hoyoku N 2007 Fucoxanthin, a natural carotenoid, induces G1 arrest and GADD45 gene expression in human cancer cells *In Vivo* **21** 305–9

[120] Food and Agricultural Organization of the United Nations and World Health Organization 2001 *Health and Nutritional Properties of Probiotics in Food Including Powder Milk with Live Lactic Acid Bacteria* (Geneva: World Health Organization)

[121] Tanasienko O A, Cheremshenko N L, Titova G P, Potebnya M G, Gavrilenko M M, Nagorna S S and Kovalenko N K 2005 Elevation of the efficacy of antitumor vaccine prepared on the base of lectines from *B. subtilis* B-7025 upon its combined application with probiotics *in vivo Exp. Oncol.* **27** 336–8

[122] Cheng M, Qian L, Shen G, Bian G, Xu T, Xu W, Shen G and Hu S 2014 Microbiota modulates tumoral immune surveillance in lung through a γδT17 immune cell-dependent mechanism *Cancer Res.* **74** 4030–41

[123] Zheng G Q, Kenney P M and Lam L K 1992 Anethofuran, carvone, and limonene: potential cancer chemopreventive agents from dill weed oil and caraway oil *Planta Med.* **58** 338–41

[124] Kapoor I P, Singh B, Singh G, De Heluani C S, De Lampasona M P and Catalan C A 2010 Chemistry and antioxidant activity of essential oil and oleoresins of black caraway (*Carum bulbocastanum*) fruits *J. Sci. Food Agric.* **90** 385–90

[125] Naderi-Kalali B, Allameh A and Rasaee M J 2005 Suppressive effects of caraway (*Carum carvi*) extracts on 2,3,7,8-tetrachloro-dibenzo-p-dioxin-dependent gene expression of cytochrome P450 1A1 in the rat H4IIE cells *Toxicology* **19** 373–7

[126] Cope K, Seifried H, Seifried R, Milner J, Kris-Etherton P and Harrison E H 2009 A gas chromatography–mass spectrometry method for the quantitation of N-nitrosoproline and

N-acetyl-S-allylcysteine in human urine: application to a study of the effects of garlic consumption on nitrosation *Anal. Biochem.* **394** 243–8

[127] Mei X, Lin X, Uu J Z, Lin X Y, Song P J, Hu J F and Liang X J 1989 The blocking effect of garlic on the formation of A'-nitrosoproline in humans *Acta Nutrimenta Sin.* **11** 141–6

[128] Milner J A 2001 Mechanisms by which garlic and allyl sulfur compounds suppress carcinogen bioactivation: garlic and carcinogenesis *Adv. Exp. Med. Biol.* **492** 69–81

[129] Wu C C, Sheen L Y, Chen H W, Kuo W W, Tsai S J and Lii C K 2002 Differential effects of garlic oil and its three major organosulfur components on the hepatic detoxification system in rats *J. Agric. Food Chem.* **50** 378–83

[130] Knowles L M and Milner J A 2001 Possible mechanism by which allyl sulfides suppress neoplastic cell proliferation *J. Nutr.* **131** 1061S–6S

[131] Antosiewicz J, Ziolkowski W, Kar S, Powolny A A and Singh S V 2008 Role of reactive oxygen intermediates in cellular responses to dietary cancer chemo-preventive agents *Planta Med.* **74** 1570–9

[132] Nian H, Delage B, Ho E and Dashwood R H 2009 Modulation of histone deacetylase activity by dietary isothiocyanates and allyl sulfides: studies with sulforaphane and garlic organosulfur compounds *Environ. Mol. Mutagen.* **50** 213–21

[133] Chrubasik S, Pittler M H, Roufogalis B D and Zingiberis R 2005 A comprehensive review on the ginger effect and efficacy profiles *Phytomedicine* **12** 684–701

[134] Dragan S, Nicola T, Ilina R, Ursoniu S, Kimar A and Nimade S 2007 Role of multi-component functional foods in the complex treatment of patients with advanced breast cancer *Rev. Med. Chir. Soc. Med. Nat. Iasi* **111** 877–84

[135] Takezaki T, Inoue M and Kataoka H 2003 Diet and lung cancer risk from a 14-year population-based prospective study in Japan: with special reference to fish consumption *Nutr. Cancer* **45** 160–7

[136] Voorrips L E, Brants H A, Kardinaal A F, Hiddink G J, van den Brandt P A and Goldbohm R A 2002 Intake of conjugated linoleic acid, fat, and other fatty acids in relation to postmenopausal breast cancer: the Netherlands Cohort Study on Diet and Cancer *Am. J. Clin. Nutr.* **76** 873–82

[137] Gerber M 2012 Omega-3 fatty acids and cancers: a systematic update review of epidemiological studies *Br. J. Nutr.* **107** S228–39

[138] Clarke N, Germain P, Altucci L and Gronemeyer H 2004 Retinoids: potential in cancer prevention and therapy *Expert Rev. Mol. Med.* **6** 1–23

[139] Micksche M, Cerni C, Kokron O, Titscher R and Wrba H 1977 Stimulation of immune response in lung cancer patients by vitamin A therapy *Oncology* **34** 234–8

[140] Omenn G S *et al* 1998 Antiproliferative effect of carotenoids on human colon cancer cells without conversion to retinoic acid *Nutr. Cancer* **32** 20–31

[141] Yu N, Su X, Wang Z, Dai B and Kang J 2015 Association of dietary vitamin A and beta-carotene intake with the risk of lung cancer: a meta-analysis of 19 publications *Nutrients* **7** 9309–24

[142] Galluzzi L, Vacchelli E, Michels J, Garcia P, Kepp O, Senovilla L, Vitale I and Kroemer G 2013 Effects of vitamin B6 metabolism on oncogenesis, tumor progression and therapeutic responses *Oncogene* **32** 4995–5004

[143] Johansson M, Relton C and Ueland P M *et al* 2010 Serum B vitamin levels and risk of lung cancer *JAMA* **303** 2377–85

[144] Fanidi A, Muller D C and Yuan J M *et al* 2018 Circulating folate, vitamin B6, and methionine in relation to lung cancer risk in the Lung Cancer Cohort Consortium (LC3) *J. Natl. Cancer Inst.* **110** 57–67
[145] Hartman T J, Woodson K, Stolzenberg-Solomon R, Virtamo J, Selhub J, Barrett M J and Albanes D 2001 Association of the B-vitamins pyridoxal 5′-phosphate (B[6]), B(12), and folate with lung cancer risk in older men *Am. J. Epidemiol.* **153** 688–94
[146] Wu X, Cheng J and Yang K 2016 Vitamin D-related gene polymorphisms, plasma 25-hydroxy-vitamin D, cigarette smoke and non-small cell lung cancer (NSCLC) risk *Int. J. Mol. Sci.* **17** 1597
[147] Muller D C, Hodge A M and Fanidi A *et al* 2018 No association between circulating concentrations of vitamin D and risk of lung cancer: an analysis in 20 prospective studies in the Lung Cancer Cohort Consortium (LC3) *Ann. Oncol.* **29** 1468–75
[148] Chen G C, Zhang Z L, Wan Z, Wang L, Weber P, Eggersdorfer M, Qin L Q and Zhang W 2015 Circulating 25-hydroxy-vitamin D and risk of lung cancer: a dose–response meta-analysis *Cancer Causes Control* **26** 1719–28
[149] Wei H, Jing H, Wei Q, Wei G and Heng Z 2018 Associations of the risk of lung cancer with serum 25-hydroxyvitamin D level and dietary vitamin D intake: a dose–response PRISMA meta-analysis *Medicine* **97** e12282
[150] Zhang L, Wang S, Che X and Li X 2015 Vitamin D and lung cancer risk: a comprehensive review and meta-analysis *Cell. Physiol. Biochem.* **36** 299–305
[151] Feng Q, Zhang H, Dong Z, Zhou Y and Ma J 2017 Circulating 25-hydroxyvitamin D and lung cancer risk and survival: a dose-response meta-analysis of prospective cohort studies *Medicine (Baltimore)* **96** e8613
[152] Liu J, Dong Y, Lu C, Wang Y, Peng L, Jiang M, Tang Y and Zhao Q 2017 Meta-analysis of the correlation between vitamin D and lung cancer risk and outcomes *Oncotarget* **8** 81040–51
[153] Narita S, Saito E and Sawada N *et al* 2018 Dietary consumption of antioxidant vitamins and subsequent lung cancer risk: The Japan Public Health Center-based prospective study *Int. J. Cancer* **142** 2441–60
[154] Yong L C, Brown C C, Schatzkin A, Dresser C M, Slesinski M J, Cox C S and Taylor P R 1997 Intake of vitamins E, C, and A and risk of lung cancer: The NHANES I Epidemiologic Followup Study: First National Health and Nutrition Examination Survey *Am. J. Epidemiol.* **146** 231–43
[155] Lee D H and Jacobs D R 2005 Interaction among heme iron, zinc, and supplemental vitamin C intake on the risk of lung cancer: Iowa Women's Health Study *Nutr. Cancer* **52** 130–7
[156] Luo J, Shen L and Zheng D 2014 Association between vitamin C intake and lung cancer: a dose-response meta-analysis *Sci. Rep.* **4** 6161
[157] Takata Y, Shu X O, Yang G, Li H, Dai Q, Gao J, Cai Q, Gao Y T and Zheng W 2013 Calcium intake and lung cancer risk among female non-smokers: a report from the Shanghai Women's Health Study *Cancer Epidemiol Biomarkers Prev.* **22** 50–7
[158] Zhou W, Park S, Liu G, Miller D P, Wang L I, Pothier L, Wain J C, Lynch T J, Giovannucci E and Christiani D C 2005 Dietary iron, zinc, and calcium and the risk of lung cancer *Epidemiology* **16** 772–9

[159] Li K, Kaaks R, Linseisen J and Rohrmann S 2011 Dietary calcium and magnesium intake in relation to cancer incidence and mortality in a German prospective cohort (EPIC-Heidelberg) *Cancer Causes Control* **22** 1375–82

[160] Mahabir S, Forman M R, Dong Y Q, Park Y, Hollenbeck A and Schatzkin A 2010 Mineral intake and lung cancer risk in the NIH-American Association of Retired Persons Diet and Health Study *Cancer Epidemiol. Biomarkers Prev.* **19** 1976–83

[161] Cobanoglu U, Demir H, Sayir F, Duran M and Mergan D 2010 Some mineral, trace element and heavy metal concentrations in lung cancer *Asian. Pac. J. Cancer Prev.* **11** 1383–8

[162] Patrick L 2004 Selenium biochemistry and cancer: a review of the literature *Altern. Med. Rev.* **9** 239–58

[163] Shiau R J, Chen K Y, Wen Y D, Chuang C H and Yeh S L 2010 Genistein and beta-carotene enhance the growth-inhibitory effect of trichostatin A in A549 cells *Eur. J. Nutr.* **49** 19–25

[164] Wu T C, Yang Y C, Huang P R, Wen Y D and Yeh S L 2012 Genistein enhances the effect of trichostatin A on inhibition of A549 cell growth by increasing expression of TNF receptor-1 *Toxicol. Appl. Pharmacol.* **262** 247–54

[165] National Center for Biotechnology Information PubChem Compound Summary for CID 65064, Epigallocatechin gallate, PubChem https://pubchem.ncbi.nlm.nih.gov/compound/Epigallocatechin-Gallate (Accessed 19 July 2023)

[166] Sadava D, Whitlock E and Kane S E 2007 The green tea polyphenol, epigallocatechin-3-gallate inhibits telomerase and induces apoptosis in drug-resistant lung cancer cells *Biochem Biophys Res Commun.* **360** 233–7

[167] Tanasienko O A, Cheremshenko N L, Titova G P, Potebnya M G, Gavrilenko M M, Nagorna S S and Kovalenko N K 2005 Elevation of the efficacy of antitumor vaccine prepared on the base of lectines from B. subtilis B-7025 upon its combined application with probiotics in vivo *Exp Oncol.* **27** 336–8

[168] Vétizou M *et al* 2015 Anticancer immunotherapy by CTLA-4 blockade relies on the gut microbiota *Science* **350** 1079–84

[169] Bachoual R, Talmoudi W, Boussetta T, Braut F and El-Benna J 2011 An aqueous pomegranate peel extract inhibits neutrophil myeloperoxidase in vitro and attenuates lung inflammation in mice *Food Chem Toxicol.* **49** 1224–8

[170] Agarwal S and Rao A V 2000 Tomato lycopene and its role in human health and chronic diseases *CMAJ* **163** 739–44

[171] Serkova M I, Urtenova M A, Tkachenko E I, Avalueva E B, Orlov S V, Ivanov S V, Orishak E A and Skazyvaeva E V 2013 On the possibilities of correction of changes of the gastrointestinal tract microbiota in patients with lung cancer treated receiving chemotherapy *Eksp Klin Gastroenterol.* **2013** 15–20

[172] Yesil-Celiktas O, Sevimli C, Bedir E and Vardar-Sukan F 2010 Inhibitory effects of rosemary extracts, carnosic acid and rosmarinic acid on the growth of various human cancer cell lines *Plant Foods Hum Nutr.* **65** 158–63

IOP Publishing

Phytochemicals as an Epigenetic Modifier in Cancer Prevention

Nidhi Puranik, Deepa Yadav and Sangeeta Shukla

Chapter 5

Polyphenols and their metabolites: a molecular regulator at the epigenetic level in cancer protection

Alibha Rawat, N Ganesh and Gresh Chander

Epigenetics is the branch of science that deals with the heritable mechanisms that do not involve any changes in the genomic DNA sequence and are able to modulate gene expression. The mechanisms by which the gene expressions are modulated are DNA methylation and histone. The epigenome is concerned with regulating gene expression by encoding critical information. Because of the rapid advancement in the field of epigenetics during the last few decades, various studies are increasingly filling the gap in knowledge regarding the relevance of these mechanisms. In addition to explaining the mechanisms, these studies have explained possible associations between these epigenetic modifications and disease development including cancer. A number of epigenetic biomarkers are being identified in various types of cancers. These biomarkers are a potential target for therapeutic interventions. These discoveries have opened the gate for many herbal and phytochemical compounds to find application as anti-cancer therapeutic agents with a potential to modify epigenetic signatures. One such group of phytochemicals that are extensively being studied are the polyphenols. As per various studies, these compounds have anti-cancer properties and one of their mechanisms of action is their ability to modify epigenetic signals and thus they have a huge role to play in cancer development and management.

5.1 Introduction

Epigenetic studies have taken a priority in today's genomic era and have found applications in cancer studies and give amazing results in throwing light on the role of various dietary agents like polyphenols in cancer management by modifying epigenetic patterns. It has been found in many studies that polyphenols can actually

doi:10.1088/978-0-7503-5252-9ch5

reverse the adverse effect of epigenetic regulation by modifying DNA methylation and histone modification, and the other tools of genetic regulations that affect cancer development like microRNA expression or altering the enzymatic activity involved with tumor suppressor genes and/or oncogenes, thus altering the outcome. These outstanding results have generated immense interest in the scientific and medical fraternity towards polyphenols and their metabolites as potential anti-cancer agents that can prevent and/or treat cancer. In other words, polyphenols and their metabolites with their epigenetic modifications mechanisms have found application in cancer diagnostics and therapeutics as well as possibly in cancer prevention.

5.2 Polyphenols and their metabolites

Polyphenols are secondary metabolites that are common in the plant kingdom. They carry one or more hydroxyl groups. The major types of polyphenols that exist in nature with a broad range of biological activities are chalcones, xanthones, and flavonoids and they are chemically diverse polyphenols. Polyphenols are classified on the basis of the number of phenol rings that they contain and of the structural elements that bind these rings to one another. They are broadly divided in four classes; **phenolic acids, flavonoids, stilbenes and lignans**.

5.3 Chemical structure of four classes of polyphenols

The chemical structures of these polyphenols are shown in figure 5.1.

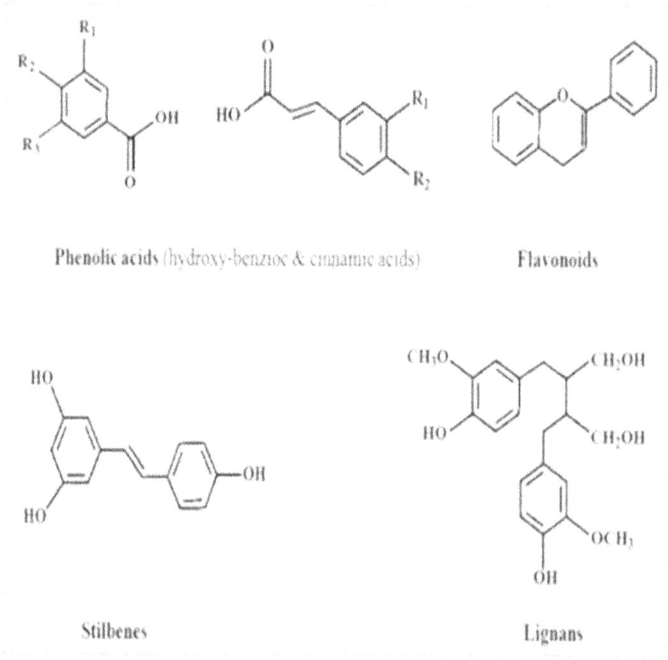

Figure 5.1. Chemical structure of polyphenols.

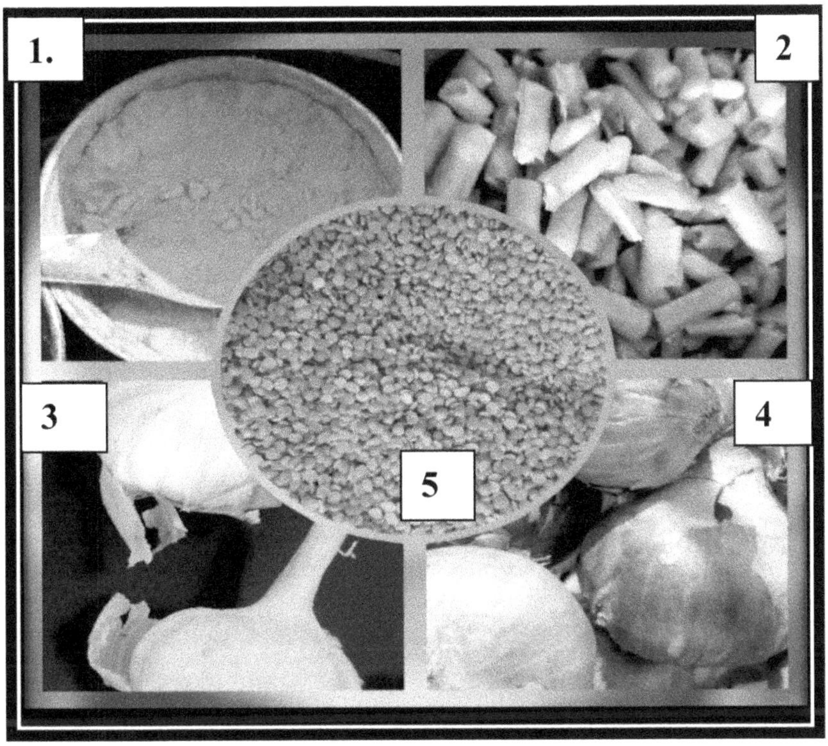

Figure 5.2. Food sources of polyphenols.

5.4 Food sources of polyphenols:

Some of the most common sources of polyphenols are the widely consumed commodities like fruit and vegetables, tea such as green tea and black tea, chocolate etc. Some other significant suppliers of certain polyphenols are herbs, nuts, spices, and algae. Some specific polyphenols are found in specific foods like flavanones and found specifically in citrus fruit, isoflavones in soya, phloridzin in apples; and polyphenols are also found in fruit, vegetables and cereals etc [1] (figure 5.2).

5.5 Medicinal properties of polyphenols

In recent decades, polyphenols have attracted worldwide attention for their medicinal properties. A number of supportive studies have demonstrated the benefits of consuming polyphenols for maintaining good health. However, there are over 8000 polyphenols, and their full health impacts have not yet been adequately described [2]. Various animal studies and epidemiological studies have shown that polyphenols have antioxidant and anti-inflammatory characteristics. These properties may help prevent or treat obesity, cancer, neurological illnesses, and cardiovascular disease [3]. Furthermore, some have issued a warning that excessive use could have negative consequences, especially when compounds are ingested alone rather than as part of a food product [4, 5]. Current polyphenol

Table 5.1. The Most archetypal polyphenols, and their plant bases.

Utmost archetypal polyphenols and their plant bases		
S. No.	Polyphenols	Plant bases
1.	Oleuropein	Seeds of olive, and olive oil
2.	Curcumin	Turmeric
3.	Licopen	Vitamin C containing fruits and i.e., papaya, tomatoes, watermelon strawberries, cherries, pomegranate, orange
4.	Epigallocatechin gallate	Raspberries, blackberries, black, green, and white tea, apples, pecans, hazelnuts, peaches, pistachios avocados, and onions
5.	Resveratrol	Berries, blueberries, and red grapes

studies are mostly based on animal studies and epidemiologic studies. There is evidence from both animal and human research that polyphenols' anti-inflammatory and antioxidant capabilities may be used to treat or prevent a wide range of non-communicable disorders [3, 6]. According to recent research, eating diets high in polyphenols over the long run may offer protection against many diseases including malignancies, heart disease, type 2 diabetes, GI issues, lung disorders and neurological conditions [7–9].

Plants generate polyphenols, which are thought to be very important functional foods in our diet. Based on the different chemical components they possess, they are categorized into a variety of classes. Stilbenes, lignans, flavonoid content, and phenolic acids make up the four main categories of polyphenols. Their impact on health has been studied by various *in vivo* and *in vitro* research work. Polyphenols remove reactive oxygen species (ROS), which are responsible for a number of ailments and also shield the body from environmental stimuli. Tea, chocolate, fruit and vegetables all contain polyphenols that may be beneficial to human health. For example, cocoa flavan-3-ols have been linked to a lower rate of diabetes, heart attack, and strokes. Dietary polyphenols also aid in reducing systemic inflammation, insulin resistance, blood pressure, and lipid profiles. Resveratrol and the flavonoid quercetin have both been related to better cardiovascular health. A bidirectional relationship between dietary polyphenols and the gut flora may, at least in part, be responsible for their ability to have therapeutic benefits. This is due to the fact that polyphenols are known to alter the composition of the gut microbiota in ways that improve people's health. In particular, polyphenols are transformed into bioactive molecules with therapeutic benefits by the gut flora. Based on results from *in vivo* and *in vitro* experimental trials, the antioxidant, cytotoxicity, anti-inflammatory, antihypertensive, and anti-diabetic properties of polyphenols are detailed in this study [10] (table 5.1).

5.5.1 Polyphenols as a neurodegenerative modulatory agent

Polyphenols are also known to have a protective role against neurological disorders like Parkinson's, Huntington's, and Alzheimer's. Resveratrol, which is included in three to four glasses of wine per day, has been linked to an 80% reduction in the prevalence of depression and dementia, according to a study conducted [11]. Further epidemiological data revealed that drinking red wine on a monthly or weekly basis was linked to a lower risk of neurodegenerative illnesses, whereas beers and spirits were not [12]. Epigallocatechin gallate (EGCG), a family of polyphenols, was demonstrated in animal tests to effectively suppress a neurotoxic known to trigger Parkinson's-like illness [13]. An important polyphenol EGCG can trigger signaling pathways and guard neurons [14]. Another very useful polyphenol component, curcumin, has many medicinal values including a protective role in Alzheimer's disease in the Indian population according to a study. In a research of senior South Asian volunteers, those who frequently eat curry had improved cognitive performance compared to those who seldom do so [15]. After correcting for other characteristics like alcohol use and physical exercise, a prospective study indicated that Japanese elderly people who take herbal tea containing polyphenols show low incidence of cognitive problems when compared to non-drinkers [16].

5.6 Anticancer properties of polyphenols

Cancer is defined as a collection of intricate processes that include defective cell death, uncontrolled cell growth, and physiologic alterations in the cells. These processes frequently lead to the development of malignant tumors that metastasize and invade other tissues [17]. A class of primarily natural, water-soluble chemical molecules is known as polyphenols. Globally, the prevalence of cancer and mortality are both rising quickly [18]. Over the past 10–15 years, there has been constant evaluation and meta-analysis of the link between polyphenol intake and the risk of developing cancer. In a meta-analysis of trials, it was seen that isoflavones can lower the risk of stomach cancer to about 19% [19]. Several epidemiological research studies have demonstrated that consuming soy products lowers the breast cancer rate [20]. In another cohort and case-control, it was demonstrated that isoflavone and flavonol intake was associated with an decrease in ovarian and endometrial malignancies risk to about 30% [21]. Various supportive studies have indicated the lower risk of cancers like colorectal cancer and prostate cancer by consumption of high intake of total soy plants. Similarly, studies show that flavonoids had positive impacts on lung carcinogenic effects, according to case-control research conducted in Canada [22, 23] (figure 5.3).

These mechanisms involved in exerting anti-cancer effects include modification of signaling pathway and/or apoptotic induction by these polyphenolic compounds. The activities of enzymes involved in tumor cell proliferation are also regulated by polyphenols. In addition, they have free radical scavenging properties that can protect cells against free radicals damage and polyphenols can modulate immune system response.

There are several cancer preventive mechanisms exerted by polyphenols, including apoptotic induction, oxidation prevention, and/or estrogenic/anti-estrogenic activity. They have stimulating effects on the immune system as well as effects on

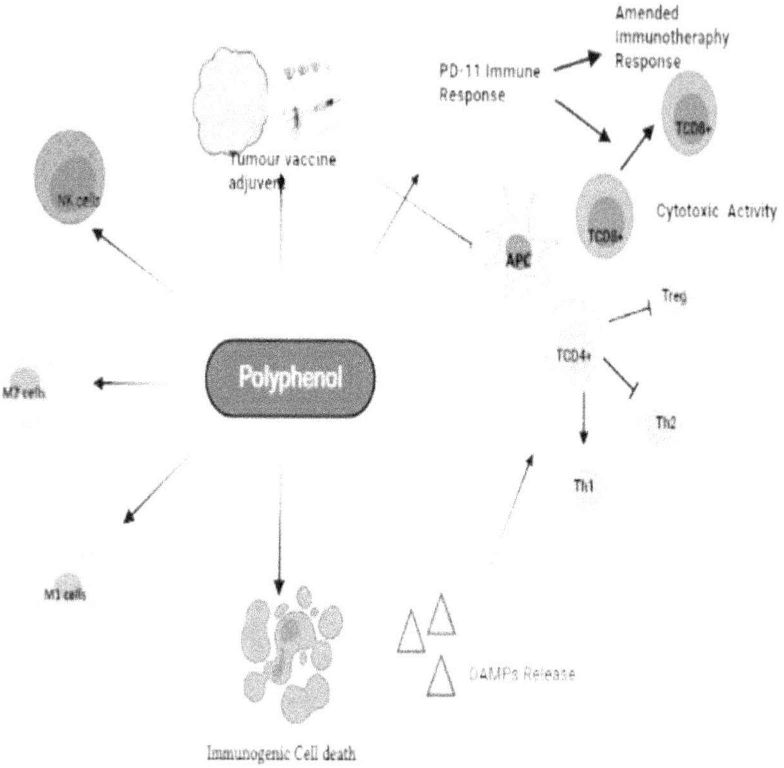

Figure 5.3. The immunoregulatory function of polyphenols in cancer immunity.

the cellular signaling system. A study done by Shen *et al* [24], showed the effects of polyphenols in gene expression and cellular signaling cascades.

5.7 Epigenetic regulation of gene expression

The word 'epigenetic' describes factors beyond the genetic code. Thus, epi-genetics is the science of genetics that is concerned with DNA sequences that have a regulatory role to play in gene expression and not a coding role. In other words, whether genes will be turned on or off is determined and regulated by epigenetic changes that are modifications to DNA. These modifications changes the way the gene expresses without changing the DNA sequence. Thus, epigenome is the modifications that regulate the expression of the genes within a complete genome.

These epigenetic modifications will be explained in detail in the following sections.

5.7.1 DNA methylation mechanism

DNA methylation is the process in which a methyl group is added to specific places on the DNA, where it blocks the proteins that attach to DNA to 'read' the gene thus rendering it off. Demethylation on the other hand is a process in which methyl group is removed and that in turn turns the genes 'on' as it is exposed for 'reading.'

The pyrimidine ring in the cytosine (C) is also modified to transfer epigenetic information as part of the genetic code [25]. Methylation of the fifth position of cytosine (5mC) has a very significant impact on genome stability, gene expression, and development, which is a highly conserved epigenetic modification of DNA that is found in most prokaryotic and eukaryotic models. About 70%–80% of CpG sites throughout the genome show methylation of DNA.

Epigenetic regulations regulate some processes that are fundamental to human development such as maintaining pluripotency and altering promoter accessibility and affecting transcription and translation, thus altering gene expression.

Epigenetic regulations influence the production of proteins in cells by determining which genes are turned on or off; this ensures that only required proteins are produced. For example, proteins of a particular type of tissues like bone tissues are not produced in other types of tissue such as muscle tissues. One interesting fact about epigenetic modification is that it can vary from individual to individual, tissues to tissues in an individual or even cells to cells in an individual. Environmental factors like diet and pollutants can impact the epigenome, and epigenetic modifications can be inherited through the generations as well as maintained from cell to cell and here lies its significance. It can be reversed by well regulatory dietary modifications and counter affecting the bad effects (figures 5.4 and 5.5).

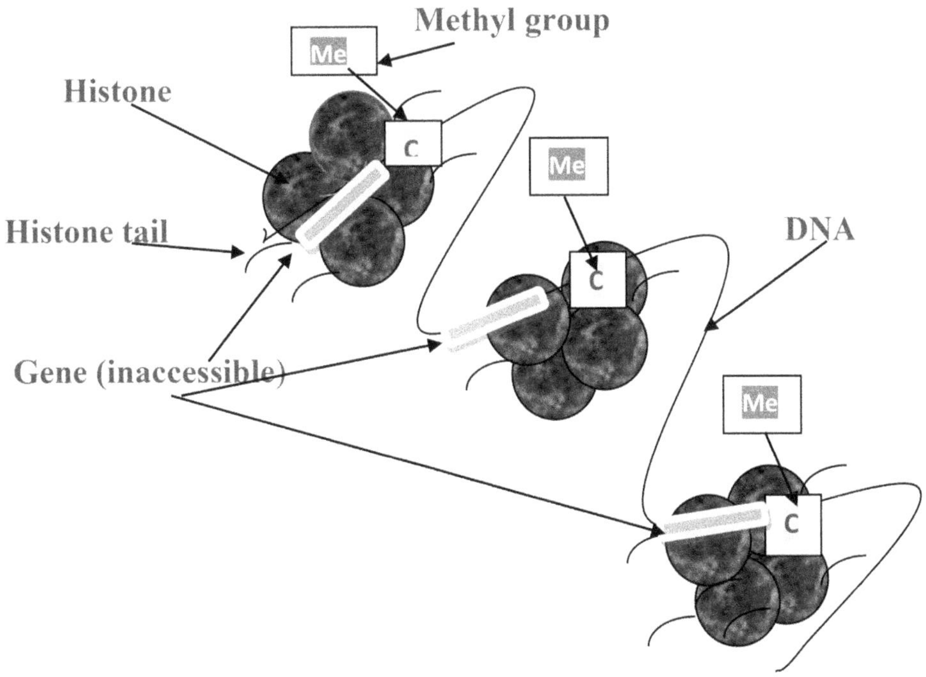

Figure 5.4. DNA methylation.

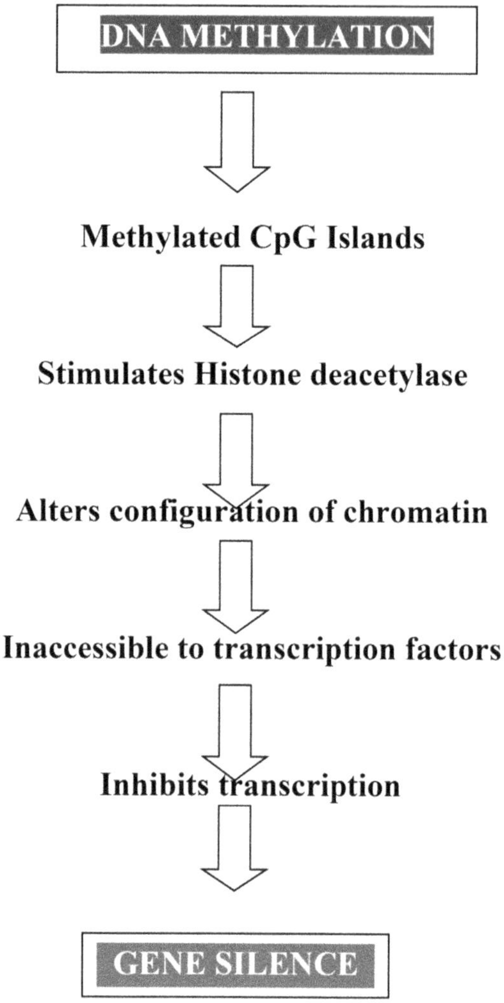

Figure 5.5. Flow chart for mechanism of DNA methylation in gene regulation.

5.7.2 Histone modification

DNA wraps around proteins called histones giving chromosomes their shape. DNA when wrapped tightly around histones cannot be read by the proteins rendering them 'off' while DNA not wrapped around histones is turned 'on.' Another epigenetic modification is done by adding or removing chemical groups and rendering them 'on' or 'off'.

Thus, both the mechanisms of DNA methylation and histone acetylation cooperatively take part in epigenetic regulation. The enzymes involved in histone modification are counteractivity of histone acetyl transferases (HAT) and HDAC. In addition, histone methyltransferases (HMTs) mediate histone methylation [26].

Since these epigenetic regulations have such a pivotal role to play in gene expression, errors in any step of these processes can lead to abnormal gene activity or inactivity. These errors are a common cause of genetic disorders. Many medical conditions including cancer can be attributed to epigenetic errors.

5.7.3 Non-coding RNA

In recent years, a large number of studies have shown that non-encoding **RNAs** play a significant role in **epigenetic** modification and can regulate gene expression. Non-coding RNA is not used to make proteins, but instead used in helping gene expression by attaching to coding RNA, causing them to break down and rendering them unable to make proteins. Non-coding RNA can also turn genes 'on' or 'off' by recruiting proteins to modify histones.

5.8 Epigenetic modifications by polyphenols

It is believed that nutrition affects the epigenetic regulations of DNA methylation in several possible epigenetic pathways: one such pathway is DNA methylation. Certain dietary components are known to alter the substrates and cofactors that are necessary for proper DNA methylation; by altering enzymatic activities and several such possible mechanisms related to DNA demethylation activity. One such dietary component is the polyphenolic component which comprises several compounds such as **phenolic acids, flavonoids, stilbenes and lignans.** These compounds are known to alter epigenetic regulations by various pathways mentioned above. Other epigenetic modifications made by these dietary components are altering histone modifications and microRNA expression.

A number of studies done in the last decade have thrown light on the epigenetic regulation of cancer development and the role some dietary components play in modifying these regulations. Polyphenolic compounds are one of those prominent phytochemicals. A study done by Clark and Rager [27], reviewed studies done on the epigenetic mechanism like CpG methylation, chromatin remodeling, and regulatory/non-coding RNAs and their role in disease development and as therapeutic target. Further research needs to be done to understand the mechanisms of epigenetic mechanisms such as ubiquitination, sumoylation, RNA-and polycomb-based mechanisms.

As per Arora *et al* [28], polyphenols are potent micronutrients that can be found in large quantities in various food sources and spices. These compounds have a major role to play in disease prevention including cancer development by what is now understood to be epigenetic modifications.

Link *et al* [29] discussed the pivotal role of diet and environmental factors on epigenetic modifications. They provided a comprehensive review on the role of various dietary polyphenols. They summarized the results of various *in vivo* and *in vitro* model studies on the effects of dietary agents on the various epigenetic mechanisms including DNA methylation, histone modifications and regulation of expression of non-coding miRNAs.

Carlos-Reyes *et al* [30] discussed the role of various phytochemicals including polyphenols in anti-cancer activities by modulating epigenetic activities. These modulations have huge potential as therapeutic alternatives in cancer management and will pave way for novel biomarkers for cancer prevention.

Another supportive study for the potential of polyphenols as anti-cancer agents by Wu *et al* [31], discussed the role environmental and dietary factors play in inducing epigenetic modifications thus highlighting the potential therapeutic role of such components.

Bag and Bag [32] demonstrated the potential anti-cancer effect of tea polyphenols by epigenetic modifications. Thus, tea polyphenols can be promoted as a very commonly found and affordable agent that has anti-cancer property.

Polyphenols, which are abundantly found in foods, are easily available, cost effective and a safe bet for promoting good health. By changing DNA methylation and histone modification, polyphenols reverse unfavorable epigenetic regulation. They also control the expression of microRNAs or communicate directly with enzymes to control genes involved with cancer development like tumor suppressor genes or oncogenes. As a result, diet-targeted epigenetics for illness diagnosis and prevention will become a promising strategy [33].

The interesting point to note is that since epigenetics regulates gene expression without a corresponding alteration in DNA sequence and in contrast to hereditary changes, epigenetic modifications are reversible, making them a good target for therapeutic intervention. It is now understood that epigenetic inheritance is a crucial and important mechanism in gene regulation that plays a role in biological development. The molecular mechanisms involved in epigenetic alterations, including as DNA methylation, histone modifications, and microRNA, have been studied extensively during the past few decades. Gene transcription and silencing are systematically modulated by the combined action of these alterations and genetic polymorphisms. These studies have thus bridged the gap in knowledge regarding this biological phenomenon that can be utilized in designing therapeutic interventions with dietary polyphenols for the prevention and management of diseases like cancer (figure 5.6).

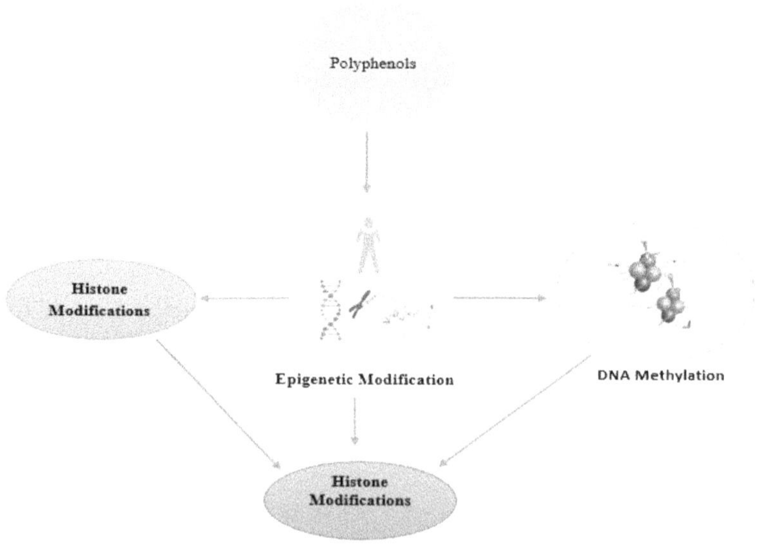

Figure 5.6. Flow chart showing anti-cancer effect of polyphenols by epigenetic modifications.

5.9 Conclusion

It can be concluded that polyphenols have huge potential in the field of cancer therapy, and various therapeutic interventions can be made using the different varieties of polyphenols available in nature, for example flavonoids like quercetin and catechins in fruits, polyphenolic amides like capsaicinoids in chili peppers. Similarly, vegetables and whole grains contain phenolic acids like lignans and stilbenes. Resveratrol is found in red wine and ellagic acid in berries.

All these are naturally available and their role in epigenetic modifications and eventually cancer management can work wonders in the field of cancer therapy and care. All the available supportive studies indicate the potential anti-cancer properties of polyphenols and their mechanism of action which can regulate the genes responsible for cancer development. These have minimal side effects and are found abundantly in nature.

Acknowledgments

We would like to extend our heartfelt acknowledgment to the management of JNCHRC, Idgah Hills, Bhopal for giving us the platform to carry out our research work and for their continued support and blessings. We would also like to thank the editing team of this book for accepting our chapter for their book, namely Dr Nidhi Puranik, Dr Deepa Yadav and Professor Sangeeta Shukla.

References

[1] D' Archivio M, Filesi C, Vari R, Scazzocchio B and Masella R 2010 Bioavaliability of the polyphenols: status and controversies *Int. J. Mol. Sci.* **11** 1321–42

[2] Lecour S and Lamont K T 2011 Natural polyphenols and cardioprotection *Mini Rev. Med. Chem.* **11** 1191–9

[3] Pérez-Jiménez J, Neveu V, Vos F and Scalbert A 2010 Identification of the 100 richest dietary sources of polyphenols: an application of the phenol-explorer database *Eur. J. Clin. Nutr.* **64** S112–120

[4] Crowe K M and Francis C 2013 Position of the academy of nutrition and dietetics: functional foods *J. Acad. Nutr. Diet.* **113** 1096–103

[5] Williamson G and Holst B 2008 Dietary reference intake (DRI) value for dietary polyphenols: are we heading in the right direction? *Br. J. Nutr.* **99** S55–58

[6] Singh A, Holvoet S and Mercenier A 2011 Dietary polyphenols in the prevention and treatment of allergic diseases *Clin. Exp. Allergy* **41** 1346–59

[7] Fraga C G, Galleano M, Verstraeten S V and Oteiza P I 2010 Basic biochemical mechanisms behind the health benefits of polyphenols *Mol. Aspects Med.* **31** 435–45

[8] Martín-Peláez S, Covas M I, Fitó M, Kušar A and Pravst I 2013 Health effects of olive oil polyphenols: recent advances and possibilities for the use of health claims *Mol. Nutr. Food Res.* **57** 760–71

[9] Xiao J B and Högger P 2015 Dietary polyphenols and type 2 diabetes: current insights and future perspectives *Curr. Med. Chem.* **22** 23–38

[10] Rana A, Samtiya M, Dhewa T, Mishra V and Aluko R E 2022 Health benefits of polyphenols: a concise review *J. Food Biochem.* **46** e14264

[11] Orgogozo J M, Dartigues J F, Lafont S, Letenneur L, Commenges D, Salamon R, Renaud S and Breteler M B 1997 Wine consumption and dementia in the elderly: a prospective community study in the Bordeaux area *Rev. Neurol (Paris)* **153** 185–92

[12] Truelsen T, Thudium D and Grønbæk M 2002 Amount and type of alcohol and risk of dementia *Neurology* **59** 1313

[13] Aquilano K, Baldelli S, Rotilio G and Ciriolo M R 2008 Role of nitric oxide synthases in Parkinson's disease: a review on the antioxidant and anti-inflammatory activity of polyphenols *Neurochem. Res.* **33** 2416–26

[14] Rossi L, Mazzitelli S, Arciello M, Capo C R and Rotilio G 2008 Benefits from dietary polyphenols for brain aging and Alzheimer's disease *Neurochem. Res.* **33** 2390–400

[15] Ng T P, Chiam P C, Lee T, Chua H C, Lim L and Kua E H 2006 Curry consumption and cognitive function in the elderly *Am. J. Epidemiol.* **164** 898–906

[16] Noguchi-Shinohara M *et al* 2014 Consumption of green tea, but not black tea or coffee, is associated with reduced risk of cognitive decline *PLoS One* **9** e96013

[17] Anjana R M *et al* 2017 Prevalence of diabetes and prediabetes in 15 states of India: results from the ICMR–INDIAB population-based cross-sectional study**5** 585–96

[18] Bray F, Ferlay J, Soerjomataram I, Siegel R L, Torre L A and Jemal A 2018 Global cancer statistics 2018: GLOBOCAN estimates of incidence and mortality worldwide for 36 cancers in 185 countries *CA. Cancer J. Clin.* **68** 394–424

[19] Grosso G, Godos J, Lamuela-Raventos R, Ray S, Micek A, Pajak A, Sciacca S, D'Orazio N, Del Rio D and Galvano F 2017 A comprehensive meta-analysis on dietary flavonoid and lignan intake and cancer risk: level of evidence and limitations *Mol. Nutr. Food Res.* **61** 1600930

[20] Messina M 2016 Impact of soy foods on the development of breast cancer and the prognosis of breast cancer patients *Complement. Med. Res.* **23** 75–80

[21] Rothwell J A, Knaze V and Zamora-Ros R 2017 Polyphenols: dietary assessment and role in the prevention of cancers *Curr. Opin Clin. Nutr. Metab Care.* **20** 512–21

[22] Christensen K Y, Naidu A, Parent M, Pintos J, Abrahamowicz M, Siemiatycki J and Koushik A 2012 The risk of lung cancer related to dietary intake of flavonoids *Nutr. Cancer* **64** 964–74

[23] Tabrez S *et al* 2013 Cancer chemoprevention by polyphenols and their potential application as nanomedicine *J. Environ. Sci. Health C: Environ. Carcinog. Ecotoxicol. Rev.* **31** 67–98

[24] Shen S Q, Zhang Y, Xiang J J and Xiong C L 2007 Protective effect of curcumin against liver warm ischemia/reperfusion injury in rat model is associated with regulation of heat shock protein and antioxidant enzymes *World J. Gastroenterol.* **13** 1953–61

[25] Zhang N 2015 Epigenetic modulation of DNA methylation by nutrition and its mechanisms in animals *Anim. Nutr.* **1** 144–51

[26] Elsheikh S E, Green A R, Rakha E A, Powe D G, Ahmed R A, Collins H M, Soria D, Garibaldi J M, Paish C E and Ammar A A *et al* 2009 Global histone modifications in breast cancer correlate with tumor phenotypes, prognostic factors, and patient outcome *Cancer Res.* **69** 3802–9

[27] Clark J and Rager J E 2020 Epigenetics: an overview of CpG methylation, chromatin remodeling, and regulatory/noncoding RNAs *Environmental Epigenetics in Toxicology and Public Health* (Amsterdam: Elsevier) Translational Epigenetics vol 22 pp 3–32

[28] Arora I, Sharma M and TollefsbolInt T O 2019 Combinatorial epigenetics impact of polyphenols and phytochemicals in cancer prevention and therapy *J. Mol. Sci.* **20** 4567

[29] Link A, Balaguer F and Goel A 2010 Cancer chemoprevention by dietary polyphenols: promising role for epigenetics *Biochem. Pharmacol.* **80** 1771–92
[30] Carlos-Reyes Á, López-González J S, Meneses-Flores M, Gallardo-Rincón D, Ruíz-García E, Marchat L A, Astudillo-de la Vega[4] H, Hernández de la Cruz O N and López-Camarillo C 2019 Dietary compounds as epigenetic modulating agents in cancer *Front. Genet.* **10** 79
[31] Wu J-C, Lai C-S, Lee P-S, Ho C-T, Liou W-S, Wang Y-J and Pan M-H 2016 Anti-cancer efficacy of dietary polyphenols is mediated through epigenetic modifications *Curr. Opin. Food Sci.* **8** 1–7
[32] Bag A and Bag N 2018 Tea polyphenols and prevention of epigenetic aberrations in cancer *J. Nat. Sci. Biol. Med.* **9** 2–5
[33] Pan M H, Lai C S, Wu J C and Ho C T 2013 Epigenetic and disease targets by polyphenols *Curr. Pharm Des.* **19** 6156–85

IOP Publishing

Phytochemicals as an Epigenetic Modifier in Cancer Prevention

Nidhi Puranik, Deepa Yadav and Sangeeta Shukla

Chapter 6

Potential role of nutritional factors in lung cancer prevention and management

Smarti Verma and Nidhi Puranik

The biggest cause of cancer-related death worldwide is lung cancer. The main reason for the disproportionate mortality from lung cancer is that it is frequently detected after it has progressed past the point at which it may be treated and is no longer responding to surgery or radiation therapy. Nutrition plays a major role in both preventing and treating lung cancer. The latter appears to be influenced by a number of things, such as cigarette smoking or particular environmental circumstances. As a result, the process of carcinogenesis requires an increase in oxidative stress. Eicosapentaenoic acid (EPA), n-3 fatty acids, polyunsaturated fatty acids (PUFAs), vegetables, fruit, white meat, and soy products are specifically stressed as significantly lowering the risk of cancer. Early nutritional management and dietary counseling effectively delay weight loss and sarcopenia in lung cancer patients. Moreover, foods with anti-inflammatory and antioxidant characteristics can prevent a number of illnesses that affect people, including lung cancer. The goal of this review is to assess the role of nutrition in lung cancer in order to give suggestions for dietary and lifestyle changes to prevent this form of cancer.

6.1 Introduction

The most prevalent form of cancer and one of the main reasons for cancer-related death is lung cancer. Over 1.8 million people die from lung cancer each year, making it the leading cause of death globally (WHO 2020). Predictions (Didkowska 2016) state that 3 million people will have this condition by the year 2035. Over 90% of occurrences of lung cancer are attributable to tobacco use, which is the main avoidable cause of the disease (Tong *et al* 1996). Chronic exposure to tobacco chemicals may cause the mutation of oncogenes like Kras and the deletion of tumor suppressor genes like p53 (Avancini *et al* 2020). Ex-smokers also have a very high

doi:10.1088/978-0-7503-5252-9ch6

risk of developing lung cancer given the relatively slow drop in instances that occurs after cessation of smoking (Gilpin and Pierce 2002, Bunn 2012). The single biggest risk factor for this illness is active smoking. In addition to air pollution, risk factors for cancer include exposure to heavy metals (cadmium, lead, nickel, and arsenic), asbestos, and other cancer-causing chemicals (Thun *et al* 2008, Smolle and Pichler 2018). Figure 6.1 displays the etiological factors linked to lung cancer. Smokers' lower levels of circulating NK cells may accelerate the development of cancer, worsening the negative effects of cancer treatment (Jung *et al* 2020).

Small-cell lung cancer (SCLC) and non-small-cell lung cancer (NSCLC) are the two forms of lung cancer based on histological images, as shown in figure 6.2. The patient's general health status, the nature of the intervention, and the likelihood of survival are all significantly influenced by the stage of lung cancer (Löfling *et al* 2021). The 15% 5 year survival rate that is now the average is significantly influenced by the type and clinical stage of the malignancy (Didkowska 2016). The 5 year survival rate for patients with early-stage cancer is 25%, compared to 1%–5% for those with advanced disease (Yang 2009).

Since it cannot be treated surgically or with chemotherapy and radiation, it is typically found at a late stage and is incurable. On a patient's well-being and capacity for everyday living, cancer, and its treatment have a substantial impact.

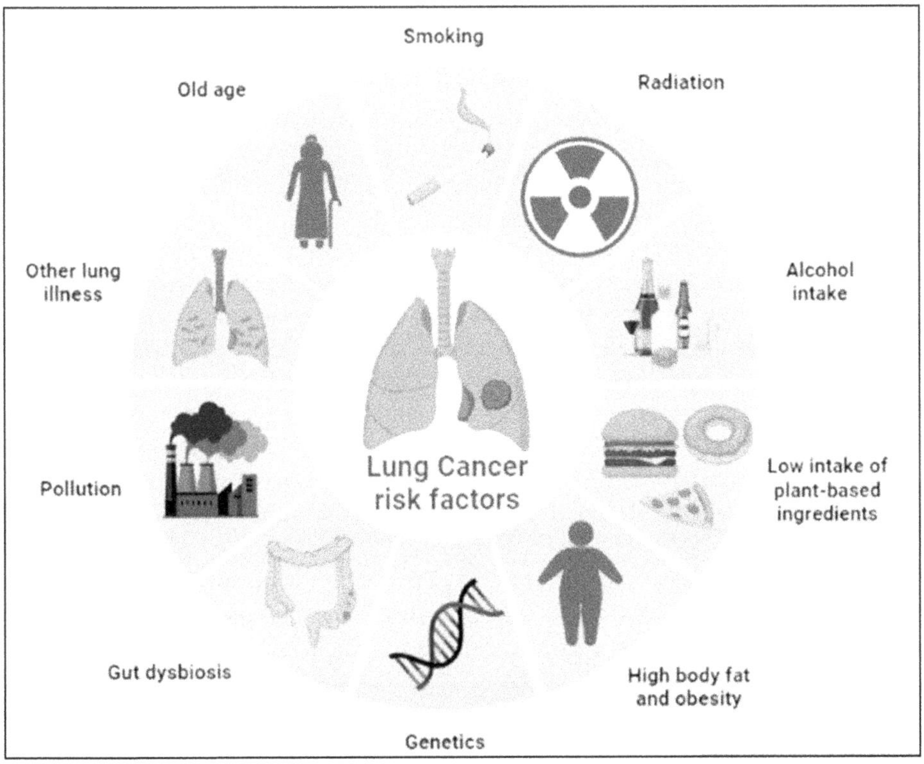

Figure 6.1. Basic risk factors of lung cancer.

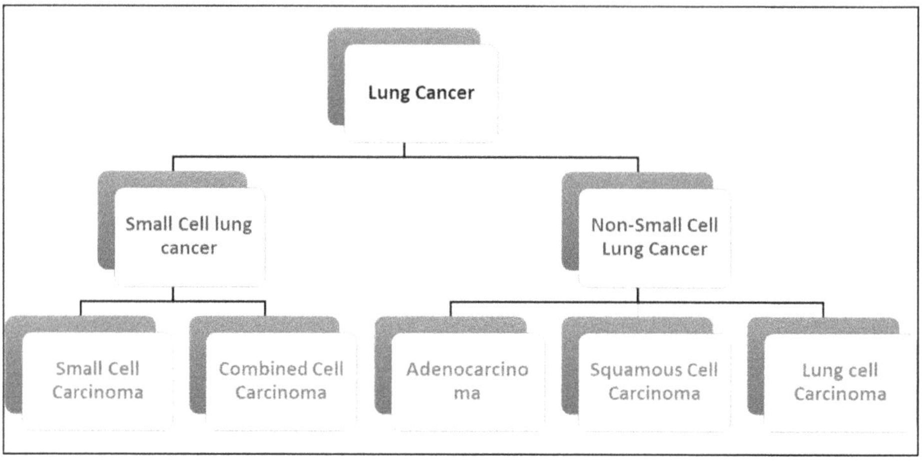

Figure 6.2. Classification of lung cancer.

The most common lung cancer symptoms are chest pain, difficulty breathing, and a persistent cough. Systemic symptoms, such as unintentional weight loss, weakness, a decreased ability to tolerate activity, and low appetite may also be present in addition to respiratory symptoms. Patients with advanced and metastatic cancer are more likely to be undernourished (Chabowski *et al* 2018). Lung cancer is brought on, among other things, by mutations linked to carcinogenic causes and manifests in the epithelial cells that line the airways. A growing body of research shows that specific foods, including grapes, pomegranates, apples, cruciferous vegetables, tomatoes, bitter melons, turmeric, ginger, saffron, garlic, chili, rosemary, soy, rice bran, corn, shiitake mushrooms, *Calvatia gigantea*, and *Thelephora ganbajun*, are important in the prevention and treatment of lung cancer. These ingestible natural products and their bioactive ingredients affect the growth and spread of cancer in a number of ways, including immunomodulation, cell apoptosis, reducing lung carcinogens, obstructing cell migration and adhesion, and making cancer cells more susceptible to anti-tumor medications (Cao *et al* 2019).

At all stages of cancer treatment, from palliative care and recuperation after treatment to preventing problems and continuous treatment (surgery, chemotherapy, and radiotherapy), eating a balanced diet and paying strict attention to nutritional management are crucial (Bagan *et al* 2013). While undergoing radiation and chemotherapy, patients can help to enhance their quality of life (QoL) and decrease their unpleasant side effects by eating enough food and maintaining a nutritious diet. Cancer treatment, whether surgical or non-surgical, is physically demanding on the body and causes catabolism, which raises the patient's requirement for protein and energy (Gupta *et al* 2010). In advanced NSCLC patients receiving chemotherapy, eicosapentaenoic acid (EPA) and polyunsaturated fatty acids (PUFA) supplementation improves physical and mental function as well as the maintenance of weight and muscle mass (Nigro *et al* 2021).

In view of the known antioxidant and anti-inflammatory properties of particular nutrients on the human body as well as previous research findings, we hypothesized that food could aid in both the prevention and treatment of cancer. It is yet unknown whether food has an impact on how people with lung cancer respond to treatment or their prognosis because research findings to date have been contradictory. Underweight NSCLC patients are apparently more likely to experience surgical complications and have a lower overall survival time. Malnutrition weakens the intercostal muscles as well as the immune system. It also increases the risk of deadly and contagious effects. Therefore, nutritional therapy is essential before, during, and after treatment response as well as during the patient's healing phase (Gibson *et al* 2013). As a result, altering one's diet in addition to quitting smoking and using tobacco may be thought of as an appealing strategy for the prevention and management of lung cancer. In this review paper, we address the utilization of particular dietary components for the prevention and treatment of lung cancer.

6.2 Malnutrition in patients with lung cancer

Prior to therapy, malnutrition is present in 26%–40% of lung cancer patients. Cancer prevention, survival prognosis, quality of life, and side effects of treatment are all negatively impacted by malnutrition, which is brought on by insufficient nutrient intake or improper absorption (Sanchez *et al* 2012). According to Kłęk *et al* (2015), BMI, which is used to evaluate nutritional status in healthy individuals, is not pertinent in oncological patients. In an investigation by Sanchez *et al* the average BMI in a patient population with NSCLC undergoing chemotherapy has been 24.8 kg m^{-2}, considered normal body weight (Sanchez *et al* 2012). Because of increased fluid retention in patients receiving intensive treatment and a lack of consideration for the possibility of compensating for disturbed metabolic processes, BMI measurement without an evaluation of malnutrition risk factors is inaccurate. Lower nutrient status in lung cancer patients correlates with their overall quality of life, especially with decreased appetite, fatigue, dyspnea, and diarrhea. The incidence of the above-mentioned symptoms could serve as an effect and a cause of malnutrition, implying that patients exhibiting these symptoms require special nutritional supervision (Xara *et al* 2011, Sanchez *et al* 2012).

Lung cancer patients may experience malnutrition as well as sarcopenia (Dunne *et al* 2019). Studies conducted by Baracos *et al* and Prado *et al* imply that all patients must be under the care of a nutritional team and urgent nutritional intervention should be considered from the beginning of treatment to maintain/increase muscle mass and prevent an increase in fat tissue (Prado *et al* 2008, Baracos *et al* 2010). Undernourished patients had a relatively short survival time and a higher risk of postoperative complications compared to those with normal nutritional status or BMI >18.5 kg m^{-2} in studies on patients awaiting lung cancer surgery (Thomas *et al* 2014). This is most likely to be due to a weakened respiratory system and immune system response caused by a lack of essential nutrients, which would result in an increased infection risk (Jagoe *et al* 2001, Fiorelli *et al* 2014). Nutritional counseling, meal planning, and supplement use are critical approaches to combating malnourishment and sarcopenia in lung cancer patients. Tanaka *et al* demonstrated that early nutritional intervention with dietary counseling in lung cancer patients undergoing chemotherapy effectively prevents weight loss and sarcopenia (Tanaka *et al* 2018). Despite nutritional counseling, many patients do not meet the recommended dietary intake (Nasrah *et al* 2020). Patients with lung cancer have been shown to benefit from a diet plan that includes meals and snacks that are high in protein and energy (Prado *et al* 2016, Leedo *et al* 2017). Therefore, it is evident that numerous components of the Mediterranean diet have beneficial antioxidant and anti-inflammatory effects, underscoring the possibility of improving chronic stress and inflammation, as well as the possible reduction in the incidence of cancer (Porro *et al* 2022).

6.3 Nutrient's role in lung cancer treatment

Building blocks like proteins, lipids, carbs, vitamins, fiber, macro- and micronutrients, etc are provided by the nutrients in the diet. Table 6.1 lists some dietary components that have anti-cancerous potential. A fatty acid called EPA has been found to have particular therapeutic advantages. The possible advantages of EPA in terms of body composition have been explained by a number of different mechanisms, including enhanced responsiveness to insulin, which promotes protein synthesis, or suppression of catabolic stimuli via control of pro-inflammatory cytokine production. EPA may alter nutrient status, body composition, and the reduction of inflammation (Pappalardo *et al* 2015, Ravasco *et al* 2018). According to several research, $n - 3$ fatty acids help maintain muscle mass while avoiding muscle loss with few negative side effects (Arends *et al* 2017). In order to reduce the risk of cancer, vegetables, fruit, white meat, and soy products are explicitly noted as being very beneficial (Sun *et al* 2016, Wang *et al* 2019). The most likely causes of immune system dysfunction and cancer growth include oxidative stress, a unique microenvironment inside the lung tissue altered by carcinogenic agents, and a reduced prealbumin level, which is also utilized as a sign of nutritional status (Allin *et al* 2009). The basic role of nutritional diet in lung cancer prevention and management is shown in figure 6.3.

6.3.1 Role of probiotics/prebiotics in lung cancer

Because microbiota now plays a crucial role in controlling both the emergence of cancer and the immune system's response to cancer cells, it may affect how well immunotherapy works (Ramírez-Labrada *et al* 2020). The lungs' microbiome, which is no longer thought to be sterile, is also connected to lung health. The development of lung cancer and the establishment of pulmonary metastases from other early-stage malignancies are linked to the lung microbiome, which is why it is gaining more attention (Ramírez-Labrada *et al* 2020). The primary cross-talk for this communication occurs between the gut and lungs, and alteration of the structure and function of the gut microbiota affects pulmonary immunological homeostasis, increasing susceptibility to disease. Gut dysbiosis affects the onset and progression of lung cancer via genotoxicity, systemic inflammation, and impaired

Table 6.1. A list of common nutritional factors used in cancer management.

Nutritional factors	Common examples	Role	References
Probiotics/ prebiotics	Yogurt, cheese, supplements, probiotics in capsules or in other forms	Probiotics are supposed to be linked with immunomodulation of gut microbiota	Sharma *et al* (2018), Pizzo (2022
Vitamins	Vitamins A (vegetables and milk), C (fruit), and E (vegetable oils, seed and nuts)	Have antioxidant property, reduced oxidative stress, DNA damage and attenuated other deleterious changes in cell	Didier *et al* (2023)
Dietary fibers	Vegetables (broccoli, onion, cucumber, bean sprout, tomato juice etc); fruits (papaya orange, apple, strawberries, grapes, melon, watermelon, peach, kiwifruit, pineapple etc)	Related to anti-inflammatory response in cancer cell	Cai *et al* (2022)
Fatty acid	Seaweed, flaxseeds, and chia seeds	SCFAs and PUFAs to improve the outcome of immunotherapeutic approaches	Westheim *et al* (2022)
Amino acids and Protein	Dietary essential amino acids (EAA)	Dietary free EAA are very efficient in inducing anabolism in advanced cancer	Engelen *et al* (2015)
Antioxidants	Vitamins, phenolics, flavonoids and carotenoids	Reduce oxidative stress; induced apoptosis	Luo *et al* (2022), Marino *et al* (2023)
Anti-inflammatory	Ginger, garlic tomatoes, olive oil, green leafy vegetables, and nuts	Decreases the incidence and recurrence of various cancers, and can improve the prognosis for patients	Rayburn *et al* (2009)
Minerals	Zinc, potassium, Iron and calcium and magnesium	Reduced risk of LC	Muka *et al* (2017), Xu *et al* (2021)

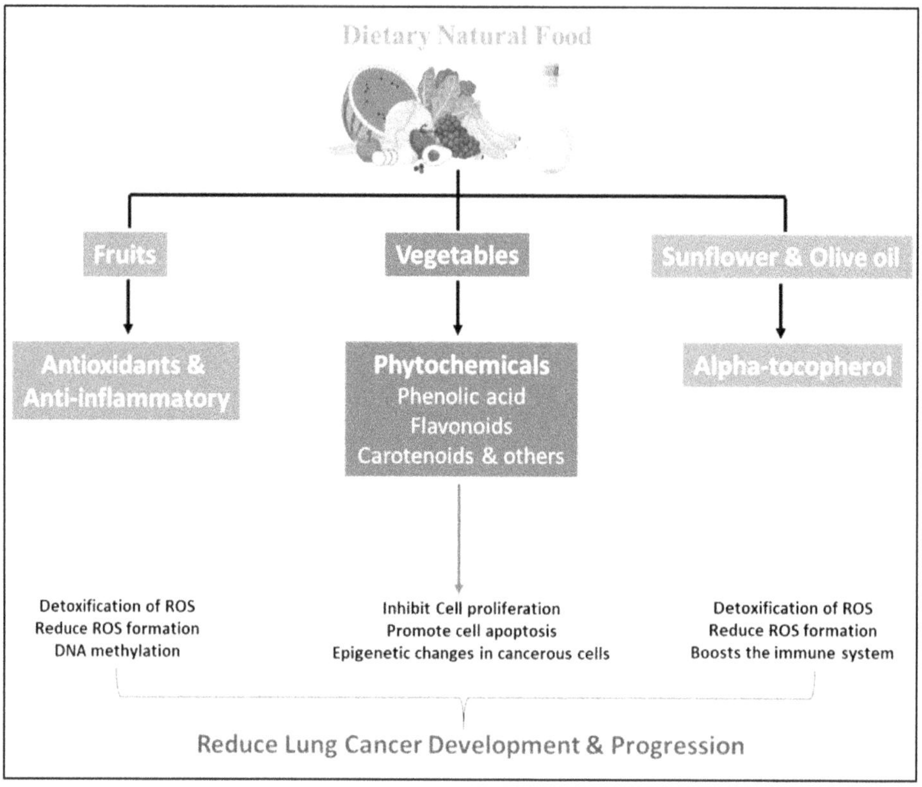

Figure 6.3. Role of dietary natural food in lung cancer treatment and management.

immunosurveillance (Liu *et al* 2021). The 'gut-lung axis' refers to the cross-talk between the microbiota of the gut and the microbiota of the lungs, which can affect pulmonary health (Keely *et al* 2012). Profiling of the intestinal and pulmonary microbiota may identify symbiotic characteristics linked to immunotherapy success and delayed tumor growth (Wang *et al* 2020). *Veillonella*, *Megasphaera*, *Cyanobacteria* (Apopa *et al* 2018), *Streptococcus*, and *Neisseria* (Liu *et al* 2018, Liu *et al* 2018), are commonly detected in lung cancer patients.

6.3.2 Role of vitamins and minerals in lung cancer

Carotene, vitamins C and E, selenium, and zinc are components that shield immune system cells from reactive oxygen species (ROS), which are particularly prone to them (DyMarska *et al* 2013). According to Zagrodzki (2004), selenium deficiency affects the immune system's ability to fight off bacterial and viral infections, lowers the activity of T lymphocytes, macrophages, and natural killer cells, and interferes with the creation of prostaglandins and immunoglobulins. In addition to reducing the total number of B-lymphocytes, zinc deficiency interferes with chemotaxis, natural killer cells, and macrophage phagocytic capacity. Immune response suppression can be modified by vitamin D, whose receptors are present on macrophages, monocytes, dendritic cells, and active T- and B-lymphocytes (Krzysik *et al* 2007). Vitamin A and carotene's antioxidant activity, stimulation of detoxification enzymes, and inhibition of cellular growth may all be connected. According to Yu *et al* (2015), this may have a big impact on preventing lung cancer. In addition, vitamin A and, carotene play a role in DNA methylation and DNA damage. It's possible that vitamin A and carotene's antioxidant action, stimulation of detoxification enzymes, and prevention of cellular proliferation are all connected (Cooper *et al* 1999) and may significantly contribute to preventing lung cancer (Luo *et al* 2014). By preventing proliferation, vitamin C causes cell cycle arrest and apoptosis in lung cancer cell lines. Clinical studies suggest that large intravenous doses of vitamin C may be used in combination with chemotherapy to decrease its negative effects or increase its efficacy (Polanski *et al* 2023). Vitamin D exhibits antiproliferative properties in a variety of lung cancer epithelial cell lines (Norton and O'connell 2012). Dietary vitamin E consumption lowers the chance of developing lung cancer, and higher dietary vitamin E intake may lower that risk by 14.2% (Chen *et al* 2015). Lung cancer patients had significantly lower levels of lutein, zeaxanthin, carotene, retinol, and tocopherol in their blood as compared to healthy individuals (Goodman *et al* 2003). These substances serve to prevent DNA damage, support the smooth operation of the eyes, and have antioxidant characteristics (Arigony *et al* 2013). Malnutrition in lung cancer patients may benefit from supplementation with certain nutrients that are particularly effective. However, it is important to exercise caution when going beyond the recommended daily dosage because of the possible toxicity of retinoids on the liver and skin, as well as their capacity to interfere with coagulation (vitamin E) and cause diarrhea (vitamin C) (Prasad 2003).

6.3.3 Role of protein and amino acids in lung cancer

For individuals with lung cancer to recover fully from surgery, protein-rich diet supplements may be essential (Kiss and Curtis 2022). The appropriate activation and operation of cytotoxic T-cells and memory cells depend on nitric oxide, arginine, and cysteine as well as an adequate protein intake (Domagała-Kulawik and Osińska 2014). Additionally, these components are required for tissue repair. According to Schlemmer *et al* (2015) and Posthauer (2006), the amino acids cysteine and methionine are involved in the formation of collagen and connective tissue. Additionally, the endogenic production of ornithine and arginine depends on glutamine. Because it is the primary energy source for quickly dividing cells like enterocytes and immune system cells, glutamine is a crucial part of the healing process (Schlemmer *et al* 2015). Ajouz *et al* (2019) have shown that branched-chain amino acids and their metabolites, such as β-hydroxy methylbutyrate (HMB), a metabolite of the branched-chain amino acid leucine, are potential nutritional components that can promote muscle protein synthesis and decrease protein breakdown. In patients with NSCLC who showed no indications of malnutrition, Kaya *et al* (2016) studied the effects of arginine, omega-3 fatty acids, and nucleotide supplementation before surgical treatment (Kaya *et al* 2016).

6.3.4 Role of polyunsaturated fatty acids enriched diets in lung cancer

Changes in diet can reduce inflammation, which plays a significant role in the genesis of cancer. In fact, according to Shivappa *et al* (2019), inflammation and nutrition are substantial risk factors for a range of cancers, including lung cancer. Animal studies have shown that PUFAs have anti-inflammatory and anti-tumor properties (Luu *et al* 2018). The Shanghai Women's Health Study (SWHS) and Shanghai Men's Health Study (SMHS), two population-based cohort studies with a combined total of 121 970 individuals, investigated the association between certain dietary PUFA intakes and the risk of developing lung cancer (Zheng *et al* 2005, Shu *et al* 2015). Total dietary fatty acid intake, saturated fatty acid intake, and monounsaturated fatty acid intake do not significantly enhance the risk of lung cancer. The adverse link between PUFA intake and the ratio of $n-3$ to $n-6$ PUFAs and the risk of lung cancer, particularly in never-smokers, is, however, intriguing. This discovery highlights the significant public health impact of PUFAs on people with lung cancer. These PUFA effects seem to be based on molecular mechanisms that are anti-inflammatory and antioxidative, both of which can improve the nutritional status of cancer patients (Gu *et al* 2015, Meital *et al* 2019, Oppedisano *et al* 2020).

6.3.5 Role of fibers-enriched diet in lung cancer

The prevention of cancer has long been linked to high fiber intake (Marmot 2018). These many health benefits appear to be mediated through the modulation of the gut microbiota and modification of metabolic pathways brought on by fiber (Yang *et al* 2020). The incidence of lung cancer was found to be inversely connected to fruit consumption when compared to vegetable consumption, according to Bradbury *et al* (2014); however, this correlation with fruit consumption is only apparent in smokers. According to a study by Büchner *et al* on the impact of fruit and vegetables on 1830 incident cases of lung cancer, increasing the amount of fruit and vegetable diet by 100 g/day was associated with a lower risk of lung cancer (Büchner *et al* 2010). Additionally, Baldrick *et al* (2012), who discovered favorable benefits in ex-smokers consuming a diet high in fibers from legumes via anti-inflammatory pathways, demonstrated that alternate fiber sources do not impact favorable results.

6.3.6 Anti-inflammatory and antioxidant in lung cancer

It is widely believed that eating a diet rich in fruit and vegetables can prevent a variety of diseases in people (Cena *et al* 2020). Antioxidants are abundant in plants and make up the majority of the human diet (Pandey *et al* 2009). Common antioxidants taken from the natural diet with their antioxidant properties are presented in table 6.2. The effect of oxidative stress is reduced by antioxidants to prevent lung cancer, as shown in figure 6.4. For instance, phenols are molecules with an attached –OH group to a benzene ring that are effective ROS scavengers. Food flavonoids have been shown to protect against a variety of tumor types, including lung, gastric, hepatic, prostate, and ovarian tumors (Romagnolo and Selmin 2012,

Table 6.2. A list of common antioxidants with their antioxidant property.

Vitamin	Chief plant source	Antioxidants property	References
Vitamin A (Retinoic Acid)	Sweet potatoes and carrots	Incredibly effective singlet oxygen quenchers that reduce lipid peroxidation by serving as antioxidants that break chains	Kim *et al* (2021)
Vitamin C (Ascorbic Acid)	Citrus fruits, strawberries, tomatoes, broccoli and potatoes	Neutralize the cell's free radicals and serve as a vitamin E regenerator	Villagran *et al* (2021)
Vitamin E (α-Tocopherol, Tocotrienol)	Vegetable oils, whole grains, fortified cereals, seeds, and nuts	To prevent membrane oxidation, lipid radicals created by the lipid peroxidation chain reaction are interacted with	Hajibabaei (2016), Yang *et al* (2020)
Zinc	Nuts	Zinc supplementation enhances the anti-cancer activity of docetaxel in NSCLS via inducing apoptosis	Kocdor *et al* (2015)
Selenium	Whole grains	Utilize a number of potential mechanisms to stop the development of lung cancer and their effects on various stages of carcinogenesis	Elassal *et al* (2014)
Flavonoids	Tea, green tea, citrus fruits, red wine, onion and apples	By modulating redox homeostasis, increasing apoptosis, acting as pro-apoptotic factors and survival genes, halting cell cycle progression and autophagy, and reducing cell proliferation and invasiveness, natural flavonoids suppress lung cancer	Nath *et al* (2023)
Carotenoids	Sweet potatoes, carrots, tomatoes, brussels sprouts, winter squash and broccoli	According to *in vitro* study, carotenoids function via the PI3K/AKT/mTOR, ERK-MAPK, and PPAR pathways and cause apoptosis via IFNs, RAR, and PPAR, which are p53 mediators in lung cancer signaling. Positive results from studies using cell lines and animal models were obtained	Varghese *et al* (2023)
Phenolics	Fruit, vegetables, legumes, and cereals	a cancer cell line's development and trigger apoptosis	Muller *et al* (2019)

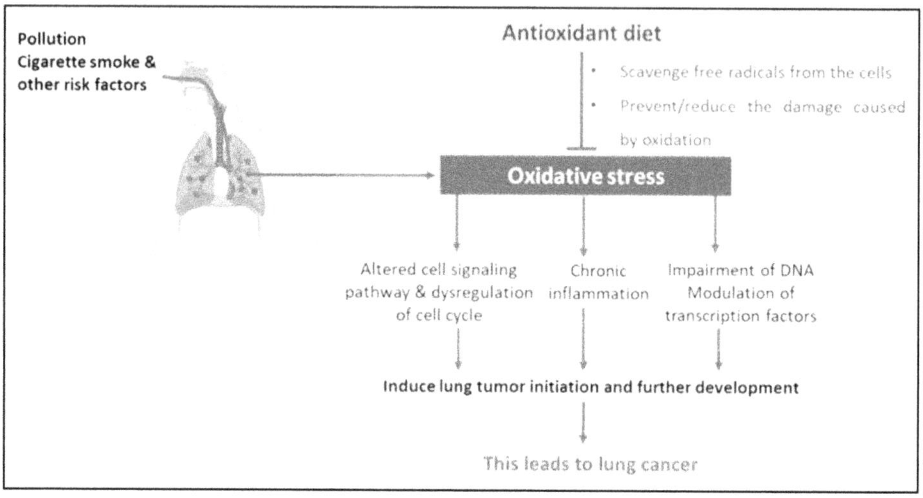

Figure 6.4. An overview of an antioxidant diet in the prevention of lung cancer.

Turati *et al* 2015), among others, by shielding DNA from free radical damage (Russo *et al* 2000), most likely through metal ion chelation. Copper or iron-complexed flavonoids reduce the generation of ROS (Arif *et al* 2015). According to studies by Nani *et al* (2015), Del *et al* (2013), Ghiselli *et al* (1998), Godos *et al* (2017), and others, phenols can be found in foods including olive oil, whole grains, fruit, vegetables, nuts, tea, coffee, and red wine.

Due to the presence of conjugated double bonds in carotenoids, these substances can accept electrons from reactive species and thereby reduce ROS (Rutz *et al* 2016). Vitamin E or vitamin C, as well as beta-carotene, are lipophilic antioxidants that may offer significantly more advantages than a single antioxidant (Stahl *et al* 2005). In human dermal fibroblast (FEK4) cells exposed to UV radiation, investigations have shown that beta-carotene inhibits the production of the heme oxygenase-1 gene (El-Agamey *et al* 2004, Rao and Rao 2007). Another carotenoid called lycopene is mainly present in tomatoes (Agarwal *et al* 2000). It has been shown to be a potent antioxidant against the ROS generated by cigarette smoke in addition to having an impact on redox-sensitive cellular targets like protein kinase, protein tyrosine phosphatase (PTP), MAPK, and transcription factors (Kaulmann *et al* 2014).

Another pharmacological and bioactive substance is curcumin, which is well-known for its antioxidant and anti-inflammatory properties as well as for its potent reactivity to peroxyl radicals. Curcumin, a substance produced from turmeric, may one day be used to treat cancers of the bowel, skin, and colon as well as to prevent them (Marchiani *et al* 2014). Additionally, it stops BV2 microglial cells (LPS-stimulated) from producing the pro-inflammatory cytokines IL-6 and TNF (Panaro *et al* 2020). According to Porro *et al* (2019), curcumin inhibits the COX-2 and STAT signaling pathways. Furthermore, it neutralizes free radicals and encourages the production of antioxidant enzymes (Menon *et al* 2007, Benameur *et al* 2021).

Phytoestrogens and glucosinolate hydrolysis products are also recognized as possible micronutrients in fruit and vegetables that may help prevent lung cancer (Keck *et al* 2004, Brennan *et al* 2005). Accordingly, dietary antioxidants and vitamin and mineral nutritional supplements are used by cancer patients to reduce inflammation and infection (Moyad 2001), cancer growth (Gonzalez *et al* 2005), mutation (Hochstein *et al* 1988), and malignant cell proliferation, among other effects. They are also used to induce differentiation (Lee *et al* 2003) and de-differentiation (Kang *et al* 1999), among other effects. Also connected to pain relief is this supplementation (Luo *et al* 1998, Riordan *et al* 2003).

6.4 Physical activity and lung cancer prevention

Physical activity has been cited as a risk-lowering factor and a non-pharmacological disease management strategy in the context of lung cancer, improving chemotherapy response, prognosis, and survival (Thune *et al* 1997, Tardon *et al* 2005, Friedenreich *et al* 2020, Yang *et al* 2020). It is undeniable that individuals with lung cancer can benefit from home-based exercise in terms of their symptoms and quality of life (Hoffman *et al* 2014). On the other side, a significant risk of functional capacity loss is associated with physical inactivity. Inflammation has been demonstrated to decrease with exercise and physical activity (Cole *et al* 2018), and exercise and physical activity have also been shown to activate molecular signaling pathways that support muscle mass growth and enhance advantageous metabolic changes (Hardee *et al* 2019). By activating natural killer cells, lymphocytes, and dendritic cells, exercise can raise the levels of pro-inflammatory cytokines in the cancer micro-environment, suppressing the progression of cancer (Koelwyn *et al* 2015). These pathways, at least in part, account for the anti-cancer advantages of exercise. Another significant mechanism of action for the beneficial effects of exercise is the modulation of angiogenesis (Kwak *et al* 2018, Avancini *et al* 2019).

6.5 Conclusion

The great majority of people with lung cancer have an advanced disease that is incurable with the available treatment options. As a result, there is a critical need for efficient chemopreventive treatments for lung cancer. A balanced diet is necessary for optimum health and is crucial while unwell. Effective lung cancer treatment depends on giving patients the nutrients they require to operate normally. The existence of a malignant tumor in the body affects the patient's dietary requirements and capacity to consume and absorb nutrients.

Due to the constant activation of the body's immune system and the protracted duration of the illness, food must contain all essential elements in the proper proportions, including carbohydrates, proteins, fats, vitamins, and micro- and macronutrients. Even if it is unlikely to be able to cure the disease, a nutritious diet is a crucial component of the treatment for cancer patients. Its major goal is to stop cancer-related undernutrition and weight loss. Starting at the moment of diagnosis, a balanced diet can strengthen the immune system, lessen the negative effects of radiation therapy, chemotherapy, or immunotherapy, and decrease the risk of perioperative complications. These goods could offer effective options for treating and preventing lung cancer. This research reveals that consuming foods rich in anti-inflammatory and antioxidant substances on a regular basis may reduce the risk of developing lung cancer.

Acknowledgments

The authors thank their respective organizations and the head of the Department to provide the necessary facilities to write a book chapter.

References

Agarwal S and Rao A V 2000 Tomato lycopene and its role in human health and chronic diseases *CMAJ* **163** 739–44

Ajouz H, Garcia A M and Barbul A 2019 Role of β-hydroxy β-methylbutyrate (HMB) in cancer cachexia/sarcopenia *J. Nutr. Oncol.* **4** 1–8

Allin K H, Boisen S E and Nordestgaard B G 2009 Baseline C-reactive protein is associated with incident cancer and survival in patients with cancer *J. Clin. Oncol.* **27** 2217–24

Apopa P L *et al* 2018 PARP1 is up-regulated in non-small cell lung cancer tissues in the presence of the cyanobacterial toxin microcystin *Front. Microbiol.* **9** 1757

Arends J, Bachmann P, Baracos V, Barthelemy N, Bertz H, Bozzetti F, Fearon K, Hütterer E, Isenring E and Kaasa S *et al* 2017 ESPEN guidelines on nutrition in cancer patients *Clin. Nutr.* **36** 11–48

Arif H, Rehmani N, Farhan M, Ahmad A and Hadi S M 2015 Mobilization of copper ions by flavonoids in human peripheral lymphocytes leads to oxidative DNA breakage: a structure activity study *Int. J. Mol. Sci.* **16** 26754–69

Arigony A L V, de Oliviera I M, Machado M, Bordin D L, Bergter L, Prá D and Henriques J A 2013 The influence of micronutrients in cell culture: a reflection on viability and genomic stability *BioMed. Res. Int.* 597282 PMID: 23781504

Avancini A, Pala V, Trestini I, Tregnago D, Mariani L, Sieri S, Krogh V, Boresta M, Milella M and Pilotto S *et al* 2020 Exercise levels and preferences in cancer patients: a cross-sectional study *Int. J. Environ. Res. Public Health* **17** 5351

Avancini A, Sartori G, Gkountakos A, Casali M, Trestini I, Tregnago D, Bria E, Jones L W, Milella M and Lanza M *et al* 2019 Physical activity and exercise in lung cancer care: will promises be fulfilled? *Oncologist* **25** e555–69

Bagan P, Berna P, De Dominicis F, Pereira J C, Mordant P, De La Tour B, Le Pimpec-Barthes F and Riquet M 2013 Nutritional status and postoperative outcome after pneumonectomy for lung cancer *The Ann. Thorac. Surg.* **95** 392–6

Baldrick F R, Elborn J S, Woodside J V, Treacy K, Bradley J M, Patterson C C, Schock B C, Ennis M, Young I S and McKinley M C 2012 Effect of fruit and vegetable intake on oxidative stress and inflammation in COPD: a randomised controlled trial *Eur. Respir. J.* **39** 1377–84

Baracos V E, Reiman T, Mourtzakis M, Gioulbasanis I and Antoun S 2010 Body composition in patients with non-small cell lung cancer: a contemporary view of cancer cachexia with the use of computed tomography image analysis *Am. J. Clin. Nutr.* **91** 1133S–7S

Benameur T, Soleti R, Panaro M A, La Torre M E, Monda V, Messina G and Porro C 2021 Curcumin as prospective anti-aging natural compound: focus on brain *Molecules* **26** 4794

Bradbury K E, Appleby P N and Key T J 2014 Fruit, Vegetable, and fiber intake in relation to cancer risk: findings from the european prospective investigation into cancer and nutrition (EPIC) *Am. J. Clin. Nutr.* **100** 394S–8S

Brennan P, Hsu C C, Moullan N, Szeszenia-Dabrowska N, Lissowska J, Zaridze D, Rudnai P, Fabianova E, Mates D and Bencko V 2005 Effect of cruciferous vegetables on lung cancer in patients stratified by genetic status: a mendelian randomisation approach *Lancet* **366** 1558–60

Büchner F L, Bueno-de-Mesquita H B, Ros M M, Overvad K, Dahm C C, Hansen L, Tjønneland A, Clavel-Chapelon F, Boutron-Ruault M-C and Touillaud M *et al* 2010 Variety in fruit and vegetable consumption and the risk of lung cancer in the european prospective investigation into cancer and nutrition *Cancer Epidemiol. Biomark. Prev. Publ. Am. Assoc. Cancer Res. Cosponsored Am. Soc. Prev. Oncol.* **19** 2278–86

Bunn P A 2012 Worldwide overview of the current status of lung cancer diagnosis and treatment *Arch. Path. Lab. Med.* **136** 1478–81

Cai H, Sobue T, Kitamura T, Ishihara J, Murai U, Sawada N, Iwasaki M, Yamaji T, Inoue M and Tsugane S 2022 Dietary fibre intake is associated with reduced risk of lung cancer: a Japan public health centre-based prospective study (JPHC) *Int. J. Epidemiol.* **51** 1142–52

Cao S Y, Li Y, Meng X, Zhao C N, Li S, Gan R Y and Li H B 2019 Dietary natural products and lung cancer: effects and mechanisms of action *J. Funct. Foods* **52** 316

Cena H and Calder P C 2020 Defining a healthy diet: evidence for the role of contemporary dietary patterns in health and disease *Nutrients* **12** 334

Chabowski M, Polański J, Jankowska-Polańska B, Janczak D and Rosińczuk J 2018 Is nutritional status associated with the level of anxiety, depression and pain in patients with lung cancer? *J. Thorac. Dis.* **10** 2303–10

Chen G, Wang J, Hong X, Chai Z and Li Q 2015 Dietary vitamin E intake could reduce the risk of lung cancer: evidence from a meta-analysis *Int. J. Clin. Exp. Med.* **8** 6631

Cole C L, Kleckner I R, Jatoi A, Schwarz E M and Dunne R F 2018 The role of systemic inflammation in cancer-associated muscle wasting and rationale for exercise as a therapeutic intervention *JCSM Clin. Rep.* **3** e00065

Cooper D A, Eldridge A L and Peters J C 1999 Dietary carotenoids and lung cancer: a review of recent research *Nutr. Rev.* **57** 133–45

Del Rio D, Rodriguez-Mateos A, Spencer J P E, Tognolini M, Borges G and Crozier A 2013 Dietary (poly) phenolics in human health: structures, bioavailability, and evidence of protective effects against chronic diseases *Antioxid. Redox Signal.* **18** 1818–92

Didier A J, Stiene J, Fang L, Watkins D, Dworkin L D and Creeden J F 2023 Antioxidant and anti-tumor effects of dietary vitamins A, C, and E *Antioxidants* **12** 632

Didkowska J, Wojciechowska U, Mańczuk M and Łobaszewski J 2016 Lung cancer epidemiology: contemporary and future challenges worldwide *Ann. Transl. Med.* **4** 50

Domagała-Kulawik J and Osińska I 2014 Immune alterations in lung cancer—the new therapeutic approach *Pneumol. Alergol. Pol.* **82** 286–99

Dunne R F, Loh K P, Williams G R, Jatoi A, Mustian K M and Mohile S G 2019 Cachexia and sarcopenia in older adults with cancer: a comprehensive review *Cancers* **11** 1861

Dymarska E, Grochowalska A and Krauss H 2013 The influence of nutrition on immune system. Immunomodulation by fatty acids, vitamin, minerals and antioxidants *Now Lek.* **82** 222–31

El-Agamey A, Lowe G M, McGarvey D J, Mortensen A, Phillip D M, Truscott T G and Young A J 2004 Carotenoid radical chemistry and antioxidant/pro-oxidant properties *Arch. Biochem. Biophys.* **430** 37–48

Elassal G, Samy H, Said M and Elbatrawy S 2014 Significance of selenium levels in non-small cell lung cancer patients: a comparative study *Egypt. J. Chest Dis.Tuberc* **63** 1019–23
Engelen M P, Safar A M, Bartter T, Koeman F and Deutz N E 2015 High anabolic potential of essential amino acid mixtures in advanced nonsmall cell lung cancer *Ann. Oncol* **26** 1960–6
Fiorelli A, Vicidomini G, Mazzella A, Messina G, Milione R, di Crescenzo V G and Santini MEPITHOR Group 2014 The influence of body mass index and weight loss on outcome of elderly patients undergoing lung cancer resection *Thorac Cardiovasc Surg.* **62** 578–87
Friedenreich C M, Ryder-Burbidge C and McNeil J 2020 Physical activity, obesity and sedentary behavior in cancer etiology: epidemiologic evidence and biologic mechanisms *Mol. Oncol.* **15** 790–800
Ghiselli A, Nardini M, Baldi A and Scaccini C 1998 Antioxidant activity of different phenolic fractions separated from an Italian red wine *J. Agric. Food Chem.* **46** 361–7
Gibson G J, Loddenkemper R, Sibille Y and Lundback B 2013 The European lung white book: respiratory health and disease in Europe *Eur. Respir. J.* **42** 559–63
Gilpin E A and Pierce J P 2002 Demographic differences in patterns in the incidence of smoking cessation: United States 1950–1990 *Ann. Epidemiol.* **12** 141–50
Godos J, Sinatra D, Blanco I, Mulè S, La Verde M and Marranzano M 2017 Association between dietary phenolic acids and hypertension in a mediterranean cohort *Nutrients* **9** 1069
Gonzalez M J, Miranda-Massari J R, Mora E M, Guzmán A, Riordan N H, Riordan H D, Casciari J J, Jackson J A and Román-Franco A 2005 Orthomolecular oncology review: ascorbic acid and cancer 25 years later *Integr. Cancer Ther.* **4** 32–44
Goodman G E, Schaffer S, Omenn G S, Chen C and King I 2003 The association between lung and prostate cancer risk, and serum micronutrients: results and lessons learned from beta-carotene and retinol efficacy trial *Cancer Epidemiol. Biomarkers Prev.* **12** 518–26
Gu Z, Shan K, Chen H and Chen Y Q 2015 N-3 polyunsaturated fatty acids and their role in cancer chemoprevention *Curr. Pharmacol. Rep.* **1** 283–94
Gupta D and Lis C G 2010 Pretreatment serum albumin as a predictor of cancer survival: a systematic review of the epidemiological literature *Nutr. J.* **9** 69
Hajibabaei K 2016 Antioxidant properties of vitamin E *Ann. Res. Antioxid* **1** e22
Hardee J P, Counts B R and Carson J A 2019 Understanding the role of exercise in cancer cachexia therapy *Am. J. Lifestyle Med.* **13** 46–60
Hochstein P and Atallah A S 1988 The nature of oxidants and antioxidant systems in the inhibition of mutation and cancer *Mutat. Res.* **202** 363–75
Hoffman A J, Brintnall R A, von Eye A, Jones L W, Alderink G, Patzelt L H and Brown J K 2014 Home-based exercise: promising rehabilitation for symptom relief, improved functional status and quality of life for post-surgical lung cancer patients *J. Thorac. Dis.* **6** 632–40
Jagoe R T, Goodship T H and Gibson G J 2001 The influence of nutritional status on complications after operations for lung cancer *Ann. Thorac. Surg.* **71** 936–43
Jung Y S, Park J H, Park D I, Sohn C I, Lee J M and Kim T I 2020 Impact of smoking on human natural killer cell activity: a large cohort study *J. Cancer Prev.* **25** 13–20
Kang J H, Shi Y M and Zheng R L 1999 Effects of ascorbic acid on human hepatoma cell proliferation and redifferentiation *Zhongguo Yao Li Xue Bao* **20** 1019–24
Kaulmann A and Bohn T 2014 Carotenoids, inflammation, and oxidative stress-implications of cellular signaling pathways and relation to chronic disease prevention *Nutr. Res.* **34** 907–29

Kaya S O, Akcam T I, Ceylan K C, Samancılar O, Ozturk O and Usluer O 2016 Is preoperative protein-rich nutrition effective on postoperative outcome in non-small cell lung cancer surgery? A prospective randomized study *J. Cardiothorac. Surg.* **11** 14

Keck A S and Finley J W 2004 Cruciferous vegetables: cancer protective mechanisms of glucosinolate hydrolysis products and selenium *Integr. Cancer Ther.* **3** 5–12

Keely S, Talley N J and Hansbro P M 2012 Pulmonary-intestinal cross-talk in mucosal inflammatory disease *Mucosal Immunol.* **5** 7–18

Kim J A, Jang J H and Lee S Y 2021 An updated comprehensive review on vitamin A and carotenoids in breast cancer: mechanisms, genetics, assessment, current evidence, and future clinical implications *Nutrients* **13** 3162

Kiss N and Curtis A 2022 Current insights in nutrition assessment and intervention for malnutrition or muscle loss in people with lung cancer: a narrative review *Adv. Nutr.* **13** 2420–32

Kłęk S, Jankowski M, Kruszewski W J, Fijuth J, Kapała A, Kabata P, Wysocki P, Krzakowski M and Rutkowski P 2015 Clinical nutrition in oncology: Polish recommendations *Oncol. Clin. Prakt.* **11** 172–88

Kocdor H, Ates H, Aydin S, Cehreli R, Soyarat F, Kemanli P, Harmanci D, Cengiz H and Kocdor M A 2015 Zinc supplementation induces apoptosis and enhances antitumor efficacy of docetaxel in non-small-cell lung cancer *Drug Des. Devel. Ther.* **9** 3899

Koelwyn G J, Wennerberg E, Demaria S and Jones L W 2015 Exercise in regulation of inflammation-immune axis function in cancer initiation and progression *Oncology* **29** 908–20, 922

Krzysik M, Biernat H and Grajeta H 2007 The influence of chosen nutrients on immune system functioning. Part II. Immunomodulatory effects of vitamins and trace elements on the human body *Adv Clin Exp Med.* **1** 123–33

Kwak S-E, Lee J-H, Zhang D and Song W 2018 Angiogenesis: focusing on the effects of exercise in aging and cancer *J. Exerc. Nutr. Biochem.* **22** 21–6

Lee J Y, Chang M Y, Park C H, Kim H Y, Kim J H, Son H, Lee Y S and Lee S H 2003 Ascorbate-induced differentiation of embryonic cortical precursors into neurons and astrocytes *J. Neurosci. Res.* **73** 156–65

Leedo E, Gade J, Granov S, Mellemgaard A, Klausen T W, Rask K and Astrup A 2017 The effect of a home delivery meal service of energy- and protein-rich meals on quality of life in malnourished outpatients suffering from lung cancer: a randomized controlled trial *Nutr. Cancer* **69** 444–53

Liu H X, Tao L L, Zhang J, Zhu Y G, Zheng Y, Liu D, Zhou M, Ke H, Shi M M and Qu J M 2018 Difference of lower airway microbiome in bilateral protected specimen brush between lung cancer patients with unilateral lobar masses and control subjects *Int. J. Cancer* **142** 769–78

Liu X *et al* 2021 The role of gut microbiota in lung cancer: from carcinogenesis to immunotherapy *Front. Oncol.* **11** 720842

Liu Y *et al* 2018 Lung tissue microbial profile in lung cancer is distinct from emphysema *Am. J. Cancer Res.* **8** 1775

Löfling L, Bahmanyar S, Kieler H, Lambe M and Wagenius G 2021 Temporal trends in lung cancer survival: a population-based study *Acta Oncol.* **61** 625–31

Luo J, Shen L and Zheng D 2014 Association between vitamin C intake and lung cancer: a dose-response meta-analysis *Sci. Rep.* **4** 6161

Luo M, Zhou L, Huang Z, Li B, Nice E C, Xu J and Huang C 2022 Antioxidant therapy in cancer: rationale and progress *Antioxidants* **11** 1128

Luo G, Xie Z Z, Liu F Y and Zhang G B 1998 Effects of vitamin C on myocardial mitochondrial function and ATP content in hypoxic rats *Zhongguo Yao Li Xue Bao* **19** 351–5

Luu H N, Cai H, Murff H J, Xiang Y-B, Cai Q, Li H, Gao J, Yang G, Lan Q and Gao Y-T *et al* 2018 A prospective study of dietary polyunsaturated fatty acids intake and lung cancer risk *Int. J. Cancer* **143** 2225–37

Marchiani A, Rozzo C, Fadda A, Delogu G and Ruzza P 2014 Curcuminandcurcumin-likemolecules: fromspice to drugs *Curr. Med. Chem.* **21** 204–22

Marino P, Pepe G, Basilicata M G, Vestuto V, Marzocco S, Autore G, Procino A, Gomez-Monterrey I M, Manfra M and Campiglia P 2023 Potential role of natural antioxidant products in oncological diseases *Antioxidants* **12** 704

Marmot M 2018 Diet, cancer, and NCD prevention *Lancet Oncol.* **19** 863–4

Meital L T, Windsor M T, Perissiou M, Schulze K, Magee R, Kuballa A, Golledge J, Bailey T G, Askew C D and Russell F D 2019 Omega-3 fatty acids decrease oxidative stress and inflammation in macrophages from patients with small abdominal aortic aneurysm *Sci. Rep.* **9** 12978

Menon V P and Sudheer A R 2007 Antioxidant and anti-inflammatory properties of curcumin *Adv. Exp. Med. Biol.* **595** 105–25

Moyad M A 2001 Results and lessons from clinical trials using dietary supplements for cancer: direct and indirect investigations *Semin. Urol. Oncol.* **19** 232–46

Muka T, Kraja B, Ruiter R, Lahousse L, De Keyser C E, Hofman A, Franco O H, Brusselle G and Stricker B H 2017 Dietary mineral intake and lung cancer risk: the Rotterdam Study *Eur. J. Nutr.* **56** 1637–46

Muller A G, Sarker S D, Saleem I Y and Hutcheon G A 2019 Delivery of natural phenolic compounds for the potential treatment of lung cancer *DARU J. Pharm. Sci.* **27** 433–49

Nani A, Belarbi M, Ksouri-Megdiche W, Abdoul-Azize S, Benammar C, Ghiringhelli F, Hichami A and Khan N A 2015 Effects of polyphenols and lipids from *Pennisetum glaucum* grains on T-cell activation: modulation of Ca^{2+} and ERK1/ERK2 signaling *BMC Complement. Altern. Med.* **15** 426

Nasrah R, Van Der Borch C, Kanbalian M and Jagoe R T 2020 Defining barriers to implementation of nutritional advice in patients with cachexia *J. Cachexia. Sarcopenia Muscle* **11** 69–78

Nath R, Das C, Kityania S, Nath D, Das S, Choudhury M D, Patra J K and Talukdar A D 2023 Natural flavonoids in the prevention and treatment of lung cancer: a pharmacological aspect *Comb. Chem. High Throughput Screen* **26** 863–79

Nigro E, Perrotta F, Scialò F, D'Agnano V, Mallardo M, Bianco A and Daniele A 2021 Food, nutrition, physical activity and microbiota: which impact on lung cancer? *Int. J. Environ. Res. Public Health* **18** 2399

Norton R and O'Connell M A 2012 Vitamin D: potential in the prevention and treatment of lung cancer *Anticancer Res.* **32** 211–21

Oppedisano F, Macrì R, Gliozzi M, Musolino V, Carresi C, Maiuolo J, Bosco F, Nucera S, Caterina Zito M and Guarnieri L *et al* 2020 The anti-inflammatory and antioxidant properties of n–3 PUFAs: their role in cardiovascular protection *Biomedicines* **8** 306

Panaro M A, Corrado A, Benameur T, Paolo C F, Cici D and Porro C 2020 The emerging role of curcumin in the modulation of TLR-4 signaling pathway: focus on neuroprotective and anti-rheumatic properties *Int. J. Mol. Sci.* **21** 2299
Pandey K B and Rizvi S I 2009 Plant polyphenols as dietary antioxidants in human health and disease *Oxid. Med. Cell Longev.* **2** 270–8
Pappalardo G, Almeida A and Ravasco P 2015 Eicosapentaenoic acid in cancer improves body composition and modulates metabolism *Nutrition* **31** 549–55
Pizzo F, Maroccia Z, Hammarberg Ferri I and Fiorentini C 2022 Role of the Microbiota in lung cancer: insights on prevention and treatment *Int. J. Mol. Sci.* **23** 6138
Polański J, wiątoniowska-Lonc N, Kołaczyńska S and Chabowski M 2023 Diet as a factor supporting lung cancer treatment—a systematic review *Nutrients* **15** 1477
Porro C *et al* 2022 The potential role of nutrition in lung cancer establishment and progression *Life* **12** 270
Porro C, Cianciulli A, Trotta T, Lofrumento D D and Panaro M A 2019 Curcumin regulates anti-inflammatory responses by JAK/STAT/SOCS signaling pathway in BV-2 microglial cells *Biology* **8** 51
Posthauer M E 2006 The role of nutrition in wound care *Adv. Skin Wound Care* **19** 43–52 PMID: 16477165
Prado C M, Lieffers J R, McCargar L J, Reiman T, Sawyer M B, Martin L and Baracos V E 2008 Prevalence and clinical implications of sarcopenic obesity in patients with solid tumours of the respiratory and gastrointestinal tracts: a population-based study *Lancet Oncol.* **9** 629–35
Prado C M, Cushen S J, Orsso C E and Ryan A M 2016 Sarcopenia and cachexia in the era of obesity: clinical and nutritional impact *Proc. Nutr. Soc.* **75** 188–98
Prasad K N 2003 Antioxidants in cancer care: when and how to use them as an adjunct to standard and experimental therapies *Expert Rev. Anticancer Ther.* **3** 903–15
Ramírez-Labrada A G, Isla D, Artal A, Arias M, Rezusta A, Pardo J and Gálvez E M 2020 The influence of lung microbiota on lung carcinogenesis, immunity, and immunotherapy *Trends Cancer* **6** 86–97
Rao A V and Rao L G 2007 Carotenoids and human health *Pharmacol. Res.* **55** 207–16
Ravasco P, Lavriv D and Neves P 2018 Should omega-3 be used in cancer cachexia? *Clin. Nutr. ESPEN* **25** 18–25
Rayburn E R, Ezell S J and Zhang R 2009 Anti-inflammatory agents for cancer therapy *Mol. Cell. Pharm.* **1** 29
Riordan H D, Hunninghake R B, Riordan N H, Jackson J J, Meng X, Taylor P, Casciari J J, González M J, Miranda-Massari J R and Mora E M *et al* 2003 Intravenous ascorbic acid: protocol for its application and use *Health Sci. J.* **22** 287–90
Romagnolo D F and Selmin O I 2012 Flavonoids and cancer prevention: a review of the evidence *J. Nutr. Gerontol. Geriatr* **31** 206–38
Russo A, Acquaviva R, Campisi A, Sorrenti V, Giacomo C D, Virgata G, Barcellona M L and Vanella A 2000 Bioflavonoids as antiradicals, antioxidants and DNA cleavage protectors *Cell Biol. Toxicol.* **16** 91–8
Rutz J K, Borges C D, Zambiazi R C, da Rosa C G and da Silva M M 2016 Elaboration of microparticles of carotenoids from natural and synthetic sources for applications in food *Food Chem.* **202** 324–33
Sanchez-Lara K, Turcott J G, Juarez E, Guevara P, Núñez-Valencia C, Oñate-Ocaña L F, Flores D and Arrieta O 2012 Association of nutrition parameters including bioelectrical impedance

and systemic inflammatory response with quality of life and prognosis in patients with advanced non-small-cell lung cancer: a prospective study *Nutr. Cancer* **64** 526–34

Schlemmer M, Suchner U, Schäpers B, Duerr E M, Alteheld B, Zwingers T, Stehle P and Zimmer H G 2015 Is glutamine eficiency the link between inflammation, malnutrition, and fatigue in cancer patients? *Clin. Nutr.* **34** 1258–65

Sharma A, Viswanath B and Park Y S 2018 Role of probiotics in the management of lung cancer and related diseases: an update *J. Funct. Foods* **40** 625–33

Shivappa N, Wang R, Hébert J R, Jin A, Koh W-P and Yuan J M 2019 Association between inflammatory potential of diet and risk of lung cancer among smokers in a prospective study in Singapore *Eur. J. Nutr.* **58** 2755–66

Shu X-O, Li H, Yang G, Gao J, Cai H, Takata Y, Zheng W and Xiang Y-B 2015 Cohort profile: the shanghai men's health study *Int. J. Epidemiol.* **44** 810–8

Smolle E and Pichler M 2018 Non-smoking-associated lung cancer: a distinct entity in terms of tumor biology, patient characteristics and impact of hereditary cancer predisposition *Cancers* **11** 204

Stahl W and Sies H 2005 Bioactivity and protective effects of natural carotenoids *Biochim. Biophys. Acta.* **1740** 101–7

Sun Y, Li Z, Li J, Li Z and Han J 2016 A healthy dietary pattern reduces lung cancer risk: a systematic review and meta-analysis *Nutrients* **8** 134

Tanaka N, Takeda K, Kawasaki Y, Yamane K, Teruya Y, Kodani M, Igishi T and Yamasaki A 2018 Early intensive nutrition intervention with dietary counseling and oral nutrition supplement prevents weight loss in patients with advanced lung cancer receiving chemotherapy: a clinical prospective study *Yonago Acta Med.* **61** 204–12

Tardon A, Lee W J, Delgado-Rodriguez M, Dosemeci M, Albanes D, Hoover R and Blair A 2005 Leisure-time physical activity and lung cancer: a meta-analysis *Cancer Causes Control* **16** 389–97

Thomas P A, Berbis J, Falcoz P E, Le Pimpec-Barthes F, Bernard A, Jougon J, Porte H, Alifano M and Dahan MEPITHOR Group 2014 National perioperative outcomes of pulmonary lobectomy for cancer: the influence of nutritional status *Eur. J. Cardiothorac. Surg.* **45** 652–19

Thun M J *et al* 2008 Lung cancer occurrence in never-smokers: an analysis of 13 cohorts and 22 cancer registry studies *PLoS Med.* **5** e185

Thune I and Lund E 1997 The influence of physical activity on lung-cancer risk: a prospective study of 81,516 men and women *Int. J. Cancer* **70** 57–62

Tong L, Spitz M R, Fueger J J and Amos C A 1996 Lung carcinoma in former smokers *Cancer* **78** 1004–10 PubMed: 8780538

Turati F, Rossi M, Pelucchi C, Levi F and La Vecchia C 2015 Fruit and vegetables and cancer risk: a review of southern European studies *Br. J. Nutr.* **113** 102–10

Varghese R, Efferth T and Ramamoorthy S 2023 Carotenoids for lung cancer chemoprevention and chemotherapy: promises and controversies *Phytomedicine* **116** 154850

Villagran M, Ferreira J, Martorell M and Mardones L 2021 The role of vitamin C in cancer prevention and therapy: a literature review *Antioxidants* **10** 1894

Wang C, Yang T, Guo X and Li D 2019 The associations of fruit and vegetable intake with lung cancer risk in participants with different smoking status: a meta-analysis of prospective cohort studies *Nutrients* **11** 1791

Wang J, Yang H-R, Wang D-J and Wang X-X 2020 Association between the gut microbiota and patient responses to cancer immune checkpoint inhibitors *Oncol. Lett.* **20** 342

Westheim A J, Stoffels L M, Dubois L J, Van Bergenhenegouwen J, Van Helvoort A, Langen R C, Shiri-Sverdlov R and Theys J 2022 Fatty acids as a tool to boost cancer immunotherapy efficacy *Front. Nutr.* **9** 1168

WHO 2020 *Fact Sheets-Cancer* 19th August 2020 (https://who.int/news-room/fact-sheets/detail/cancer)

Xara S, Amaral T F and Parente B 2011 Undernutrition and quality of life in non-small-cell lung cancer patients *Rev. Port. Pneumol.* **17** 153–8

Xu X, Wei W, Xu J, Huang J, Li L, Han T, Qi J, Sun C, Li Y and Jiang W 2021 The association of minerals intake in three meals with cancer and all-cause mortality: the US National Health and Nutrition Examination Survey, 2003–2014 *BMC Cancer* **21** 1–4

Yang C S, Luo P, Zeng Z, Wang H, Malafa M and Suh N 2020 Vitamin E and cancer prevention: studies with different forms of tocopherols and tocotrienols *Mol. Carcinog* **59** 365–89

Yang P 2009 Epidemiology of lung cancer prognosis: quantity and quality of life *Methods Mol. Biol.* **471** 469–86

Yang M, Liu L, Gan C-E, Qiu L-H, Jiang X-J, He X-T and Zhang J-E 2020 Effects of home-based exercise on exercise capacity, symptoms, and quality of life in patients with lung cancer: a meta-analysis *Eur. J. Oncol. Nurs. Off. J. Eur. Oncol. Nurs. Soc.* **49** 101836

Yang Q, Liang Q, Balakrishnan B, Belobrajdic D P, Feng Q-J and Zhang W 2020 Role of dietary nutrients in the modulation of gut microbiota: a narrative review *Nutrients* **12** 381

Yu N, Su X, Wang Z, Dai B and Kang J 2015 Association of dietary vitamin A and β-carotene intake with the risk of lung cancer: a meta-analysis of 19 publications *Nutrients* **7** 9309–24

Zagrodzki P 2004 Selenium and the immune system *Postępy Hig. Med. Dośw.* **58** 140–9

Zheng W, Chow W-H, Yang G, Jin F, Rothman N, Blair A, Li H-L, Wen W, Ji B-T and Li Q *et al* 2005 Thc Shanghai womcn's health study: rationale, study design, and baseline characteristics *Am. J. Epidemiol.* **162** 1123–31

Chapter 7

Plant flavonoids and cancer chemoprevention: their role in epigenetic regulations

Neha Sharma, Pallavi Singh Chauhan and Rajesh Singh Tomar

DNA methylation, histone modification, and RNA non-coding regulation are examples of epigenetics. Epigenetics is a physiological regulatory modification that affects gene expression without altering the DNA sequence. Dysregulation of normal epigenetic processes can result in abnormal gene expression, as has been demonstrated in many disorders, including cancer. Recent discoveries in histone modification, non-coding RNA processes and DNA methylation involved in gene expression patterns in tumor cells have led to a paradigm shift in cancer diagnosis and treatment. The search for chemicals that can modify the altered epigenetic landscape of tumor cells and take advantage of therapeutic capability for malignant tumors is accelerating. Flavonoids are naturally occurring phenolic molecules found in a variety of phytochemicals that can affect epigenetic processes. The development of epigenetic drugs and the combined treatment of malignant tumors requires accurate knowledge of flavonoid-mediated epigenetic changes. The reversible nature of epigenetic alterations implicates the mechanisms involved in cancer prevention, with the fact that epigenetic problems are considered to be a symptom of cell carcinogenesis and malignant events that affect tumor progression and drug resistance. Clinicians consider that it can be an important target for treatment. Epidemiological and preclinical studies, on the other hand, show that the epigenome is constantly being reprogrammed by natural organic chemicals and the environment, indicating that natural substances can be used to influence epigenetics in cancer treatment. Flavonoids in herbs, vegetables, fruit and tea are not produced by the human body, but can be taken on a regular basis. The epigenetic anti-cancer effects of flavonoids need further investigation due to their natural and food source origin, no side effects, and their extraordinary biological activity. On the other hand, epidemiological and preclinical studies have shown that the epigenome is constantly being reprogrammed by natural organic chemicals and the environment, indicating that natural substances can be used to influence epigenetics in cancer treatment.

doi:10.1088/978-0-7503-5252-9ch7

7.1 Introduction

An epigenetics change occurs in cells during early differentiation stages and is steadily inherited without changes in nucleotide sequences. They are often referred to as physical level changes in gene expression [1, 2]. Epigenetic modifications are necessary for the healthy development of cells, but when they are deregulated they can cause numerous diseases, such as cancer. The control of gene expression through epigenetics is exhibited through broadly three routes, i.e., DNA methylation (chromatin remodeling), effect of non-coding RNAs and histone modifications [3] (figure 7.1).

It has been reported that in 2020 only approximately 19.3 million new cancer cases were reported globally that caused nearly 10 million deaths; a decline in cancer

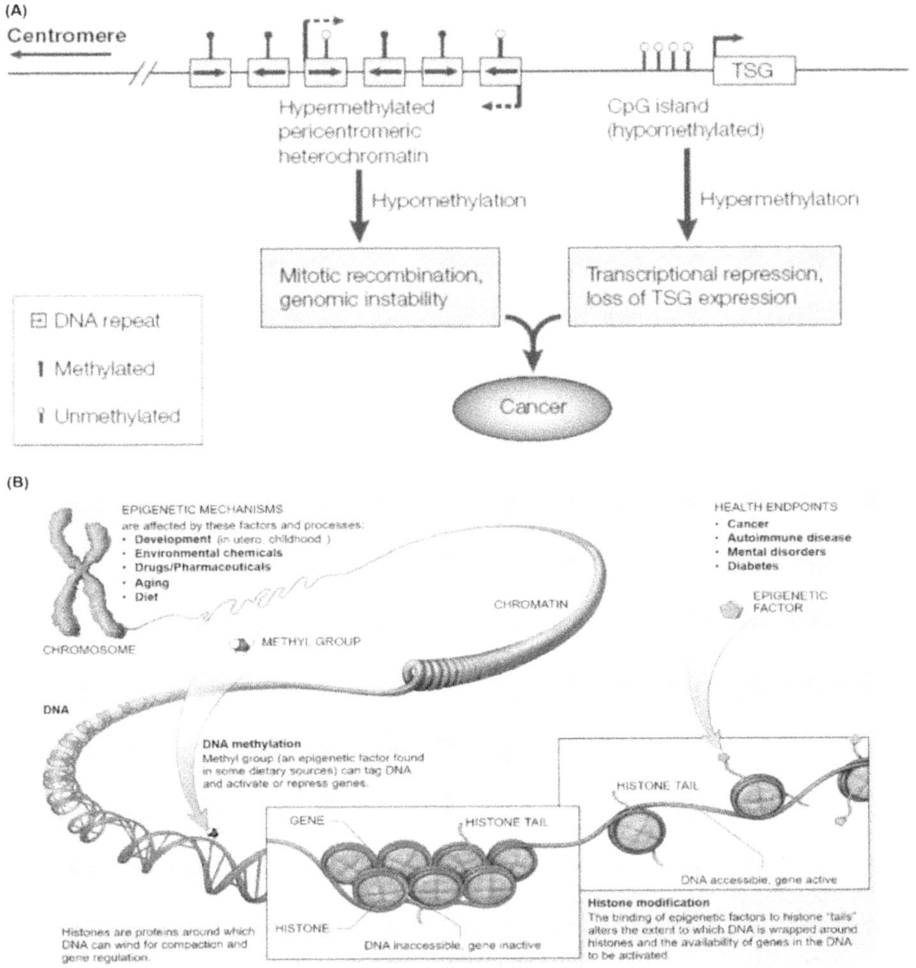

Figure 7.1. DNA methylation and its role in transcriptional inactivation and cancer (A) and histone modification (B). Reproduced from [4], copyright (2020) CC BY 4.0.

associated deaths has been observed since 1991 and was reducing by 31% to 2018 [5]. The multistage process of carcinogenesis includes a series of events, such as epigenetic and genetic changes, that initiate, promote, and progress cancer. Chemoprevention is a method to use safe natural substances, synthetic chemicals, or their mixtures to combat the progression of multistage carcinogenesis. In recent years, chemoprevention has been possible through diet modification, which includes addition of more plant-based food in the diet. This strategy has been recognized as one of the most effective and potentially cost-effective methods to decrease the risk of cancer [6]. Cancer treatments generally involve multiple therapy and approaches including use of chemotherapeutic agents, radiotherapy, immunotherapy etc, which have shown a lot of promise in cancer treatment [7]. In recent years, application of epigenetic modulators has been used to treat aberrant epigenetic modifications in cancer cells, and some other approaches such as chimeric antigen receptor-engineered T cells (CAR-T cells) have also been confirmed as a very effectual strategy in handling malignancies of B-cells [8].

The contemporary methods of cancer treatment using radiation and chemotherapeutic agents have vast side effects on patients; therefore, there is a pressing requirement to explore alternative medicines with no or minimal side effects. Phytochemicals are considered as most appropriate and most suitable in this standard, and could be a potential agent for exploring anti-cancer properties for their effective use as a potential anti-cancer drug. Anti-carcinogenic components in plant-based foodstuffs are known to prevent cancer through several methods, including antioxidant and immunomodulatory actions. It is interesting to note that phytochemicals have been shown to influence epigenetic processes via DNA methyltransferases (DNMTs) and histone deacetylases (HDACs) [9]. The key class of phytochemicals known as flavonoids play a role in modulating the cancer-related gene expression pattern [10]. Flavonoids are naturally occurring polyphenols that are present in a wide variety of plant-based foods, including vegetables, tea, fruit, and most medicinal plants [6]. This chapter focuses on the role of plant flavonoids epigenetic regulations and various strategies and processes of cancer treatments.

7.2 Epigenetics of cancer

Although every cell in the body has the same set of genes, how the genome is read and manifests itself during various embryonic stages, cellular differentiation, and lineage commitment in adult tissues is controlled by epigenetic information. To influence the function and level of gene expression without altering the nucleotide sequence, epigenetic information is stored as covalent modifications of chromatin factors, which change the original chromatin environment, affect DNA accessibility, and provide docking/recognition sites for regulatory proteins. Epigenetic changes are comparatively meiotically and/or mitotically inheritable, letting gene trait work be inherited by the next generation to maintain cellular identity and lineage fidelity [11].

Epigenetic mechanisms are necessary for natural development and preservation of tissue-exact gene expression patterns in mammals. Malignant cellular transformation and altered gene function can result from epigenetic mechanisms being disrupted. Universal transformations in the epigenetic geography are an authentication of cancer [12]. The metamorphosis of normal cells into cancer cells involves epigenetic differences and in most of the cases it is preceded by inheritable mutations [13]. Among the key methods involved in epigenetic regulation are association with histone variations, nucleosome positioning, DNA variations and non-coding RNAs. These processes have a major impact on cellular homeostasis [14] (table 7.1).

7.3 Epigenetics modulators: Flavonoids

7.3.1 Dietary flavonoids

Traditional knowledge and scientific evidence suggest that medicinal plants are rich in physiologically active compounds that can be used for treating a range of ailments, including cancer [15]. In the 1940s, nitrogen mustards and folic acid antagonists were used in the first effort to create chemotherapeutic medicine. Flavonoid research has made great strides in the discovery of anti-cancer drugs capable of killing cancer cells by inducing apoptosis [16]. Plants are an inexhaustible source of phytochemicals, or phytochemicals, that are increasingly being used to fight cancer. For example, structural complexity, lack of significant side effects, affordability, chemical diversity, and unique biological activity make plant polyphenols attractive candidates for new therapies [17]. Flavonoids have limited bioavailability and depend on esterification, subclass, molecular weight, glycosylation, and structure [18]. For example, when humans ingest the food flavonoid quercetin (250–500 mg), a dose of 1% is obtained, eventually entering the circulatory system and plasma concentrations peak in the low nanomolar range (20 nM) [19]. Flavonoids are often converted by Phase II and hydrolases in the liver, colon and small intestine to conjugated metabolites such as o-glucuronides, sulfates, and o-methyl esters. After being metabolized by either intestinal-level de-glycosylation processes or carrier transport, quercetin glycosides have been shown to be better absorbed than equivalent aglycones and higher plasma concentrations are observed [20]. In normal cells, these low levels of flavonoids should not interfere with the cell cycle process. Several substances, including 3-hydroxyflavon, luteolin, and apigenin, cause significant cytotoxicity and increase ROS production at high doses [21]. They can even cause cell destruction by inducing the cell death system of healthy cells [22] (figure 7.2).

7.3.2 Hormetic effects of dietary flavonoids

If you are considering phytochemicals as a dietary enhancement for the restraint or management of cancer, however, there are several flavonoids and polyphenols that exhibit hormesis properties and can be sufficiently dangerous. Hormesis is a biphasic dose–response phenomenon characterized by stimulating effect of a low-dose compound on a biotic procedure or phenotype but exhibits adverse effect of a high-dose on a biological process or phenotype [83]. U-shaped biphasic response

Table 7.1. List of epigenetic changes [12].

S. No.	Types of epigenetic changes	Mechanism	Role and regulations	Additional information
1	**DNA methylation**			
	DNA methylation especially in CpG dinucleotides. CpG islands are preferentially located at the 5′ end of genes and occupy ~60% of human gene promoters	CpG dinucleotide cytosine residues undergo covalent modification	Regulation of gene expression and chromatin architecture	Inheritably gene silencing and non-coding genomic regions
2	**Histone modification**			
	Histone proteins in nucleosome core	Histone proteins N-terminal tails undergoes a type of posttranslational covalent changes including ubiquitylation, methylation, acetylation, and phosphorylation on particular residues	Regulate essential biological functions like replication, repair, and transcription	Various kinds of cells exhibit specific patterns of histone modifications, which are considered to be essential for determining cellular identity
3	**Nucleosome positioning**			
	Nucleosome-free regions (NFRs) present at the 5′ and 3′ ends of genes are thought to provide the sites for assembly and disassembly of the transcription machinery	Non-covalent nucleosome remodeling and replacement of canonical histone proteins with specialized histone variants	Play an important role in chromatin structure and gene regulatory functions	Loss of a nucleosome directly upstream of the transcription start site is tightly correlated with gene activation
4	**Non-coding RNAs**			
	miRNAs are small, ~22 nt or non-coding RNAs expressed in a tissue-specific manner	Target messenger RNA is degraded or its translation inhibited as a result of sequence-specific base pairing between miRNAs and the 3′ untranslated sections of the target messenger RNA in the RNA-induced silencing complex	Control cell proliferation, apoptosis and differentiation	miRNAs can modulate epigenetic regulatory mechanisms inside the cell by targeting enzymes responsible for DNA methylation and histone modifications

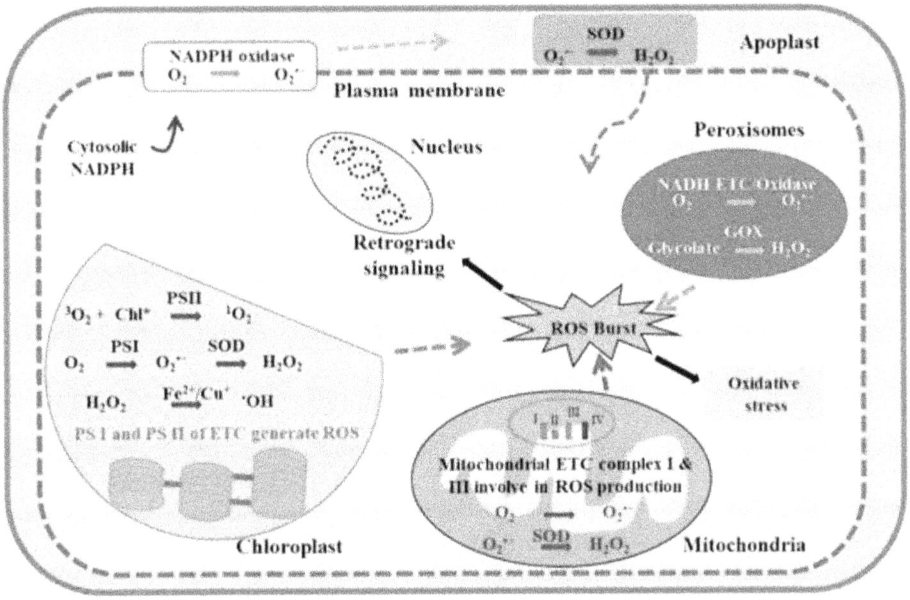

Figure 7.2. Abiotic stresses induced the production of ROS in different plant cell organelles which either initiate signaling (retrograde) or cause oxidative stress [23]. Figure reprinted with permission from Dr Mohammad Israil Ansari.

results from the benefits of adaptation to mild magnitude of the cellular stress level. However, increased stressor intensity (e.g., increased level of dietary flavonoids), the reaction is no longer compensating for the stressor, leading to adverse effects, and the treatment is harmful [24].

To explain this concept for instance resveratrol improves heart health by improving ventricular recovery after ischemia and encouraging the expression of survival-promoting and anti-apoptotic proteins that may reduce after a heart attack. On the other hand, high doses of resveratrol promote cardiomyocyte apoptosis and increase infarct size [25].

In the context of cancer development and progression, resveratrol exhibits some distinct properties like stimulating tumor growth of different histological origins and stages at low doses, but promotes apoptosis of cancer cells at high doses. Among the flavonoids and polyphenols in the diet, resveratrol is not as a rule but an exception, and some others such as genistein, apigenin, luteolin, and kaempferol all show hormonal effects and promote the development of cancer at low doses [26]. Administer cans, which have been shown to inhibit tumor growth at high doses. Similarly, the cancer-preventing effect of quercetin is dose-dependent, with low doses acting primarily as antioxidants and high concentrations acting as antioxidants that may increase chromosomal instability [27].

In addition, the cumulative or synergistic effects of many dietary flavonoids or polyphenols at very low concentrations are not expected to have harmful or toxic effects on the biological system. However, hormesis effects can be detrimental to people taking supplements and therefore should not be undermined. There are also potential confounders in clinical trials where patients are taking over-the-counter dietary supplements that modify drug clearance, and cellular responses. Organic is not always secure in all dosages and combinations. Therefore, more research is needed on the dose-related chemoprophylaxis effects of flavonoids.

7.3.3 Damage of cellular DNA

Flavonoids have been shown to provide health advantages in humans and animals in studies conducted over a decade in cell cultures, animals, and human populations. They may be used to fight a variety of diseases, including cancer, because they are abundantly found in our food, such as fruit, vegetables, teas, and wine, all of which have powerful antioxidative, estrogenic regulating, and antibacterial properties. Apoptotic, angiogenesis, invasion processes, cell cycle arrest and metastasis are all possible inhibitors of cancer growth [28].

Apigenin is a flavone discovered in a variety of pharmaceutical plants and vegetables, with *Petroselinum crispum* L and *Lycopodium clavatum* L. (club moss) [29]. (Parsley) and *Apium graveolens* L. (celery) have been shown to protect against UVB-induced inflammatory diseases and DNA damage. Apigenin has antiproliferative properties that result in cell cycle arrest and death in cancer models, according to recent *in vitro* and *in vivo* studies. Apigenin has been shown to protect DNA from UVB-induced ROS and DNA damage in skin cells and mice by eliminating the cyclobutane ring, inhibiting ROS production, and down-regulating NFB [30–33]. Biologically active compounds like apigenin [32], catechins [34] etc showed potent ROS capture capacity in human cancer cells and showed G1 cell cycle arrest through the regulation of CDK2 kinase. A population experiment of ovarian cancer patients has shown that apigenin reduces flavonoid development and DNA damage [33] in ovarian tumours. Oxidative damage is the major cause of radiation-induced skin injury (RISI) which is commonly seen in cancer patients [35, 36]. It was also reported that curcumin and selenium L-methionine compounds protect against RISI. [37]

Apigenin showed potent ROS capture capacity in human bladder cancer T24 cells and diploid fibroblasts and showed G1 cell cycle arrest through the regulation of CDK2 kinase. A population experiment of ovarian cancer patients has shown that apigenin reduces flavonoid development and DNA damage in ovarian tumors. Apigenin can protect endothelial cells from inflammation caused by lipopolysaccharide (LPS). Apigenin inhibits the formation of reactive oxygen species (ROS) and the expression of caspase 3, thereby preventing DNA damage [38–40]. Apigenin causes DNA damage/apoptosis in cancer cells by activating the phosphorylation of ATM and H2AX and down-regulating the cell cycle and DNA repair genes. In malignant glioma cells, apigenin has also been shown to reduce DNA damage by cell proliferation regulators, inhibiting casein kinase 2, NFB activators and DNA damage mediators [41].

In many cancer models, the antioxidant flavan-3ol epigallocatechin gallate (EGCG) activates repair mechanisms and stops DNA damage. The most prevalent catechin and well-known antioxidant in green tea, EGCG, is a free radical scavenger [42]. After irradiation with an x-ray linear accelerator and overexpressing heme oxygenase 1, EGCG was found to protect skin cells (HO1). In these HaCaT keratinocytes, EGCG reduces phosphorylation of H2AX lesions [43]. In human peripheral blood samples collected from adult volunteers before and after ingesting 540 ml of green tea, EGCG provided protection against UVR-induced DNA damage [44]. In addition, EGCG has been shown to exert radioregulatory effects on the plasmid DNA of the pBR322 plasmid and the DNA of mouse splenocytes when exposed to gamma rays [45]. In PC12 rat pheochromocytoma cells, luteolin, a flavone found in salviatomentosamil (balsam sage) and many other plants, prevents oxidative stress generated SSB [46]. Luteolin showed apoptotic properties in CH27 cells of human squamous cell carcinoma of the lung, and was found to have increased 'S' phase cell cycle arrest and DNA damage [47]. In many cancer cells, luteolin stimulates the endogenous apoptotic pathway by causing DNA damage and p53. luteolin promotes apoptosis of breast cancer cells and prostate by blocking fatty acid synthase, mainly, enzymes that are lipid-producing and overexpressed in numerous human malignancies [48]. There is chemoprophylaxis activity and related mechanisms of luteolin in the neoplastic mouse cell line JB6P + and the hairless SKH1 mouse model. Luteolin has been shown to inhibit or block the growth of cancer cells *in vitro* and *in vivo*, protect DNA from carcinogenic stimuli, and induce cell cycle arrest and death through internal and external signaling pathways [49]. In addition, luteolin produces ROS, initiates DNA damage, activates ATR/Chk2/p53 signaling, inhibits NFkB signaling, activates p38, and depletes anti-apoptotic proteins [50]. This causes apoptosis in multidrug-resistant cancer cells. The flavonols quercetin glycosides found in apples, onions and garlic have been shown to cause DNA damage to cancer cells [51]. Quercetin is structurally similar to kaempferol and luteolin, but has been shown to cause significant damage to normal mammalian DNA. However, quercetin has been shown to defend Caco-2 human epithelial colorectal adenocarcinoma cells from hydrogen peroxide (H_2O_2)-induced DNA damage by increasing the DNA repair pathway through the regulation of DNA repair enzymes [52]. In rats, intraperitoneal injection of quercetin protected kidney and bladder tissue from radiation-induced DNA damage. In rats, free radical capture and antioxidant capacity reduce myeloperoxidase and caspase 3 activity and reduce DNA protection [53]. In normal human breast cancer cells of MCF10A, the quercetin metabolite kercetin 3-O-glucuronide is potent against binding of norepinephrine to 2-adrenergic receptors by reducing DNA damage caused by 4-hydroxyestradiol and norepinephrine therapy [54]. It was found to show a positive inhibitory effect. In HT1080 human fibrosarcoma cells, quercetin reduces the phosphorylation of H2AX and p53 [55]. Glutathione (GSH) levels in the blood were restored in rats given chrysin, [56]. which suppresses DNA fragmentation caused by methylmercury (MeHg+) [57]. In the brain, kidney, and liver tissues of rats treated with D-galactose, chysin lowers redox status abnormalities such as superoxide dismutase, catalase, glutathione peroxidase, and GSH. Chrysin was found to protect male albino rats against the oxidative stress produced by N-nitro-Lariginine methyl ester in another study [58]. It has been demonstrated that the isoflavones daidzein and genistein, which are present in plants like *Glycine max* L. (soybean) and *Pueraria mirifica* L. (Kwao Krua), shield skin cells from DNA damage brought on by UV irradiation [59]. They effectively reduce the cyclo-oxygenase-2 and DNA-damage-inducible (Gadd45) genes in skin samples after treatment. The synergistic impact of genistein and daidzein when administered together, however, produced significantly higher photoprotective properties than either chemical alone [60].

Malvidin-3-O-glucoside is a key ingredient of dietary anthocyanins, particularly in red wine. By decreasing ROS generation and apoptotic proteins, malvidin-3-O-glucoside protects endothelial cells against peroxynitrite-induced apoptosis [61]. In endothelial cells, malvidin-3-O-glucoside treatment increases the expression of proapoptotic proteins. Malvidin was also reported to protect DNA from, cisplatin, procarbazine, and cyclophosphamide-induced DNA damage in mice. Malvidin had a dose–response protecting effect against cyclophosphamide-induced chromosomal damage in 30 min pretreated mice [62].

A flavanone called hesperetin, which is also present in oranges, cherries, grapefruit, and tomatoes possesses anti-inflammatory, anti-carcinogenic, neuroprotective, and antioxidant, characteristics [63]. As evidenced by the comet and TUNEL tests, it protects rats from doxorubicin-induced oxidative stress by decreasing DNA fragmentation. Dietary polyphenols such as genistein, guggulsterone emodin, and ellagic acid, have also been shown to play a role in cancer cell cycle and apoptosis control [64]. Naringenin, a different flavanone found in orange peel, was found to have the power to break DNA and induce apoptosis in HaCaT immortalized keratinocytes and other cancer cells [65].

Plant common extracts rich in flavonoids (quercitrin, rutin isoquercitrin, and quercetin) obtained from the leaves of *Scutia buxifolia* L. protect cultured human lymphocytes against chromosomal damage by maintaining mitotic index and genomic stability in the presence of H_2O_2 [66]. *Gynostemma pentaphylla* (Southern Ginseng), an antioxidant-rich herb, was discovered to protect human endothelium cells from cholesterol-induced DNA damage by preventing excessive ROS generation during atherosclerosis. It also prevents H2AX and other PI3K proteins from being phosphorylated, providing DNA protection [67].

In isolated human blood leukocytes, flavonoid-rich extracts from the rhizomes of *Podophyllum hexandrum* L. (Himalayan May Apple) were shown to prevent DNA damage and trigger DNA repair pathways [68]. During DNA DSBs, the active components were discovered to have the ability to block H2AX and P53BP1 phosphorylation. It also increases the levels of DNA-PKcs and Ku80, which help to protect DNA from radiation and aid DNA repair processes [69].

Withania somnifera L. (Ashwagandha), a common Ayurvedic herb, was recently shown to buffer brain DNA damage caused by H_2O_2 oxidative stress in glioblastoma and neuroblastoma cells by down-regulating -H2AX and DSBs proteins like Rad51, 53BP1, and others [70]. Antioxidant-rich herb *Nigella sativa* L. An ethanolic extract was found to protect Swiss albino mice against radiation-induced DNA damage [71]. Orally administered *N. sativa* ethanolic extract protected mice from oxidative damage to the liver, and spleen as determined by lipid peroxidation and antioxidant enzyme activity [72].

Pollen extracts from *Crataegus pinnatifida* L. (Chinese hawberry) have been shown to protect mouse lymphocytes against DNA damage caused by H_2O_2. It also has a high total phenolic content, total flavonoid content, and significant free radical scavenging activity, all of which might explain the protective benefits found [73].

7.4 Anticancerous agent: plant flavonoids

Flavonoids' capacity to decrease fatty acid synthase activity is linked to their capability to induce apoptosis in cancer cells. In oral squamous cell carcinoma, methanolic extracts of *Gracilaria tenuistipitata*, a genus of red algae, were shown to exhibit anti-cancer action [74]. By increasing, mitochondrial depolarization ROS production, and DNA damage, the extract causes apoptotic cell death. It also causes cancer cells to die by increasing phosphorylation of γ-H2AX and DSBs [75].

The herbal remedy for breast cancer and fever, *Fagonia cretica* L. (Virgin's Mantle), also causes apoptosis in MCF-7 and MDA-MB-231 breast cancer cells by producing -H2AX, DNA damage, cell cycle arrest, and p53 expression. In the absence of p53, *F. cretica* extract causes apoptosis through the production of FOXO3a (transcription factor) [74].

The mammalian target of rapamycin (mTOR) is a serine/threonine kinase signaling protein that affects cell development, proliferation, apoptosis, and cancer, among other intracellular and extracellular pathways. Most cancer cells had mTOR expression levels that were unregulated, leading in cell proliferation. Plant polyphenols are important in blocking a variety of kinases, including mTOR signaling cascades, which are used as a cancer prevention therapy method [76].

Piceatannol is a polyphenol found in berries, sugar cane peanuts, and grapes that inhibits serine/threonine kinases and tyrosine naturally and has been discovered to control mTOR signaling in prostate cancer cells with DNA damage and death. By decreasing CDK activity, additionally, it stops the cell cycle and reduces the proliferation of DU145 and CaP prostate cancer cells. According to a recent study (NHEK), piceatannol protected Burkitt's lymphoma (Raji) and healthy human epidermal keratinocytes from H_2O_2-induced DNA damage but was not involved in DNA repair pathways [77].

Fisetin, a flavonol, inhibited AKT/mTOR signaling in human multiple melanoma cells and myeloma, effectively controlling cell growth. Fisetin suppressed colony formation in A549 lung cancer cells by inhibiting the Akt or mTOR pathways and decreasing PI3K protein levels. Phytochemicals including, butein, capsaicin and boswellic acid have been shown to inhibit PI3K, Akt, and mTOR signaling in cancer cells, and are addressed in more depth elsewhere [78].

Excessive synthesis of ROS and poor DNA repair and antioxidants processes can damage cellular macromolecules, cause chromosomal instability, genetic mutation, and/or cell growth regulation, and possibly lead to cancer. ROS such as superoxide radicals, hydrogen peroxide, hydroxyl radicals, singlet oxygen, peroxyl radical, peroxynitrite, and nitric oxide can be produced by mitochondria, peroxisomes, inflammatory cell activation, and exogenous sources such as medications and industrial chemicals [79].

Antioxidant-rich foods can help to reduce ROS generation and protect cells and tissues from damage. A significant variety of plant-derived flavonoids have been investigated as possible novel sources of natural antioxidants, with the ability to decrease DNA damage caused by ROS in diverse cells [80].

The antioxidant activities of flavonoids is the most well-known characteristic. Because these phenolic compounds may scavenge free radicals and decrease oxidative stress, they can delay, slow, or prevent oxidation [81].

The antioxidant properties of resveratrol were altered by the upregulation of ROS scavengers and phase II enzymes like catalase, glutathione reductase, glutathione peroxidase, selenophosphate synthase 2, thioredoxin reductase, and NAD(P)H: quinone oxidoreductase-1. During pregnancy, resveratrol ingestion protects both the mother and the fetus against toxicity caused by environmental contaminants. Berries are rich in antioxidant phytochemicals, particularly anthocyanins, as well as ellagitannins, flavan-3-ols, procyanidins, flavonols, and hydroxybenzoate derivatives. They were discovered to be useful in the treatment of cardiovascular illnesses, age-related oxidative stress, inflammatory reactions, and a variety of degenerative diseases [82].

Inedible berry components can scavenge ROS and minimize oxidative DNA damage, as well as activate antioxidant enzymes, limit carcinogen-induced DNA adduct formation, and improve DNA repair. Strawberry bioactive components are well known to be potent antioxidants, and extracts have been demonstrated to protect skin from H_2O_2-induced damage by enhancing mitochondrial activity. A cool-climate berry crop called haskap (*Lonicera caerulea* L.) is rich in polyphenols like anthocyanins (cyanidin-3-O-glucoside, cyanidin-3-Orutinoside, peonidin-3-O-glucoside, and cyanidin-3,5-diglucoside), hydroxycinnamic acids (chlorogenic acid, 3,5-dicaffeoylquinic acid) [83].

Due to various ingredients and antioxidant capabilities, haskap is used as a source of natural health products. In SKH1 mice, oral treatment with anthocyanin-rich haskap extract provided radioprotective properties and UVB protection by regulating antioxidant enzyme activity and reducing DNA damage. UVB exposure causes oxidation of the erythrocyte membrane protected by haskap anthocyanins. Recent studies have shown that haskap methanol extract has polyphenol-dependent anti-inflammatory properties [84].

Both *in vitro* and *in vivo* tests have shown that kiwifruit, which is rich in vitamin C and other antioxidants, protects against oxidative DNA damage. In human lymphocytes, ingestion of kiwifruit increases resistance to H_2O_2-induced oxidative DNA damage [85]. It induces a base excision repair mechanism in rats after three weeks of oral administration. Supplementing Korean smokers with an eight week green vegetable drink (Angelica egg-based juice) shows protection against DNA damage to peripheral lymphocytes and shows that green vegetable drinks have anti-cancer effects. In addition, a study of six native purple leafy vegetables from Taiwan rich in flavonoids, anthocyanidins, and flavonols found that they protect lymphocyte DNA from H_2O_2 toxicity. These results add to the increased evidence suggesting that dietary polyphenols play an important role in protecting DNA from a variety of external and internal stimuli [86].

7.5 Current challenges

Antioxidants, cell cycle regulation, free radical capture, anti-estrogen effects, protein epigenetic activity and tyrosine kinase inhibition are just a few of the biological effects of flavonoids. While phytochemicals have many advantages, they also have certain drawbacks. Flavonoids have anti-cancer properties in many respects, and their lack of specificity can make drug delivery difficult. It is also a therapeutically important factor to consider when using phytochemicals. In addition, due to the hierarchical interaction and reversibility of epigenetic networks, flavonoids can cause deviations in efficiency and expected results when regulating epigenetic modifications in multiple dimensions [87]. This is a problem that other epigenetic medicines in use also face. However, flavonoids, based on various experimental studies, are believed to have important preclinical benefits in regulating cancer epigenetics. On the other hand, the widespread biological activity of flavonoids should not be used to dismiss research and treatment of the disease. Rather, the underlying process needs to be further investigated to take full advantage of its unique therapeutic potential [88].

Even with the recent significant advances in clinical flavonoid research focused on tumor epigenetics, there are currently insufficient data on therapeutic applicability. Various plants, including flavonoids, are currently in clinical trials due to many problems, including poor bioavailability. Fortunately, scientists have begun to tackle this problem by combining flavonoids with other plant compounds and anti-cancer drugs to enhance their anti-cancer effects, or by using nanodrug carrier technology to develop the pharmacokinetic properties of flavonoids. We are proposing feasible treatments such as increasing the number of patients. Determining the most effective flavonoid dose is an important element of basic and clinical research, as the doses used in cell cultures and animal models are not physiological and therefore may not be estimated in humans [89].

7.6 Conclusion and future prospects

In recent years, several studies have shown epigenetics of dysfunction in several types of cancer. Flavonoids are powerful epigenetic regulators that are widely consumed around the world. According to *in vivo* and *in vitro* studies, flavonoids can reduce cancer by repairing defective epigenetics and interfering with histone modification, DNA methylation and non-coding RNA expression. Flavonoids are highly effective when taken alone or as an adjunct therapy. Despite some obstacles, flavonoids have a bright future in terms of applicability. Moreover, comprehensive research on epigenetic dimensional changes targeted by flavonoids needs to be done in the future. Furthermore, extensive clinical examinations are required to determine the impacts of flavonoids on cancer and the utility of flavonoid use in a therapeutic environment.

References

[1] Weinhold B 2006 Epigenetics: the science of change *Environ. Health Perspect.* **114** A160–7
[2] Cheedipudi S, Genolet O and Dobreva G 2014 Epigenetic inheritance of cell fates during embryonic development *Front. Genet.* **5** 19
[3] Egger G, Liang G, Aparicio A and Jones P A 2004 Epigenetics in human disease and prospects for epigenetic therapy *Nature* **429** 457–63
[4] Ahmed A A and Essa M E 2020 Epigenetic alterations in female urogenital organs cancer: premise, properties, and perspectives *Sci. Afr.* **7** e00318
[5] Siegel R L, Miller K D, Fuchs H E and Jemal A 2021 Cancer statistics, 2021 *CA A. Cancer J. Clin.* **71** 7–33
[6] George V C, Dellaire G and Rupasinghe H P V 2017 Plant flavonoids in cancer chemoprevention: role in genome stability *J. Nutr. Biochem.* **45** 1–14
[7] Yu W-D, Sun G, Li J, Xu J and Wang X 2019 Mechanisms and therapeutic potentials of cancer immunotherapy in combination with radiotherapy and/or chemotherapy *Cancer Lett.* **452** 66–70
[8] Wang X, Waschke B C, Woolaver R A, Chen S M Y, Chen Z and Wang J H 2020b HDAC inhibitors overcome immunotherapy resistance in b-cell lymphoma *Protein Cell* **11** 472–82
[9] Shukla S, Meeran S M and Katiyar S K 2014 Epigenetic regulation by selected dietary phytochemicals in cancer chemoprevention *Cancer Lett.* **355** 9–17
[10] Busch C, Burkard M, Leischner C, Lauer U M, Frank J and Venturelli S 2015 Epigenetic activities of flavonoids in the prevention and treatment of cancer *Clin. Epigenet* **7** 64
[11] Roberti A, Valdes A F and Torrecillas R *et al* 2019 Epigenetics in cancer therapy and nanomedicine *Clin. Epigenet.* **11** 81
[12] Sharma S, Kelly T K and Jones P A 2010 Epigenetics in cancer *Carcinogenesis* **31** 2–36
[13] Brower V 2011 Epigenetics: unravelling the cancer code *Nature* **471** S12–3
[14] Zhang L, Lu Q and Chang C 2020 Epigenetics in health and disease *Adv. Exp. Med. Biol.* **1253** 3–55
[15] Ahmad S, Zahiruddin S, Parveen B, Basist P, Parveen A, Parveen R and Ahmad M 2021 Indian medicinal plants and formulations and their potential against COVID-19—preclinical and clinical research *Front. Pharmacol.* **11** 2470
[16] Kopustinskiene D M, Jakstas V, Savickas A and Bernatoniene J 2020 Flavonoids as anticancer agents *Nutrients.* **12** 457
[17] Hano C and Tungmunnithum D 2020 Plant polyphenols, more than just simple natural antioxidants: oxidative stress, aging and age-related diseases *Medicines* **7** 26
[18] da Silva G B, Manica D, Moreno M and Bagatini M D 2022 The potential of the purinergic system as a therapeutic target of natural compounds in cutaneous melanoma *Purinergic System* (London: InTech Open)
[19] Dabeek W M and Marra M V 2019 Dietary quercetin and kaempferol: bioavailability and potential cardiovascular-related bioactivity in humans *Nutrients* **11** 2288
[20] Zhang H, Hassan Y I, Liu R, Mats L, Yang C, Liu C and Tsao R 2020 Molecular mechanisms underlying the absorption of aglycone and glycosidic flavonoids in a Caco-2 BBe1 cell model *ACS Omega* **5** 10782–93
[21] Liu W N, Shi J, Fu Y and Zhao X H 2019 The stability and activity changes of apigenin and luteolin in human cervical cancer Hela cells in response to heat treatment and Fe^{2+}/Cu^{2+} addition *Foods* **8** 346
[22] Kumari R and Jat P 2021 Mechanisms of cellular senescence: cell cycle arrest and senescence associated secretory phenotype *Front. Cell Dev. Biol.* **9** 485

[23] Sachdev S, Ansari S A, Ansari M I, Fujita M and Hasanuzzaman M 2021 Abiotic stress and reactive oxygen species: generation, signaling, and defense mechanisms *Antioxidants* **10** 277
[24] Jiang W, Xia T, Liu C, Li J, Zhang W and Sun C 2021 Remodeling the epigenetic landscape of cancer—application potential of flavonoids in the prevention and treatment of cancer *Front. Oncol.* **11** 2331
[25] Singh R B, Watanabe S and Isaza A A (ed) 2022 *Functional Foods and Nutraceuticals in Metabolic and Non-Communicable Diseases* (New York: Academic)
[26] Agathokleous E, Kitao M and Calabrese E J 2019 Hormesis: a compelling platform for sophisticated plant science *Trends Plant Sci.* **24** 318–27.
[27] Ma Y, Dias M C and Freitas H 2020 Drought and salinity stress responses and microbe-induced tolerance in plants *Front. Plant Sci.* **11** 1750
[28] Dyck G J, Raj P, Zieroth S, Dyck J R and Ezekowitz J A 2019 The effects of resveratrol in patients with cardiovascular disease and heart failure: a narrative review *Int. J. Mol. Sci.* **20** 904
[29] Fares J, Fares M Y, Khachfe H H, Salhab H A and Fares Y 2020 Molecular principles of metastasis: a hallmark of cancer revisited *Signal Transduct Target Ther.* **5** 1–7
[30] Shankar E, Goel A, Gupta K and Gupta S 2017 Plant flavone apigenin: an emerging anticancer agent *Curr. Pharmacol. Rep.* **3** 423–6.
[31] Manzano C M, Nakahata D H and de Paiva R E 2022 Revisiting metallodrugs for the treatment of skin cancers *Coord. Chem. Rev.* **462** 214506
[32] Korga-Plewko A, Michalczyk M, Adamczuk G, Humeniuk E, Ostrowska-Lesko M, Jozefczyk A, Iwan M, Wojcik M and Dudka J 2020 Apigenin and hesperidin downregulate DNA repair genes in MCF-7 breast cancer cells and augment doxorubicin toxicity *Molecules* **25** 4421
[33] Hussein U K *et al* 2021 CK2α/CSNK2A1 Induces resistance to doxorubicin through sirt6-mediated activation of the dna damage repair pathway *Cells* **10** 1770
[34] Musial C, Kuban-Jankowska A and Gorska-Ponikowska M 2020 Beneficial properties of green tea catechins *Int. J. Mol. Sci.* **21** 1744
[35] Xue J, Yu C, Tang Y, Mo W, Tang Z, Sheng W, Jiao Y, Zhu W and Cao J 2021 NF-E2-related factor 2 (Nrf2) ameliorates radiation-induced skin injury *Front. Oncol.* **11** 680058
[36] Reddy A T, Lakshmi S P, Prasad E M, Varadacharyulu N C and Kodidhela L D 2020 Epigallocatechin gallate suppresses inflammation in human coronary artery endothelial cells by inhibiting NF-κB *Life Sci.* **258** 118136
[37] Bagheri H, Rezapour S, Najafi M, Motevaseli E, Shekarchi B, Cheki M and Mozdarani H 2018 Protection against radiation-induced micronuclei in rat bone marrow erythrocytes by curcumin and selenium L-methionine *Iran. J. Med. Sci.* **43** 645
[38] Wang H R, Pei S Y, Fan D X, Liu Y H, Pan X F, Song F X, Deng S H, Qiu H B and Zhang N 2020 Luteolin protects pheochromocytoma (PC-12) cells against Aβ25-35-induced cell apoptosis through the ER/ERK/MAPK signalling pathway *Evid. Based Complem. Altern. Med.* **2020** 2861978
[39] Khan A U, Dagur H S, Khan M, Malik N, Alam M and Mushtaque M 2021 Therapeutic role of flavonoids and flavones in cancer prevention: current trends and future perspectives *Eur. J. Med. Chem. Rep.* **3** 100010
[40] Fernández L P, Gomez de Cedron M and Ramírez de Molina A 2020 Alterations of lipid metabolism in cancer: implications in prognosis and treatment *Front. Oncol.* **10** 2144

[41] Raina R, Pramodh S, Rais N, Haque S, Shafarin J, Bajbouj K, Hamad M and Hussain A 2021 Luteolin inhibits proliferation, triggers apoptosis and modulates Akt/mTOR and MAP kinase pathways in HeLa cells *Oncol Lett.* **21** 1

[42] Shi T and Dansen T B 2020 Reactive oxygen species induced p53 activation: DNA damage, redox signaling, or both? *Antioxid. Redox Signal.* **33** 839–59

[43] Salehi B *et al* 2020 Therapeutic potential of quercetin: new insights and perspectives for human health *ACS Omega* **5** 11849–72

[44] Owumi S E, Lewu D O, Arunsi U O and Oyelere A K 2021 Luteolin attenuates doxorubicin-induced derangements of liver and kidney by reducing oxidative and inflammatory stress to suppress apoptosis *Hum. Exp. Toxicol.* **40** 1656–72

[45] Elhady S S, Abdelhameed R F, Mehanna E T, Wahba A S, Elfaky M A, Koshak A E, Noor A O, Bogari H A, Malatani R T and Goda M S 2022 Metabolic profiling, chemical composition, antioxidant capacity, and *in vivo* hepato- and nephroprotective effects of sonchus cornutus in mice exposed to cisplatin *Antioxidants* **11** 819

[46] Yamazaki S, Sakakibara H, Takemura H, Yasuda M and Shimoi K 2014 Quercetin-3-O-glucronide inhibits noradrenaline binding to α2-adrenergic receptor, thus suppressing DNA damage induced by treatment with 4-hydroxyestradiol and noradrenaline in MCF-10A cells *J. Steroid Biochem. Mol. Biol.* **143** 122–9

[47] Gong C, Yang Z, Zhang L, Wang Y, Gong W and Liu Y 2018 Quercetin suppresses DNA double-strand break repair and enhances the radiosensitivity of human ovarian cancer cells via p53-dependent endoplasmic reticulum stress pathway *Onco Targets Ther.* **11** 17

[48] Stompor-Gorący M, Bajek-Bil A, Machaczka M and Chrysin J 2021 Perspectives on contemporary status and future possibilities as pro-health agent *Nutrients* **13** 2038

[49] Baetas J, Rabaça A, Gonçalves A, Barros A, Sousa M and Sá R 2019 Protective role of N-acetylcysteine (NAC) on human sperm exposed to etoposide *Basic Clin. Androl.* **29** 1–9

[50] Veerappan R and Malarvili T 2019 Chrysin pretreatment improves angiotensin system, cGMP concentration in L-NAME induced hypertensive rats *Indian J. Clin. Biochem.* **34** 288–95

[51] Juliana C, Lister I N, Girsang E, Nasution A N and Widowati W 2020 Antioxidant and elastase inhibitor from black soybean (*Glycine max* L.) and its compound (daidzein) *J. Biomed Transl. Res.* **6** 11–4

[52] Kim I S 2021 Current perspectives on the beneficial effects of soybean isoflavones and their metabolites for humans *Antioxidants* **10** 1064

[53] Salehi B *et al* 2020 The therapeutic potential of anthocyanins: current approaches based on their molecular mechanism of action *Front. Pharmacol.* **11** 1300

[54] Bigoniya P, Warathe A and Singh C S 2019 Protective action of picroliv isolated from Picrorhiza kurroa against radiation clastogenecity on mice and cyclophosphamide-induced cytotoxicity in *Allium cepa* root *J. Radiat. Cancer Res.* **10** 58

[55] Pontifex M G, Malik M M, Connell E, Müller M and Vauzour D 2021 Citrus polyphenols in brain health and disease: current perspectives *Front Neurosci.* **15** 115

[56] Alaswad H A, Mahbub A A, Le Maitre C L and Jordan-Mahy N 2021 Molecular action of polyphenols in leukaemia and their therapeutic potential *Int. J. Mol. Sci.* **22** 3085

[57] Pourzand C, Albieri-Borges A and Raczek N N 2022 Shedding a new light on skin aging, iron-and redox-homeostasis and emerging natural antioxidants *Antioxidants* **11** 471

[58] Farcas A D, Mot A C, Zagrean-Tuza C, Ticolea M, Sevastre B, Kulak M, Silaghi-Dumitrescu R and Parvu A 2019 Remarkable rutin-rich hypericum capitatum extract

exhibits anti-inflammatory effects on turpentine oil-induced inflammation in rats *BMC Complement. Altern. Med.* **19** 1–3

[59] Su C, Li N, Ren R, Wang Y, Su X, Lu F, Zong R, Yang L and Ma X 2021 Progress in the medicinal value, bioactive compounds, and pharmacological activities of *Gynostemma pentaphyllum Molecules* **26** 6249

[60] Anand U *et al* 2022 Podophyllum hexandrum and its active constituents: novel radioprotectants *Biomed. Pharmacother.* **146** 112555

[61] Huang R X and Zhou P K 2020 DNA damage response signaling pathways and targets for radiotherapy sensitization in cancer *Signal Transduct. Target. Ther.* **5** 1–27

[62] Swift M L, Beishline K, Flashner S and Azizkhan-Clifford J 2021 DSB repair pathway choice is regulated by recruitment of 53BP1 through cell cycle-dependent regulation of Sp1 *Cell Rep.* **34** 108840

[63] Hannan M *et al* 2021 Black cumin (*Nigella sativa* L.): a comprehensive review on phytochemistry, health benefits, molecular pharmacology, and safety *Nutrients* **13** 1784

[64] Abd Rashid N, Abd Halim S A, Teoh S L, Budin S B, Hussan F, Ridzuan N R and Jalil N A 2021 The role of natural antioxidants in cisplatin-induced hepatotoxicity *Biomed. Pharmacother.* **144** 112328

[65] Wu M, Liu L, Xing Y, Yang S, Li H and Cao Y 2020 Roles and mechanisms of hawthorn and its extracts on atherosclerosis: a review *Front. Pharmacol.* **11** 118

[66] Gamal-Eldeen A M, Raafat B M, Alrehaili A A, El-Daly S M, Hawsawi N, Banjer H J, Raafat E M and Almehmadi M M 2022 Anti-hypoxic effect of polysaccharide extract of brown seaweed *Sargassum dentifolium* in tongue squamous cell carcinoma *Front. Nutri.* **9** 854780

[67] Zhao H, Zhuang Y, Li R, Liu Y, Mei Z, He Z, Zhou F and Zhou Y 2019 Effects of different doses of X-ray irradiation on cell apoptosis, cell cycle, DNA damage repair and glycolysis in HeLa cells *Oncol Lett.* **17** 42–54

[68] Jiang D, Xu J, Liu S, Nasser M I, Wei W, Mao T, Liu X, Zou X, Li J and Li X 2021 Rosmanol induces breast cancer cells apoptosis by regulating PI3K/AKT and STAT3/JAK2 signaling pathways *Oncol. Lett.* **22** 1–3

[69] Zou Z, Tao T, Li H and Zhu X 2020 mTOR signaling pathway and mTOR inhibitors in cancer: progress and challenges *Cell. Biosci.* **10** 1

[70] Liu Q, Cao Y, Zhou P, Gui S, Wu X, Xia Y and Tu J 2018 Panduratin A inhibits cell proliferation by inducing G0/G1 phase cell cycle arrest and induces apoptosis in breast cancer cells *Biomol. Therap.* **26** 328

[71] Hutcheson R L, Chakravorty A and Sugden B 2021 Burkitt lymphomas evolve to escape dependencies on Epstein–Barr virus *Front Cell. Infect. Microbiol.* **10** 835

[72] Cháirez-Ramírez M H, de la Cruz-López K G and García-Carrancá A 2021 Polyphenols as antitumor agents targeting key players in cancer-driving signaling pathways *Front. Pharmacol.* **12** 710304

[73] Nurcahyanti A D, Jap A, Lady J, Prismawan D, Sharopov F, Daoud R, Wink M and Sobeh M 2021 Function of selected natural antidiabetic compounds with potential against cancer via modulation of the PI3K/AKT/mTOR cascade *Biomed. Pharmacother.* **144** 112138

[74] Fujii J, Homma T and Osaki T 2022 Superoxide radicals in the execution of cell death *Antioxidants* **11** 501

[75] Lourenço S C, Moldão-Martins M and Alves V D 2019 Antioxidants of natural plant origins: from sources to food industry applications *Molecules* **24** 4132

[76] Viswanatha G L, Venkataranganna M V and Prasad N B 2019 Methanolic leaf extract of Punica granatum attenuates ischemia-reperfusion brain injury in Wistar rats: potential antioxidant and anti-inflammatory mechanisms *Iran. J. Basic Med. Sci.* **22** 187

[77] Wang Y, Branicky R, Noë A and Hekimi S 2018 Superoxide dismutases: dual roles in controlling ROS damage and regulating ROS signaling *J. Cell Biol.* **217** 1915–28

[78] Chang S K, Alasalvar C and Shahidi F 2019 Superfruits: phytochemicals, antioxidant efficacies, and health effects—a comprehensive review *Crit. Rev. Food Sci. Nutr.* **59** 1580–604

[79] Michalak M 2022 Plant-derived antioxidants: significance in skin health and the ageing process *Int. J. Mol. Sci.* **23** 585

[80] Česonienė L, Labokas J, Jasutienė I, Šarkinas A, Kaškonienė V, Kaškonas P, Kazernavičiūtė R, Pažereckaitė A and Daubaras R 2021 Bioactive compounds, antioxidant, and antibacterial properties of *Lonicera caerulea* berries: evaluation of 11 cultivars *Plants* **10** 624

[81] Amararathna M, Hoskin D W and Rupasinghe H V 2020 Anthocyanin-rich haskap (*Lonicera caerulea* L.) berry extracts reduce nitrosamine-induced DNA damage in human normal lung epithelial cells *in vitro Food Chem. Toxicol.* **141** 111404

[82] Gonçalves A C, Nunes A R, Falcão A, Alves G and Silva L R 2021 Dietary effects of anthocyanins in human health: a comprehensive review *Pharmaceuticals* **14** 690

[83] Kaur P, Purewal S S, Sandhu K S and Kaur M 2019 DNA damage protection: an excellent application of bioactive compounds *Bioresour. Bioprocess.* **6** 1

[84] Alhawaris A 2022 Potency of borneo endemic and typical plants as anti-cancer medicines *JKPBK* **5** 37–53

[85] Szoka L, Nazaruk J, Stocki M and Isidorov V 2021 Santin and cirsimaritin from *Betula pubescens* and *Betula pendula* buds induce apoptosis in human digestive system cancer cells *J. Cell. Mol. Med.* **25** 11085–96

[86] Kerimi A and Williamson G 2018 Differential impact of flavonoids on redox modulation, bioenergetics, and cell signaling in normal and tumor cells: a comprehensive review *Antioxid. Redox Sign.* **29** 1633–59

[87] Izzo S, Naponelli V and Bettuzzi S 2020 Flavonoids as epigenetic modulators for prostate cancer prevention *Nutrients* **12** 1010

[88] Sharifi-Rad M *et al* 2020 Lifestyle, oxidative stress, and antioxidants: back and forth in the pathophysiology of chronic diseases *Front. Physiol.* **11** 694

[89] Carlos-Reyes Á, López-González J S, Meneses-Flores M, Gallardo-Rincón D, Ruíz-García E, Marchat L A, Astudillo-De La Vega H, Hernández de la Cruz O N and López-Camarillo C 2019 Dietary compounds as epigenetic modulating agents in cancer *Front. Genet.* **10** 79

IOP Publishing

Phytochemicals as an Epigenetic Modifier in Cancer Prevention

Nidhi Puranik, Deepa Yadav and Sangeeta Shukla

Chapter 8

Targeting foremost molecular signaling pathways regulating tumor development with phytochemicals

Shiv Kumar Yadav, Nidhi Puranik and Dhananjay Yadav

Cancer is a serious medical condition that significantly lowers life expectancy and quality of life. Cancer and other chronic diseases are connected to the increased diet of fruit, vegetables, and whole grains. The nutritional approach offers preventive, non-toxic, and cost-effective cancer prevention measures. Plant-based foods have anti-cancer effects due to the presence of phytochemicals. One potential mode of action for anti-cancer phytochemicals is the control of cellular signal transduction pathways, which impacts cancer cell properties like proliferation, death, and invasion. Recent studies revealed that phytochemicals could inhibit the growth of cancer cells by targeting a wide range of cell signaling pathways at many levels, including protein activation, transcriptional or post-transcriptional control, and intercellular communication. Through the manipulation of reactive oxygen species (ROS), the mitogen-activated protein kinase (MAPK) pathway, the NF-kB pathways, and many others that are related to migration, senescence, and programmed cell death, phytochemicals control these signaling pathways of cancer. In this chapter, we go through the main molecular signaling pathways associated with cancer as well as the molecular mechanisms by which phytochemicals fight to suppress tumor development and further proliferation.

Abbreviations

ERK	Extracellular signal-regulated kinase
ROS	Reactive oxygen species
MAPK	Mitogen-activated protein kinase
PI3K	Phosphatidylinositol-3 kinase
NFkB	Protein kinase B Akt; Nuclear factor kappa B

doi:10.1088/978-0-7503-5252-9ch8

TGF	Tumor growth factor
Hh	Hedgehog
mTOR	Mammalian target of rapamycin
VEGF	Vascular endothelial growth factor
FGF	Fibroblast growth factor
AMPK	Adenosine monophosphate-activated protein kinase
Wnt	Wingless-related integration site
MMP	Matrix metalloproteinases
RCC	Renal Cell Cancer
HIF	Hypoxia-inducible factors
PDGF	Platelet-derived growth factor
EGFR	Epidermal growth factor receptor
TGF	Transforming growth factor
HGF	Hepatocyte growth factor
CSCs	Cancer stem cells
MET	Mesenchymal-epithelial transition
TCF	T-cell factor
FOXO	Forkhead box transcription factors
EGCC	Epigallocatechin gallate
CDKs	Cyclin-dependent kinases
TLRs	Toll-like receptors
NOS	Nitric oxide synthase
BCSCs	Breast cancer stem cells
TA	Tannic acid
TOPO	Topoisomerase
IKK	IB kinase
PLK1	Polo-like kinase-1
NSCLC	Non-small cell lung cancer
SNG	Sanguinarine
DATS	Diallyl trisulfide
DADS	Diallyl sulfide (DAS) and Diallyl disulfide (DADS)
XRD	X-ray powder diffraction

8.1 Introduction

The characteristic of cancer is the uncontrolled rapid and continuous division of cells. Initially, the only treatments for tumors were surgery and chemotherapy, but the identification of oncogenes and tumor suppressor genes has advanced the idea that certain proteins can be pharmacologically targeted to cure cancer. Recent advancements in multi-omics research and next-generation sequencing have further demonstrated how signaling pathways are tightly coupled to generate complex circuitries within cells that, if fully mapped, can be exploited for more accurate targeted therapies (Yip and Papa 2021). Natural goods are organic substances with biological properties that are derived from abundant natural resources like plants. Many of the medicinal medications that are currently prescribed come from natural sources such as alkaloids, taxanes, and flavonoids. To raise the therapeutic index of particular anti-neoplastic medications, natural compound chemotherapy has recently attracted more interest. Furthermore, the use of natural cancer treatments such phytochemicals, minerals, and vitamins has shown promising results in the treatment of a range of malignant tumors. To examine their synergistic efficacy with conventional anti-cancer medicines, natural substances with strong antitumor activity and minimal toxicity in healthy tissues have been suggested. The majority of earlier studies from the past three decades use *in silico*, *in vitro*, *ex vivo*, and *in vivo* investigations to show evidence of interactions between various phytochemicals and the proteins involved in signal transduction pathways (Pham *et al* 2020).

In contrast to normal cells, natural products have shown selective effects against cancer cells, but their chemical structures can also be used as models to create new medications. These medications might have fewer side effects and resistance than existing natural products. Chemoenzymatic biotransformation is one such intriguing alternative, which uses typical natural products as substrates to produce chemically varied and thoroughly described libraries of natural product derivatives (Hashem *et al* 2022). Different forms of tumors have altered cell signaling pathways. Cellular signaling pathways are intricate networks of interacting molecules that communicate with one another and control the biological functions of the cells. Cells integrate the information they get from several growth factor receptors to control a variety of cellular functions, including protein synthesis, cell motility, differentiation, architecture, and polarity. Signaling pathways control cellular growth and induce various alterations in many cell types. Numerous signaling pathways control cell motility, proliferation, and survival. Therefore, when a mutationally triggered route is inhibited, cancer cells can grow through an alternative signaling channel. MAPK, PI3K/Akt/NFkB, TGF, Hh, Notch, Wnt/catenin, and Foxo pathways are some of the most often dysregulated signaling pathways associated with breast cancer (Yousefnia *et al* 2020). HCC carcinogenesis also involves numerous molecular signaling cascades. The major signaling pathways include the VEGF pathway, MAPK/ERK pathway, Wnt/β-catenin pathway, PI3K/AKT/mTOR signaling pathway, FGF pathway, enzymes reactions generating ROS in liver cancers, and serine/threonine kinase pathway (Jain *et al* 2021, Juaid *et al* 2021). Various transcription factors, such as NF-kβ, detoxification enzymes, AMPK, and Wnt/catenin molecular activities are linked to gastrointestinal cancer (Al-Ishaq *et al* 2020). In renal cell cancer (RCC) numerous signaling pathways have been discovered. HIF, which controls the expression of target proteins like VEGF, PDGF, EGFR, and TGF, is recognized to be the mediator of hypoxic signaling. The activation of PI3K, which in turn activates Akt, via polycystin 1 and mTOR, is triggered by the binding of VEGF and PDGF to their respective receptor tyrosine kinases (Faes *et al* 2021). It has been noted that this route prevents RCC cells from apoptosis. RCC has been linked to Wnt signaling, which induces transcription by activating catenin. Papillary RCC has been linked to the HGF and receptor mesenchymal-epithelial transition (MET) (Bajalia *et al* 2022).

Natural medicine and substances produced from plants, animals, marine life, and bacteria are largely obtained from nature. Alkaloids, flavonoids, glycosides, saponins, tannins, and terpenoids, which are present in plants and have antioxidant and anti-cancer activities in numerous cancer cell lines, particularly in liver cancer cell lines, are among them (Jain *et al* 2021). It was discovered that phytochemicals can control a number of signaling networks and their constituents in cancer cells, including PI3K/Akt/mTOR, MMP-2 and MMP-9, Wnt/-catenin, PARP, MAPK, NF-kB, Caspase-3/8/9, Bax, Bcl2, Smad4, Notch1, STAT3, Nrf2, and ROS signaling (Kamdje *et al* 2014, Abdullah *et al* 2021). According to Sohel *et al* (2023), phytochemicals cause an increase in tumor inhibitor microRNAs, which have been identified as a major component of anti-breast cancer therapies (Sohel *et al* 2023). It was observed that phytochemicals decrease TNBC cell migration by altering the PI3K/AKT pathway as well as protein kinases in the MAPK and STAT pathways (Shahi Thakuri *et al* 2020). Diet is a two-way risk factor that influences the emergence of cancer. The risk of developing cancer can be decreased by a number of dietary factors, including consuming fewer calories than necessary, more whole grains, fruits, and vegetables, dietary fibers, less red meat, and less sugar. Through important participants including Nrf2, CYP450, MAPK, Akt, JAK/STAT, Wnt/-catenin, p53, NF-kB, and cancer-related miRNAs, we examine main classes of phytochemicals and their control on cell signaling transduction against carcinogenesis in this study (Chen and Liu 2018).

8.2 Molecular signaling pathways and cancer

Although the degree, mechanisms, and co-occurrence of changes in these pathways differ between specific cancers and tumor types, genetic changes in the signaling pathways that regulate cell-cycle progression, apoptosis, and cell proliferation are frequently associated with cancer. One recent study found that 57% of cancers had at least one modification that might be targeted by currently available medications, and 89% of tumors had at least one driver alteration in these pathways. Multiple targetable changes were seen in 30% of the tumors, suggesting potential for combination therapy (Sanchez-Vega *et al* 2018).

8.2.1 Fibroblast growth factor and receptor (FGFRs)

FGFRs are important in physiological processes; tissue and metabolism homeostasis, endocrine functioning, and wound healing are all mediated by FGFs. Across a wide range of tumor types, deregulation of the FGF signaling axis has been linked to oncogenesis, tumor growth, and resistance to anti-cancer therapy. The effectiveness of anti-FGFR therapy in the clinic has been inconsistent, despite the fact that several studies have suggested the abnormal FGFR signaling pathway as a viable therapeutic target in a variety of tumor types (Babina and Turner 2017). FGFR pathway is a therapeutic strategy for various cancers including pancreatic cancer (Kang *et al* 2019), urothelial cancer (Rodriguez-Vida *et al* 2015), lung cancer (Hegab *et al* 2019, Pacini *et al* 2021), breast cancer (Criscitiello *et al* 2017, Perez-Garcia *et al* 2018, Francavilla and O'Brien 2022), oral carcinogenesis (Xie *et al* 2016), and pancreatic cancer (Carter *et al* 2021).

8.2.2 Notch signaling

A crucial function in multicellular organisms' proliferation is that stem cell maintenance, cell fate specification, differentiation, and homeostasis are regulated by the notch signaling pathway, a highly conserved molecular cell signaling mechanism that also involves angiogenesis. They are crucial to the growth of the embryonic vascular system. It has been experimentally proven that notch signaling, one of the most active pathways in cancer cells, aids in cancer spreading. The notch pathway is getting more attention as a target to get rid of cancer stem cells (CSCs) since it is crucial in the connections between angiogenesis and CSC self-renewal. Cancers like leukemia have dysregulated notch signaling (Kamga *et al* 2016, McCarter *et al* 2018), breast cancer (Acar *et al* 2016, Lamy *et al* 2017), endometrial cancer (Shang *et al* 2018, Lachej *et al* 2019), prostate cancer (Soylu *et al* 2016, O'Brien and Marignol 2017), colorectal cancer (Li *et al* 2018, Pu *et al* 2021), renal cancer (Edeling *et al* 2016), gastric cancer (Yao *et al* 2017, Hibdon *et al* 2019), liver cancer (Wu *et al* 2015, Lu *et al* 2016) and lung cancer (Lim *et al* 2017). Suppression of this signaling pathway could be a good therapeutic strategy for cancer treatment (Yuan *et al* 2015, Venkatesh *et al* 2018).

8.2.3 The wingless-type (Wnt)/β-catenin signaling

The Wnt/catenin signaling pathway is a conserved signaling pathway involved in a variety of cellular processes, including cell division, invasion, motility, apoptosis, migration, tissue homeostasis, and preservation of the stem cell niche (Ghosh *et al* 2019). There is growing evidence that certain solid tumors and hematological malignancies were able to originate and progress because of disruption of the Wnt/catenin cascade. By promoting cancer stem cell renewal, cell proliferation, and differentiation, the aberrant Wnt/catenin signaling pathway plays critical roles in carcinogenesis and therapeutic response. The therapeutic promise of drugs that target Wnt/catenin signaling in cancer is highlighted by accumulating studies. In preclinical and clinical research, the catenin destruction complex, the TCF/catenin transcription complex, and the Wnt ligand/receptor interface have all been the subject of therapy (Zhang and Wang 2020). At several cellular levels, Wnt signaling is carefully controlled, and lung cancer exhibits dysregulation of this control. Consequently, it provides therapeutic targets for the creation of novel lung cancer treatment molecules (Yang *et al* 2016). Aberrant Wnt signaling is a hallmark of many cancers including liver cancer (Liu *et al* 2016, He and Tang 2020), lung cancer (Zhu *et al* 2022), breast cancer (Pohl *et al* 2017), colon cancer (Basu *et al* 2016) and prostate cancer (Murillo-Garzón and Kypta 2017).

8.2.4 BCL-2 family

A family of related proteins called BCL2 controls apoptosis in various ways. For carcinogenesis to occur, cancer cells must have the ability to prevent apoptosis (Leverson *et al* 2015). The sentinel network, which controls the mitochondrial or intrinsic apoptotic response, is made up of proteins from the BCL2 family. Recent developments in our knowledge of apoptotic signaling pathways have made it possible to recognize malignancies that are 'primed' to experience apoptosis and have revealed potential biomarkers that may indicate which tumors will experience apoptosis in response to a particular therapy. Numerous malignancies exhibit overexpression of anti-apoptotic BCL2 family proteins, which can be brought on by chromosomal translocations, gene amplification, enhanced gene transcription, and/or alterations in post-translational processing. Follicular lymphoma and diffuse large B-cell lymphoma both have elevated BCL2 expression as a result of the translocation, as was previously mentioned (Hata *et al* 2015). One of the most effective cancer treatments involves focusing on the different addictions to the anti-apoptotic BCL-2 family (Inoue-Yamauchi *et al* 2017).

8.2.5 Receptor tyrosine kinase family

An example of a receptor tyrosine kinase is the EGFR, which is essential for cell growth, migration, adhesion, differentiation, and death. This receptor has a transmembrane domain, an intracellular tyrosine kinase domain, and an extracellular ligand binding domain. The intracellular tyrosine kinase domain of the EGFR is phosphorylated after it binds to different ligands, such as EGF and TGF, through homodimerization or heterodimerization on the cell surface. Numerous downstream signal transduction pathways, including the PI3K/Akt/mTOR pathway, are activated as a result of EGFR activation (Li *et al* 2016). A MAPK signaling cascade is an example of a complex signaling cascade with numerous connecting pathways and continual crosstalk, each of which is subject to fine-tuning and switch-like activations of regulatory elements. The MAPK is frequently involved in oncogenesis, tumor development, and treatment resistance. It is one of many tightly linked signaling cascades. The several kinases in the MAPK family that are altered in cancers have given rise to a variety of targeted medications. Resistance to MAPK inhibitors is now a problem because of the numerous interactions and potential compensatory responses (Braicu *et al* 2019).

8.2.6 Foxo family

The Forkhead box transcription factors (FOXO) family is one such class of transcription factors that could be a target for the modulation of cancer. Growth factors and stress-regulated transcription factors are FOXO proteins. In quiescent or growth factor-deficient cells, FOXO proteins often dwell in the nucleus where they regulate gene transcription. When growth factors are present, they are also prone to destruction via the ubiquitin-proteasome pathway. The PI3K/AKT pathway is the most significant route interacting with FOXO in various cancer types. FOXOs play a role in carcinogenesis through the Ras-MEK-ERK, IKK, and AMPK pathways, among other significant pathways. Finding and developing effective treatments for various malignancies may result from therapeutically targeting the FOXO signaling pathway(s), but doing so calls for a deeper comprehension of how FOXO transcription factors are regulated and operate (Farhan *et al* 2017).

8.2.7 PI3K/AKT/mTOR pathway

Important biological functions like cell development, proliferation, apoptosis, etc are regulated by the PI3K/AKT/mTOR pathway. The PI3K-Akt pathway plays a critical role in cell survival and proliferation and is connected to autophagy and apoptosis. Malignant cells are encouraged to survive and grow by aberrant activation of this pathway. Inhibiting PI3K in conjunction with standard chemotherapy and medications that target other oncogenic proteins makes sense because it is one of the most frequently mutated protein kinases found in tumor cells (Issinger and Guerra 2021). Products from nature have been looked at for possible effects on the PI3K-Akt-mTOR pathway in cancer. Natural substances that have been shown to have therapeutic potential to target the PI3K-Akt-mTOR pathway include salidroside, oridonin, afrocyclamin A, vitexin, apigenin, cryptotanshinone, and curcumin. These substances are still in the preclinical development stages (Tewari *et al* 2022). The mTOR pathway may be directly or indirectly inhibited by a number of herbs and natural phytochemicals, including curcumin, resveratrol, timosaponin III, gallic acid, diosgenin, pomegranate, EGCC, genistein, and 3,3′-diindolylmethane (Tan *et al* 2014).

8.2.8 CDK and CDK pathway

One of the main cell cycle regulation routes is the cyclin/CDK system, which also includes the E2F family of transcription factors, the retinoblastoma tumor suppressor family, and CDKs (Sarkar *et al* 2021). Generally speaking, cancer cells have higher levels of overexpressed CDKs than normal cells, which explains why cancer cells divide uncontrolled. Pharmacological treatments that are successful in modifying CDK activity may lead to a reduction in the aberrant proliferation rate of cancer cells (Gallorini *et al* 2012).

8.2.9 TLR4 signaling pathway

The well-known family of pattern recognition receptors known as toll-like receptors (TLRs) is crucial to the host immune system. TLR activation causes pro-inflammatory cytokines and chemokines to be produced, which activates both innate and adaptive immunity. More research has now revealed the connection between TLRs and cancer. Among these, the TLR4 signaling pathway is linked to the development of inflammation and cancer. The function of toll-like receptors in innate immunity is significant. TLRs could have a double-edged effect on the development of tumors, their growth, induction of apoptosis, or inhibition of tumor progression in certain cancer cell types or resistance to chemotherapy. Numerous studies have demonstrated that TLR4 activation causes inflammation and carcinogenesis. Recent research has indicated that the TLR4 pathway may be inhibited by bioactive chemicals through MyD88- and TRIF-dependent signaling pathways as a result of the anti-inflammatory actions of these drugs (Chen *et al* 2018).

8.3 Reactive oxygen species and cancer

Multiple malignancies have been associated with elevated ROS generation, which has been demonstrated to play a number of roles, including activating pro-tumorigenic signaling, promoting cell survival and proliferation, and causing DNA damage and genetic instability. Contrary to popular belief, ROS can also activate anti-tumorigenic signaling, causing tumor cells to die as a result of oxidative stress. ROS are produced by NOS enzymes, which are important redox environment regulators in cells. ROS promotes cancer and cell proliferation (Chirumbolo *et al* 2018, Sundaram *et al* 2020). Figure 8.1 shows a connection between oxidative stress and metabolism in cancer cells. Different sources of generation of ROS species have been depicted in the figure, among all of which mitochondrial biochemical pathways are the major source of generation of ROS species.

In order to detoxify excess ROS, establish a redox balance, sustain pro-tumorigenic signaling, and fight apoptosis, tumor cells express higher quantities of antioxidant proteins. Because tumor cells differ from their normal counterparts in terms of their redox balance, ROS modification is recognized as a possible target for cancer therapy (Moloney and Cotter 2018).

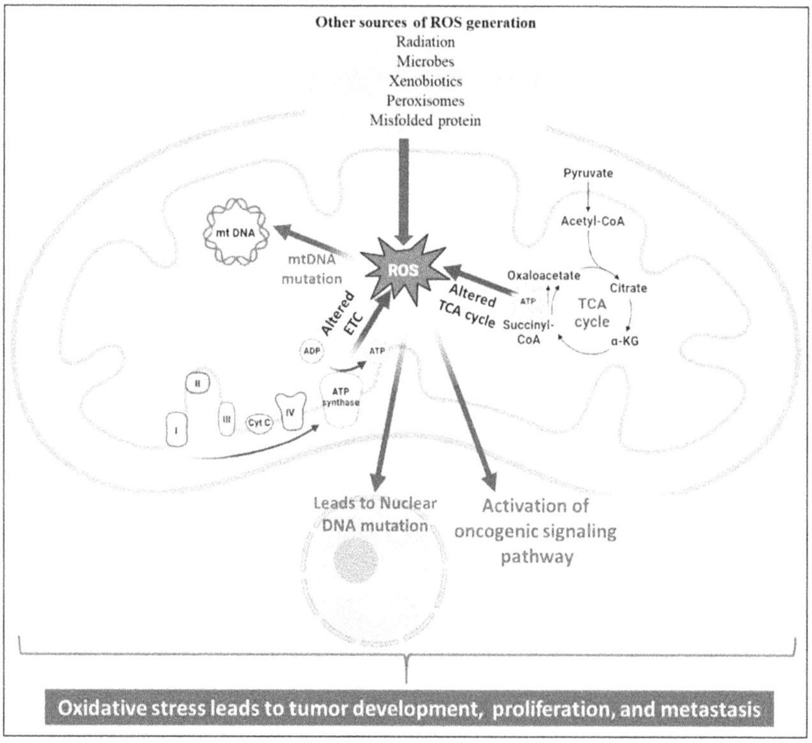

Figure 8.1. Oxidative stress generated in the mitochondria of the cell leads to tumor development, proliferation, and metastasis.

8.4 Phytochemicals

A general overview of phytochemicals, their classes, and their role in various kinds of cancer-prevented activity is given in chapter 1 in detail. In this chapter, we will discuss the role of phytochemicals in the regulation of different cell signaling pathways that have crucial roles in cell development and cell proliferation that leads to cancer or apoptosis, and autophagy that prevents cancer development. CSCs are a subpopulation of cancer cells that exhibit abnormal self-renewal, proliferation, or apoptotic control, resulting in the growth of the malignancy, the development of metastases, and resistance to therapy. Phytochemicals' anti-cancer properties also aim to target this CSC (Dandawate *et al* 2013, Dandawate *et al* 2016, Liskova *et al* 2019, Yang *et al* 2020). Most phytochemicals exhibit their pharmacologic effects in nature through a multi-targeted approach, as shown in figure 8.2; a property that is highly desirable since therapy for carcinomas invariably involves dysregulation of multiple genes and associated cell-signaling pathways at various stages of initiation, progression, and metastasis (Sun *et al* 2019). On the other hand, acquired genetic changes and microenvironment-mediated epigenetic perturbations have primarily been considered to play a significant role in neoplastic development in cancer initiation and progression. Numerous studies have been conducted to identify the genetic elements that regulate epigenetic changes (Bagla *et al* 2015).

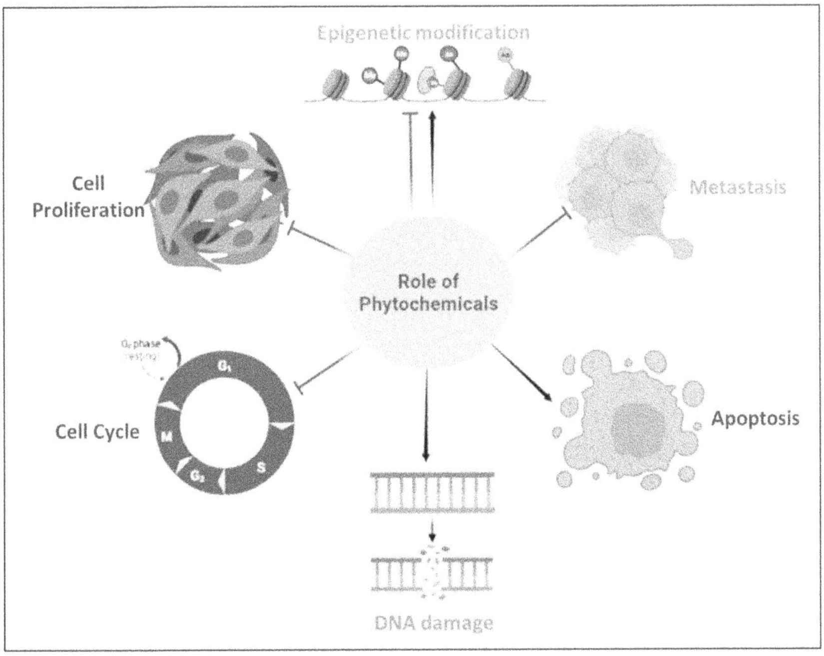

Figure 8.2. A schematic representation of the role of phytochemicals in cancer treatment and management.

8.5 Phytochemicals-based regulation of cancer signaling pathway

Biologically active substances are abundant in plants, where they can operate on a wide range of biochemical and communication pathways (Ahmed *et al* 2022). The proliferation of cancer cells can be inhibited by phytochemicals by focusing on a variety of cell signaling pathways at various levels, including protein activation, transcriptional or post-transcriptional regulation, and intercellular communication. Chen and Liu (2018) study the role of phytochemicals in cell signaling transduction including Nrf2, CYP450, MAPK, Akt, JAK/STAT, Wnt/-catenin, p53, NF-kB, and cancer-related miRNAs against carcinogenesis (Chen and Liu 2018). Recent studies examine the uniqueness and potency of therapeutic anti-cancer medicines obtained from plants. Many have been proven to have anti-cancer effects, including suppressing proteins and enzymes like CDK, PTEN, and mTOR, as well as signaling pathways including Wnt, Notch, Akt, and TRK that are connected to cancer cells (Espinosa-Sánchez *et al* 2020, Rahman *et al* 2022, Siddiqui *et al* 2022). The Inhibition of various cell cycle factors and cell signaling pathways responsible for the development and progression of different kinds of cancers are studied by various researchers, as shown in figure 8.3. The general mechanism of anti-cancerous activity of phytochemicals is depicted in figure 8.4. The most common

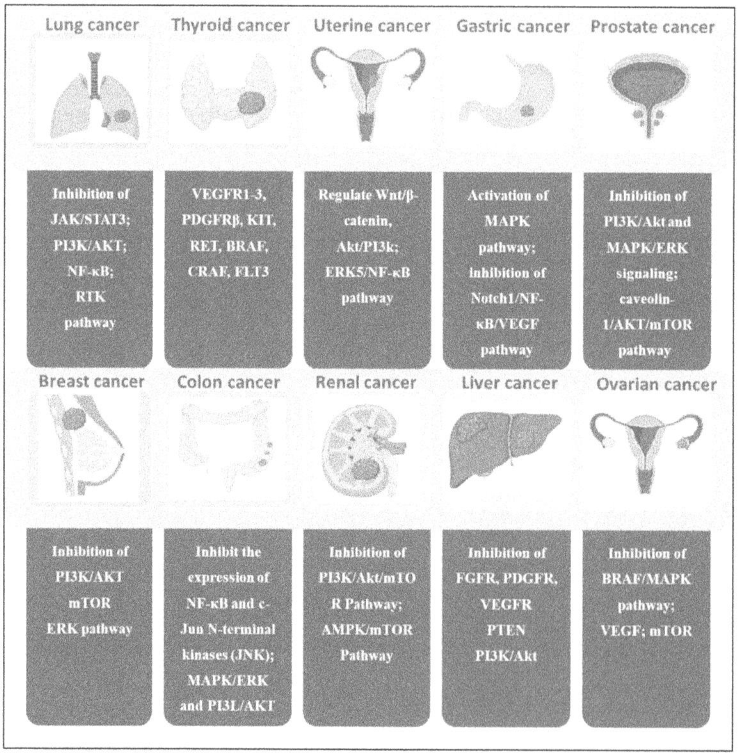

Figure 8.3. Inhibition of various cell cycle factors and cell signaling pathways responsible for tumor development and progression.

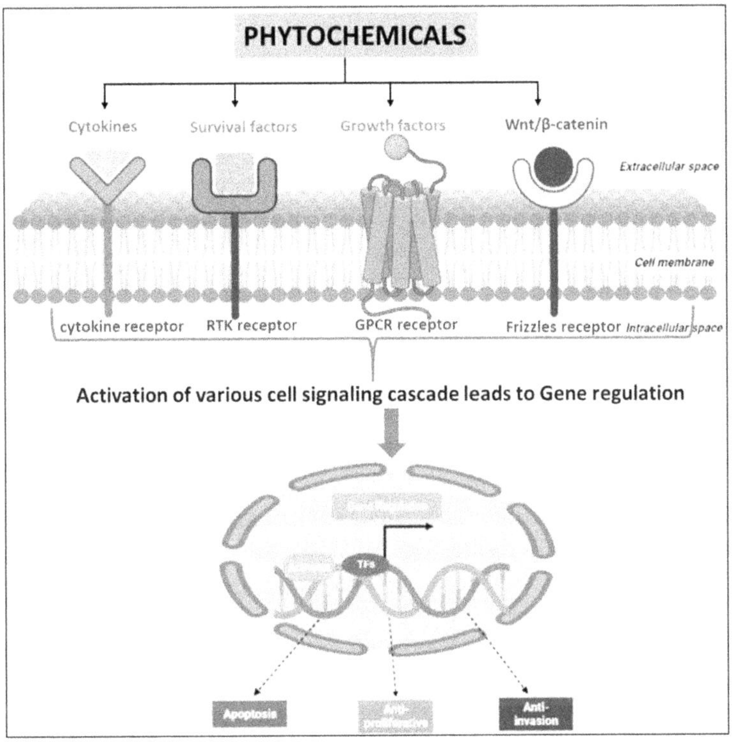

Figure 8.4. A basic schematic representation of gene regulation by phytochemicals of major signaling pathways involved in the promotion and progression of tumors.

mechanism of phytochemicals is targeting the cell signaling pathway that is responsible for cell apoptosis and inhibits cell growth and proliferation, and invasion.

8.5.1 Polyphenol

A prevalent malignancy with a dismal prognosis is breast cancer. Breast cancer stem cells (BCSCs) and CSCs are two types of heterogeneous cancer cells, and CSCs are principally responsible for tumor relapse, therapy resistance, and metastasis. Diets are known to contribute to the development of cancer. Food-derived polyphenols can reduce BCSC pathogenicity and development, suggesting that these substances and their analogs may be effective breast cancer preventatives (Gu *et al* 2020). Due to their physiological effects and structural makeup, polyphenols, which are secondary metabolites of plants, are typically involved in defense against UV radiation or aggression. Although new research has raised the possibility that polyphenols may alter several cellular pathways and hence produce a pleiotropic effect, many of the biological effects of polyphenols have previously been attributed to their antioxidant characteristics.

Polyphenol-induced cellular pathways may slow down or even stop the development of cancer in breast tissue. It is well recognized that oxidative stress changes the cellular redox status, which changes how genes are expressed by activating a number of redox-sensitive transcription factors. Cell growth and cell death are both impacted by this signaling chain. Due to oncogenic mutations that support abnormal metabolism, aggressively proliferating cancer cells produce ROS at a higher rate. It has been suggested that dietary polyphenols may be used therapeutically as chemopreventive drugs because of their capacity to alter cellular signal transduction pathways by regulating the transcription factors (Braakhuis *et al* 2016).

NF-kB controls gene expressions involved in cell survival and proliferation, drug resistance, metastasis, and angiogenesis because it is a transcription factor. Inflammation and cancer are largely influenced by the activation of NF-kB. The ingestion of polyphenols, which are frequently present in plant species, has been shown to have a deleterious impact on the NF-kB signaling pathway. They prevent NF-kB from moving into the nucleus, suppress kinase phosphorylation, and obstruct NF-kB interactions with DNA. Polyphenols suppress the inflammatory cascade, trigger apoptosis, and reduce cell proliferation and metastasis via inhibiting NF-kB (Khan *et al* 2020).

The up-regulation of tumor-suppressive genes and the down-regulation of oncogenes, the modulation of hypoxia, the formation of mammospheres, onco-inflammation, enzymatic control, and epigenetic changes in BC are just a few of the molecular mechanisms and cellular phenomena that natural compounds have been shown to affect. We discovered that phytochemicals can control a number of signaling networks and their constituents in cancer cells, including PI3K/Akt/mTOR, MMP-2 and 9, Wnt/-catenin, PARP, MAPK, NF-kB, Caspase-3/8/9, Bax, Bcl2, Smad4, Notch1, STAT3, Nrf2, and ROS signaling. They activate tumor suppressor microRNAs, which have been identified as a significant component of ani-BC therapies that are followed by phytochemical supplementation (Sohel *et al* 2023). Song X *et al* study revealed that curcumin could inhibit breast cancer cell proliferation by inducing cell cycle arrest, initiating p53-dependent apoptosis, altering the expression of signaling proteins, downregulating transcription factors, and inhibiting angiogenesis. For instance, curcumin causes p53-dependent apoptosis and stops the cell cycle in MCF-7 cells (Song *et al* 2019). Curcumin causes the creation of ROS, which upregulates the activity of Bax and caspase-3 and down-regulates the activity of MMP-2 and Bcl-2 in MCF-10A human breast epithelial cells transformed with H-Ras (Kim *et al* 2001). A study by Ravindran *et al* also demonstrated that curcumin can control various cell signaling pathways that are involved in cell proliferation, cell survival, apoptosis, mitochondrial pathways, and protein kinase (Ravindran *et al* 2009). BCSC's ability to proliferate is inhibited by curcumin, which is a significant determinant of cancer recurrence. Limiting BCSC proliferation prevents metastasis and reattachment, which ultimately prevents tumor growth (Liu and Ho 2018).

JNK, MAPK, STAT, NF-kB, and anthocyanidins are a subclass of flavonoids that have the potential to prevent colon cancer. By altering the ratio of Bax/Bcl-2 and upregulating p53 expression, apigenin promotes apoptosis. Quercetin inhibits the NF-kB signaling pathway to provide its cytotoxic anti-colorectal cancer action. In studies using animal models of colorectal cancer, EGCG was found to prevent carcinogenesis by downregulating the expression of Cox2 and the Wnt signaling pathway. As a result, various signaling pathways lead to flavonoids' strong preventive function against colorectal cancer (Hussain *et al* 2022).

Tannic acid (TA) binds to EGF-R and prevents STAT1 and STAT3 from tyrosine phosphorylation. The DNA-binding activity of STAT3/BCL-2 is inhibited as a result of this inhibition. As a result, BCl-2 expression and localization in the mitochondria decreased. Cytochrome c was released, and a caspase-based intrinsic apoptotic cascade was activated as a result of the altered expression and distribution of mitochondrial anti-pore factors. Our findings imply that TA alters the EGF-R/Jak2/STAT1/3 and P38/STAT1/p21Waf1/Cip1 and EGF-R/Jak2/STAT1/3 pathways, causing G1-arrest and intrinsic apoptosis in breast cancer (Darvin *et al* 2017).

In a study, eight flavonoids were extracted from *Tephroseris kirilowii* and characterized for their anti-cancer properties. The study revealed that three of them-isorhamnetin, genkwanin, and acacetin inhibited cell proliferation in various human cancer cell lines. In human breast cancer cells, these potent flavonoids triggered cell cycle arrest at the G2/M phase and induced apoptosis and autophagy. In human breast cancer cells, flavonoids reduce the activity of the PI3K-mediated signaling pathway, which in turn causes death and autophagy (Zhang *et al* 2018).

8.5.2 Alkaloids

Alkaloids are a broad category of substances with cyclic structures that include at least one basic nitrogen atom. The majority of the plants that contain these substances are found in the Leguminosae, Menispermaceae, Ranunculaceae, Loganiaceae, and Papaveraceae families of plants. Numerous alkaloids are well-known as powerful chemotherapeutic drugs, including camptothecin, vincristine, vinblastine, berberine, sanguinarine, evodiamine, piperine, matrine, and tetrandrine (Mondal *et al* 2019). Traditional secondary metabolites known as steroidal alkaloids are a significant family of natural chemicals found in plants, marine creatures, and invertebrates. They are a wise choice as prospective anti-cancer leads (Jiang *et al* 2016, Dey *et al* 2019). Steroidal alkaloids are chemical compounds implicated in the activation of apoptosis in particular cancer cell types, including steroidal alkaloids. By upregulating or downregulating apoptotic and autophagic proteins, they cause apoptosis or autophagy to be induced, which has anti-cancer effects. Another mechanism underpinning their anti-cancer efficacy is the interaction with CDKs, which inhibits cell cycle progression at the G0/G1 or G2/M phase. Carboline alkaloids are organic substances having a range of biochemical and psychopharmacological actions, but they have the potential to be particularly effective against cancer. Growing evidence supports the beneficial activities of β-carboline derivatives in the fight against cancer by inhibiting topoisomerase (TOPO), kinesin Eg5, telomerase, cyclin-dependent kinase (CDK), IB kinase (IKK), and polo-like kinase-1 (PLK1) in the cell cycle transition phases (Ahmad *et al* 2020). The benzylisoquinoline family of benzophenanthridine alkaloids, which includes sanguinarine, has multiple pharmacological properties that are being investigated for the treatment of several human disorders, including cancer. Accordingly, in EGFR(T790M)-containing TKI-resistant NSCLC cell lines, SNG-induced production of ROS mediates elevation of NOX3-induced EGFR degradation and death. Numerous studies demonstrate that glioma tumors and cells become resistant to apoptosis-inducing anti-cancer therapies. Curiously, SNAG has demonstrated promising anti-tumorigenic effects in human glioma cells through autophagy via ROS-induced activation of extracellular signal-regulated kinase1/2 (ERK1/2) (Pallichankandy *et al* 2015, Khan *et al* 2020).

According to a study by Gu *et al* SAN may be a possible lung cancer treatment because it decreased SPC-A1 cell proliferation and caused apoptosis in a dose-dependent way in lung cancer cells through ROS generation and ER stress (Gu *et al* 2015).

A decrease in MMP, the release of cytochrome c, the activation of caspase-9 and caspase-3, and the down-regulation of the anti-apoptotic factors XIAP and cIAP-1 are all shown to occur as a result of sanguinarine mediating ROS generation, as demonstrated by Choi and colleagues. These findings unequivocally show that ROS are involved in the initial molecular activities that lead to the sanguinarine-induced apoptotic pathway. Our findings suggest that sanguinarine-induced ROS are important mediators of MMP breakdown, which triggers the release of cytochrome c and the subsequent activation of caspase, which results in apoptosis (Choi *et al* 2008).

8.5.3 Terpenoids

The largest class of phytochemicals, terpenoids, sometimes referred to as terpenes, are found in a wide variety of plants and have a wide range of biological and metabolic functions in living systems. Compared to other living things, green plants, especially flowering plants, have an exceptionally high concentration of terpenoid chemicals. Terpenoids are a vast class of secondary metabolites that are widely distributed throughout the plant kingdom and have an isoprenoid-based structural makeup. Due to the wide variety of terpenoids and their antioxidative, anti-inflammatory, and anti-cancer effects, there is greater interest in their commercial and medicinal applications. Terpenoids are categorized into six types based on their structural similarities: monoterpenes, sesquiterpenes, diterpenes, triterpenes, tetraterpenes, and polyterpenes.

Inhibiting the early initiation and progression of tumorigenesis by inducing cell cycle arrest, tumor cell differentiation, and apoptosis, as well as suppressing angiogenesis, invasion, and metastasis in the late stages of tumor development through the regulation of various intracellular signaling pathways, are just a few of the terpenoids that have been discovered to possess anti-cancer properties. These chemicals are prospective therapeutic agents due to important advancements in the specific mechanism of their anti-cancer effect (Ansari and Akhtar 2019).

By causing mitochondrial-mediated apoptosis, G2/M phase cell cycle arrest, prevention of cell migration and invasion, and modulation of the mTOR/PI3K/AKT signaling pathway, betulin terpenoid targets OVCAR-3 human ovarian cancer cells. On OVACR-3 ovarian cancer cells, the chemical also caused G2/M phase cell cycle arrest. Additionally, it was shown that betulin might, in a concentration-dependent manner, prevent ovarian cancer cells from migrating and invading. According to the study by Yang *et al* (2021), the anti-cancer effects of the natural product betulin in OVCAR-3 human ovarian cancer cells are mediated by inducing apoptosis, arresting the cell cycle in the G2/M phase, inhibiting cell migration and invasion, and targeting the mTOR/PI3K/AKT signaling pathway (Yang *et al* 2021).

A natural substance called sanguinarine (SNG) has promising therapeutic promise against a number of malignancies. In this study, we investigated the molecular pathways that underlie SNG in NSCLC cells. Through down-regulation of the constitutively active JAK/STAT pathway in all of the NSCLC cell lines, SNG inhibited cell growth and triggered apoptosis. The JAK/STAT signaling cascade's participation was further supported by the siRNA suppression of STAT3 in NSCLC cells. The SNG therapy elevated the Bax/Bcl-2 ratio, which caused the mitochondrial membrane to leak, releasing cytochrome c and activating caspases. Additionally, we determined the anti-cancer effects of SNG through the generation of ROS, as decreasing ROS production inhibited the ability of SNG to induce apoptosis (Prabhu *et al* 2021).

In preclinical studies, the indole-2-carboxamide derivative LG25 efficiently attacked TNBC by causing cell cycle arrest and death and inhibiting the Akt/mTOR/NF-kB signaling pathway. According to our research, LG25 decreased TNBC viability in a dose-dependent way. LG25 promotes G2/M cell cycle arrest and induces cell death, according to flow cytometric and Western blot investigations. Additionally, Akt/mTOR phosphorylation and NF-kB nuclear translocation were both markedly reduced by LG25 therapy. Mice implanted with MDA-MB-231 TNBC cells verified these inhibitory actions of LG25 (Xu *et al* 2019).

8.5.4 Organosulfur compound

Garlic and its active ingredient have been shown to block angiogenesis, enhance the expression of tumor suppressor genes, cause cell cycle arrest at the G0/G1 phase and G2/M stages in cancer cells, and modulate a number of other genetic pathways (Almatroodi *et al* 2019).

In several tumor models, diallyl trisulfide (DATS), a significant organosulfur molecule produced from garlic, has demonstrated anti-carcinogenic properties. Additionally, DATS has been utilized therapeutically to treat *Helicobacter pylori* infection, the main contributor to stomach cancer. A framework for investigating DATS as a chemotherapeutic for human gastric cancer is provided by Jiang and colleagues. The study found that the DATS reduced cancer cell growth and caused cell cycle arrest in SGC-7901 cancer cells, which was accompanied by an increase in cyclin A2 and cyclin B1 expression. Additionally, DATS increased the number of apoptotic cell deaths, which resulted in an increase in cytochrome C, p53, and bax accumulations and a decrease in Bcl-2 expression. Apoptosis caused by DATS may also be mediated through mitogen-activated protein kinase (MAPK) pathways, according to the activation of JNK, ERK, and p38 phosphorylation in cells treated with DATS. In a xenograft model of gastric cancer cell SGC-7901, DATS greatly reduced tumor growth and encouraged tumor apoptosis (Jiang *et al* 2017).

Diallyl sulfide (DAS) and diallyl disulfide (DADS) possess strong antiproliferative and anti-cancer activities, according to numerous researches. By decreasing the survival of Caski cells and causing a dose-related increase in intracellular ROS generation as well as apoptosis, DAS and DADS had a strong antiproliferative effect on these cells. In Caski cells, DAS and DADS similarly caused cell cycle arrest in the G0/G1 phase, which was supported by the induction of CDK inhibitors p21WAF1/CIP1 and p27KIP1 and the up-regulation of cyclin D1 and CDK4. Additionally, DAS and DADS cause the viral oncogenes E6 and E7 to be down-regulated and the function of p53 to be restored (Ansari *et al* 2021).

From *Striga angustifolia* extracts, the organosulfur compound 5,5′-dithiobis(1-phenyl-1H-tetrazole) (COMP1) was isolated, and its structures were determined and described using single crystal x-ray powder diffraction (XRD), 13C and 1H nuclear magnetic resonance, and NMR. According to our research, COMP1 dramatically decreased breast and lung cancer cell proliferation but not that of non-malignant epithelial cells. Further investigation demonstrated that COMP1 increased lung cancer cells' cell cycle arrest and apoptosis. The mechanism by which COMP1 promotes p53 activity and suppresses mTOR signaling causes lung cancer cells to undergo cell cycle arrest and apoptosis by preventing cell proliferation. Our results imply that COMP1 may be a viable lung cancer treatment by controlling the p53/mTOR pathways (Raja *et al* 2023).

8.5.5 Nitrogen-containing compounds

A well-known and significant five-membered heterocyclic molecule with sulfur and nitrogen is called thiazole. Thiazole, a 5-membered distinctive heterocyclic motif with sulfur and nitrogen atoms, is one of the heterocyclic compounds and functions as the primary core scaffold in a number of crucial drugs. Some clinically used anti-cancer medications, including dasatinib, dabrafenib, ixabepilone, patellamide A, and epothilone, depend on the thiazole nucleus. Thiazole-containing substances have recently been created successfully as potential inhibitors of a number of biological targets, including enzyme-linked receptor(s) found on the cell membrane (i.e., polymerase inhibitors) and the cell cycle (i.e., microtubular inhibitors). Furthermore, these substances have been shown to have strong anti-cancer activity, high efficacy, and low toxicity (Sharma *et al* 2020).

Some of the synthesized compounds showed potent EGFR and HER-2 inhibition, and two series of thiazolidinone derivatives that may act as EGFR and HER-2 kinase inhibitors have been created. These thiazolidinone derivatives have high antiproliferative activity against MCF-7, according to antiproliferative assay results. Compound 12 in particular has shown significant EGFR and HER-2 inhibitory activity as well as inhibitory activity in inhibiting tumor growth, making it a potential anti-cancer agent (Lv *et al* 2010).

A summary of a few published research papers on the application of phytochemicals targeting various cell signaling pathways to inhibit tumor growth and proliferation is listed in table 8.1.

8.6 Conclusion and future prospective

Natural bioactive chemicals derived from medicinal plants have had a big impact on human health.

The identification of various new and more potent innovative bioactive pharmaceuticals derived from powerful medicinal plants was made possible by recent advancements in modern methodologies and superior instruments. This work may further contribute to the creation of formidable anti-cancer chemicals. Additionally, because of their therapeutic potential, they can be considered not only as prospective cancer treatments but also as promising and useful additional foods or nutraceuticals, which aid in both the prevention of disease and the treatment of it. Plant-based foods have anti-cancer effects in part thanks to phytochemicals. One potential mode of action for anti-cancer phytochemicals is the control of cellular signal transduction pathways, which affects cancer cell properties like proliferation, death, and invasion.

Bioactive chemicals, which are molecules that can function on a range of biochemical and signaling pathways, are abundant in plants. Recent studies examine the uniqueness and potency of therapeutic anti-cancer medicines obtained from plants. Additionally, it has been discovered that some medicinal plants and their bioactive substances have significant effects against a number of cancers, including breast cancer, lung cancer, leukemia, Hodgkin's lymphoma, follicular lymphoma, ovarian germ cell tumor, acute lymphoblastic leukemia, and others with a potential mechanism of action. Therefore, it is essential that more research into their identification or discovery be done in order to offer the public more effective and compliant medicinal treatments against cancer.

Despite the numerous significant benefits, some people are worried about the toxicity and safety of medical and herbal plants. Some therapeutic plants might cause allergies or injury to sensitive people as a whole, while in other instances, some sections of a plant may be poisonous but others may be edible. As a result, it is mandatory to conduct a toxicological evaluation of any medicinal or herbal plant in order to identify any side effects and establish the upper limits of exposure levels at which they are likely to manifest. Underestimating the toxicological difficulties brought on by using medications produced from medicinal plants could have major negative health effects (Siddiqui 2022). Despite their excellent anticancer activity, the phytochemicals are limited by their low aqueous solubility, poor bioavailability,

Table 8.1. Role of phytochemicals in cancer study as an anti-cancer agent.

Phytochemical class	Phytochemical	Cancer	Targeted signaling pathway	Study-*In vitro*/*In vivo*	Outcome	References
Alkaloid	Flavopereirine	Colorectal Cancer	P53 Signaling	*In vitro* (CRC cell lines); *In vivo* (HCT116-bearing mice)	Growth suppression	Li *et al* (2019)
	Chaetoglobosin K	Ovarian cancer	p53-dependent pathway	*In vitro* (OVCAR-3 and A2780/CP70 cell lines)	Induced preferential apoptosis and G2 cell cycle arrest	Li *et al* (2015)
	1, 4-dihydro indeno [1,2-c] Pyrazole	Cancer	p53-dependent pathway	*In vitro* (HeLa, A549, and MDA-MB-231)	Induce apoptosis	Khan *et al* (2018)
	Evodiamine	Hepatocellular cancer	NOD1	*In vitro* (SMMC-7721 and HepG2 Cells); *In vivo* (HepG2 cells containing BALB/c nude mice)	Induce apoptosis and shows inhibitory effect	Guo *et al* (2018)
	Hapalindole H	Prostate cancer	NF-κB	*In vitro* (PC-3 cell line)	Induce apoptosis	Acuña *et al* (2018)
	11-methoxytabersonine	Acute lymphoblastic leukemia	PI3K/Akt	*In vitro* (cell line MOLT-4)	Induce cell apoptosis	Wang *et al* (2022)
	Staurosporine	Hepatocellular carcinom	PI3K/Akt	*In vitro* (HepG2 cell line)	Decreased cell viability and increased cell apoptosis	Ding *et al* (2017)

	Brucine	Cervical cancer	PI3K/AKT/mTOR	*In vitro* (ME-180 cell line)	Supressed inflammation and cell proliferation	Seshadri (2021)
	Meisoindigo	Glioblastoma	PI3K/Akt	*In vitro* (glioblastoma U87 cells)	Inhibits cellular proliferation	Zhou *et al* (2021)
	Flavopereirine	Breast cancer	AKT/p38 MAPK/ ERK1/2	*In vitro* (MDA-MB-231 cells)	Induces cell cycle arrest and apoptosis	Yeh *et al* (2019)
	L20 (Calothrixin B analog)	Erythroleukemia	ROS/γ-H2AX/p38 MAPK	*In vitro* (HEL cells)	Induce cell apoptosis	Long *et al* (2021)
	Spirooxindole derivative SOID-8	Melanoma	JAK2/STAT3	*In vitro* (A2058, A375, SK-MEL-5 and SK-MEL-28)	Induce cell apoptosis	Tian *et al* (2012)
Polyphenol	Quercetin	Breast cancer	EGFR/PI3K/Akt	*In vitro* (MCF-7 and MDA-MB-231)	Induce cell apoptosis	Balakrishnan *et al* (2017)
	LYG-202	Breast cancer	PI3K/Akt	*In vitro* (MCF-7, MDA-MB-231 and MDA-MB-435 cells)	Induced apoptosis and cell cycle arrest	Zhao *et al* (2015)
	Kaempferol	Bladder cancer	(PTEN)/PI3K/Akt	*In vitro* (EJ and T24 cells)	Induced apoptosis	Xie *et al* (2013)
	Kaempferol	Cervical cancer	PI3K/AKT and telomerase pathways	*In vitro* (HeLa cell)	Induced apoptosis	Kashafi *et al* (2017)
	Flavonoid N101–2	Cervical cancer	PI3K/AKT	*In vitro* (CaSki and SiHa)	Induced apoptosis	Kim *et al* (2012)
	Apigenin	Choriocarcinoma	PI3K/AKT and ERK1/2 MAPK	*In vitro* (JAR and JEG3)	Induced apoptosis	Lim *et al* (2016)

(*Continued*)

Table 8.1. (*Continued*)

Phytochemical class	Phytochemical	Cancer	Targeted signaling pathway	Study-*In vitro*/*In vivo*	Outcome	References
	Wogonin	Leukemia	PI3K-AKT	*In vitro* (HL-60)	Induced apoptosis	Hu *et al* (2015)
	Myricetin	Pancreatic cancer	PI3K	*In vitro* (MIA PaCa-2, Panc-1 or S2–013)	Induced apoptosis	Phillips *et al* (2011)
	Artocarpin	Non-small cell lung cancer cells	MAPKs and Akt	*In vitro* (A549, H226 and H1299 cells)	Induced apoptosis	Tsai *et al* (2019)
	Hispidulin	Pancreatic cancer	PI3K/Akt/mTOR	*Ex vivo* (PANC-1, PANC-28 and BxPC-3) and *in vivo* (PANC-1 cells injected male BALB/cA)	Suppresses the angiogenesis and growth of cell	He *et al* (2011)
	Pro-EGCG	Endometrial cancer	PI3K/AKT/mTOR/HIF1α	Xenograft models	Inhibit angiogenesis	Wang *et al* (2018)
	Flavonoid	Breast cancer	PI3K/AKT/ERK	*In vitro* (MDA-MB-231 cells) and Xenograft models	Inhibits angiogenesis and metastasis	Chang *et al* (2016)
	Flavonoid glycoside	Cancer metastatic	STAT3/NF-κB/COX-2 and EGFR	*In vitro* (A549 cells)	Interrupts metastatic	Shi *et al* (2017)
	LFG-500 (synthesized)	Melanoma	PI3K/AKT/NF-κB	*In vitro* (MDA-MB-231) and *in vivo* (C57BL/6 mice B16F10 murine melanoma cells)	Inhibit cancer cell invasion	Li *et al* (2014)

Terpenoids	Corosolic acid	Colorectal cancer	Caspase-dependent pathway	*In vitro* (HCT116)	Induced apoptosis	Sung *et al* (2014)
	Zerumbone	Gastric cancer	NF-κB	*In vitro* (AGS)	Inhibiting angiogenesis	Tsuboi *et al* (2014)
	Brusatol	Nasopharyngeal carcinoma	Akt/mTOR	*In vitro* (NPC cell lines); *in vivo* (CNE-1 xenografts mouse)	Inhibited the growth of CNE-1 xenografts	Guo *et al* (2020)
	Brusatol	Acute myeloid leukemia	Nrf2 pathway	*In vitro* (HL-60 and THP-1 cells); *in vivo* (xenografts mouse)	Inhibit cell growth	Cheng *et al* (2021)
	Oleanolic acid	Bladder cancer	Akt/mTOR/S6K and ERK1/2	*In vitro* (T24 cells)	Suppresses tumor cell proliferation	Mu *et al* (2015)
	Ursolic and oleanolic acids	Lung cancer	AKT/mTOR pathways	*In vitro* (A549 cell)	Induce mitophagy	Castrejón-Jiménez *et al* (2019)
	Oleanolic acid	Cancer	ERK/Nrf2/ROS pathway	*In vitro* (A549 and PANC1); *in vivo* (BALB/c mice with A549 cells)	Induce apoptosis	Liu *et al* (2016)
	Ursolic acid	Breast cancer	Nrf2 pathway	*In vitro* (MDA-MB-231 cells)	Inhibit tumor cell proliferation	Zhang *et al* (2020)
	Dioscin	Lung cancer	PI3K/Akt and ERK and JNK	*In vitro* (A549 and H1299 cells)	Induce autophagy	Hsieh *et al* (2013)
Organosulfur compounds	Benzylic organotrisulfides	Breast cancer	Wnt/β-catenin	*In vitro* (MDA-MB-231 cells)	Tumor cell growth inhibition	Bhattacherjee *et al* (2022)
	Diallyl sulfide and diallyl disulfide	Cervical cancer	p21WAF1/CIP1 and p27KIP1	*In vitro* (Caski)		Ansari *et al* (2021)

(*Continued*)

Table 8.1. (*Continued*)

Phytochemical class	Phytochemical	Cancer	Targeted signaling pathway	Study-*In vitro*/*In vivo*	Outcome	References
					Induce apoptosis and cell cycle arrest	
	Diallyl trisulfide	Breast cancer	CCL2/MCP-1	*In vitro* (MDA-MB-231)	Inhibit breast carcinogenesis	Kanga *et al* (2021)
	Diallyl trisulfide	Breast cancer	Wnt/β-catenin pathway	*In vitro* (MCF-7 and SUM159)	Inhibit stem cell growth	Li *et al* (2018)
	Diallyl disulfide	Breast cancer	β-Catenin signaling	*In vitro* (MDA-MB-231, MDA-MB-468, and BT-549); *In vivo* (MDA-MB-231 xenograft mice)	Inhibits growth and metastatic potential	Huang *et al* (2015)
	Diallyl disulfide	Breast cancer	MMP-9	*In vitro* (MCF-7 and MDA-MB-231 cells); *In vivo* (MCF-7 and MDA-MB-231 xenograft mice)	Inhibiting the progression of cancer	Xiong *et al* (2018)

and poor penetration into cells, hepatic disposition, narrow therapeutic index, and rapid uptake by normal tissues. The efficacy of the phytochemicals in vivo studies is limited by parameters such as solubility, metabolic degradation, excretion, etc (Rizwanullah M *et al* 2018). Various approaches have now been devised to circumvent these limitations. Recently, chemical modification of phytochemicals is demonstrated to reduce some of the limitations and improve their efficacy. Similar to traditional medicines several combinatorial phytochemical formulations have shown to be more efficient. Further, phytochemicals have been reported to be even more efficient in the form of nanoparticles. However, systematic evaluation of their efficacy, mode of action in pathway modulation, usage, and associated challenges is required to be done. Furthermore, phytochemicals combined with chemotherapeutic agents could target the crosstalk among multiple signal cascades to block chemo-resistance and attenuate carcinogenic properties, and can be considered a novel and potential therapeutic strategy (Zheng Z *et al* 2022).

Acknowledgments

Authors thank their respective organizations for providing infrastructure facilities for book chapter writing.

References

Abdullah M L, Al-Shabanah O, Hassan Z K and Hafez M M 2021 Eugenol-induced autophagy and apoptosis in breast cancer cells via PI3K/AKT/FOXO3a pathway inhibition *Int. J. Mol. Sci.* **22** 9243

Acar A, Simões B M, Clarke R B and Brennan K 2016 A role for notch signalling in breast cancer and endocrine resistance *Stem Cells Int.* **2016** 2498764

Acuña U M, Mo S, Zi J, Orjala J and de Blanco E J 2018 Hapalindole H induces apoptosis as an inhibitor of NF-κB and affects the intrinsic mitochondrial pathway in PC-3 androgen-insensitive prostate cancer cells *Anticancer Res.* **38** 3299–07

Ahmad I, Fakhri S, Khan H, Jeandet P, Aschner M and Yu Z L 2020 Targeting cell cycle by β-carboline alkaloids *in vitro*: novel therapeutic prospects for the treatment of cancer *Chem. Biol. Interact.* **330** 109229

Ahmed M B, Islam S U, Alghamdi A A, Kamran M, Ahsan H and Lee Y S 2022 Phytochemicals as chemo-preventive agents and signaling molecule modulators: current role in cancer therapeutics and inflammation *Int. J. Mol. Sci.* **23** 15765

Al-Ishaq R K, Overy A J and Büsselberg D 2020 Phytochemicals and gastrointestinal cancer: cellular mechanisms and effects to change cancer progression *Biomolecules* **10** 105

Almatroodi S A, Alsahli M A, Almatroudi A and Rahmani A H 2019 Garlic and its active compounds: a potential candidate in the prevention of cancer by modulating various cell signalling pathways *Anticancer Agents Med. Chem. (Formerly Curr. Med. Chem.-Anti-Cancer Agents)* **19** 1314–24

Ansari I A, Ahmad A, Imran M A, Saeed M and Ahmad I 2021 Organosulphur compounds induce apoptosis and cell cycle arrest in cervical cancer cells via downregulation of HPV E6 and E7 oncogenes *Anticancer Agents Med. Chem. (Formerly Curr. Med. Chem.-Anti-Cancer Agents)* **21** 393–405

Ansari I A and Akhtar M S 2019 Current insights on the role of terpenoids as anticancer agents: a perspective on cancer prevention and treatment *Natural Bio-Active Compounds, Volume 2: Chemistry, Pharmacology and Health Care Practices* (Berlin: Springer) pp 53–80

Babina I S and Turner N C 2017 Advances and challenges in targeting FGFR signalling in cancer *Nat. Rev. Cancer* **17** 318–2

Bagla V P, Mokgotho M P and Mampuru L J 2015 Phytochemicals and cancer—possible molecular targets of phytochemicals in cancer prevention and therapy *Phytochemicals: Isolation, Characterisation and Role in Human Health* ed V Rao and L Rao (Books on Demand)

Bajalia E M, Azzouz F B, Chism D A, Giansiracusa D M, Wong C G, Plaskett K N and Bishayee A 2022 Phytochemicals for the prevention and treatment of renal cell carcinoma: preclinical and clinical evidence and molecular mechanisms *Cancers* **14** 3278

Balakrishnan S, Mukherjee S, Das S, Bhat F A, Raja Singh P, Patra C R and Arunakaran J 2017 Gold nanoparticles–conjugated quercetin induces apoptosis via inhibition of EGFR/PI3K/Akt–mediated pathway in breast cancer cell lines (MCF-7 and MDA-MB-231) *Cell Biochem. Funct.* **35** 217–31

Basu S, Haase G and Ben-Ze'ev A 2016 Wnt signaling in cancer stem cells and colon cancer metastasis *F1000Research* **5** 699

Bhattacherjee D, Raina K, Mandal T K, Thummer R P and Bhabak K P 2022 Targeting Wnt/β-catenin signaling pathway in triple-negative breast cancer by benzylic organotrisulfides: contribution of the released hydrogen sulfide towards potent anti-cancer activity *Free Radical Biol. Med.* **191** 82–96

Braakhuis A J, Campion P and Bishop K S 2016 Reducing breast cancer recurrence: the role of dietary polyphenolics *Nutrients* **8** 547

Braicu C *et al* 2019 A comprehensive review on MAPK: a promising therapeutic target in cancer *Cancers* **11** 1618

Carter E P, Coetzee A S, Tomas Bort E, Wang Q, Kocher H M and Grose R P 2021 Dissecting FGF signalling to target cellular crosstalk in pancreatic cancer *Cells* **10** 847

Castrejón-Jiménez N S *et al* 2019 Ursolic and oleanolic acids induce mitophagy in A549 human lung cancer cells *Molecules* **24** 3444

Chang C H, Ou T T, Yang M Y, Huang C C and Wang C J 2016 *Nelumbo nucifera* Gaertn leaves extract inhibits the angiogenesis and metastasis of breast cancer cells by downregulation connective tissue growth factor (CTGF) mediated PI3K/AKT/ERK signaling *J. Ethnopharmacol.* **188** 111–22

Chen C Y, Kao C L and Liu C M 2018 The cancer prevention, anti-inflammatory and anti-oxidation of bioactive phytochemicals targeting the TLR4 signaling pathway *Int. J. Mol. Sci.* **19** 2729

Chen H and Liu R H 2018 Potential mechanisms of action of dietary phytochemicals for cancer prevention by targeting cellular signaling transduction pathways *J. Agric. Food Chem.* **66** 3260–76

Cheng C, Yuan F, Chen X P, Zhang W, Zhao X L, Jiang Z P, Zhou H H, Zhou G and Cao S 2021 Inhibition of Nrf2-mediated glucose metabolism by brusatol synergistically sensitizes acute myeloid leukemia to Ara-C *Biomed. Pharmacother.* **142** 111652

Chirumbolo S, Bjørklund G, Lysiuk R, Vella A, Lenchyk L and Upyr T 2018 Targeting cancer with phytochemicals via their fine tuning of the cell survival signaling pathways *Int. J. Mol. Sci.* **19** 3568

Choi W Y, Kim G Y, Lee W H and Choi Y H 2008 Sanguinarine, a benzophenanthridine alkaloid, induces apoptosis in MDA-MB-231 human breast carcinoma cells through a reactive oxygen species-mediated mitochondrial pathway *Chemotherapy* **54** 279–87

Criscitiello C, Esposito A and Curigliano G 2017 Targeting FGFR pathway in breast cancer *Breast Cancer: Innovations in Research and Management* (Berlin: Springer) pp 819–22

Dandawate P, Padhye S, Ahmad A and Sarkar F H 2013 Novel strategies targeting cancer stem cells through phytochemicals and their analogs *Drug Deliv. Transl. Res.* **3** 165–82

Dandawate P R, Subramaniam D, Jensen R A and Anant S 2016 Targeting cancer stem cells and signaling pathways by phytochemicals: novel approach for breast cancer therapy *Seminars in Cancer Biology* (New York: Academic)vol 40 pp 192–208

Darvin P *et al* 2017 Tannic acid inhibits EGFR/STAT 1/3 and enhances p38/STAT 1 signalling axis in breast cancer cells *J. Cell. Mol. Med.* **21** 720–34

Dey P, Kundu A, Chakraborty H J, Kar B, Choi W S, Lee B M, Bhakta T, Atanasov A G and Kim H S 2019 Therapeutic value of steroidal alkaloids in cancer: current trends and future perspectives *Int. J. Cancer* **145** 1731–44

Ding Y, Wang B, Chen X, Zhou Y and Ge J 2017 Staurosporine suppresses survival of HepG2 cancer cells through Omi/HtrA2-mediated inhibition of PI3K/Akt signaling pathway *Tumor Biol.* **39** 1010428317694317

Edeling M, Ragi G, Huang S, Pavenstädt H and Susztak K 2016 Developmental signalling pathways in renal fibrosis: the roles of Notch, Wnt and Hedgehog *Nat. Rev. Nephrol.* **12** 426–39

Espinosa-Sánchez A, Suárez-Martínez E, Sánchez-Díaz L and Carnero A 2020 Therapeutic targeting of signaling pathways related to cancer stemness *Front. Oncol.* **10** 1533

Faes S, Demartines N and Dormond O 2021 Mechanistic target of rapamycin inhibitors in renal cell carcinoma: potential, limitations, and perspectives *Front. Cell Dev. Biol.* **9** 636037

Farhan M, Wang H, Gaur U, Little P J, Xu J and Zheng W 2017 FOXO signaling pathways as therapeutic targets in cancer *Int. J. Biol. Sci.* **13** 815

Francavilla C and O'Brien C S 2022 Fibroblast growth factor receptor signalling dysregulation and targeting in breast cancer *Open Biol.* **12** 210373

Gallorini M, Cataldi A and di Giacomo V 2012 Cyclin-dependent kinase modulators and cancer therapy *BioDrugs* **26** 377–91

Ghosh N, Hossain U, Mandal A and Sil P C 2019 The Wnt signaling pathway: a potential therapeutic target against cancer *Ann. N.Y. Acad. Sci.* **1443** 54–74

Gu S, Yang X C, Xiang X Y, Wu Y A, Zhang Y U, Yan X Y, Xue Y N, Sun L K and Shao G G 2015 Sanguinarine-induced apoptosis in lung adenocarcinoma cells is dependent on reactive oxygen species production and endoplasmic reticulum stress *Oncol. Rep.* **34** 913–9

Guo S, Zhang J, Wei C, Lu Z, Cai R, Pan D, Zhang H, Liang B and Zhang Z 2020 Anticancer effects of brusatol in nasopharyngeal carcinoma through suppression of the Akt/mTOR signaling pathway *Cancer Chemother. Pharmacol.* **85** 1097–8

Guo X X *et al* 2018 Evodiamine induces apoptosis in SMMC-7721 and HepG2 cells by suppressing NOD1 signal pathway *Int. J. Mol. Sci.* **19** 3419

Hashem S *et al* 2022 Targeting cancer signaling pathways by natural products: exploring promising anti-cancer agents *Biomed. Pharmacother.* **150** 113054

Hata A N, Engelman J A and Faber A C 2015 The BCL2 family: key mediators of the apoptotic response to targeted anticancer therapeuticsbcl2 family and targeted therapies *Cancer Discov.* **5** 475–87

He L, Wu Y, Lin L, Wang J, Wu Y, Chen Y, Yi Z, Liu M and Pang X 2011 Hispidulin, a small flavonoid molecule, suppresses the angiogenesis and growth of human pancreatic cancer by targeting vascular endothelial growth factor receptor 2-mediated PI3K/Akt/mTOR signaling pathway *Cancer Sci.* **102** 219–25

He S and Tang S 2020 WNT/β-catenin signaling in the development of liver cancers *Biomed. Pharmacother.* **132** 110851

Hegab A E *et al* 2019 Effect of FGF/FGFR pathway blocking on lung adenocarcinoma and its cancer-associated fibroblasts *J. Pathol.* **249** 193–205

Hibdon E S, Razumilava N, Keeley T M, Wong G, Solanki S, Shah Y M and Samuelson L C 2019 Notch and mTOR signaling pathways promote human gastric cancer cell proliferation *Neoplasia* **21** 702–12

Hsieh M J, Tsai T L, Hsieh Y S, Wang C J and Chiou H L 2013 Dioscin-induced autophagy mitigates cell apoptosis through modulation of PI3K/Akt and ERK and JNK signaling pathways in human lung cancer cell lines *Arch. Toxicol.* **87** 1927–37

Hu C, Xu M, Qin R, Chen W and Xu X 2015 Wogonin induces apoptosis and endoplasmic reticulum stress in HL-60 leukemia cells through inhibition of the PI3K-AKT signaling pathway *Oncol Rep.* **33** 3146–54

Huang J, Yang B, Xiang T, Peng W, Qiu Z, Wan J, Zhang L, Li H, Li H and Ren G 2015 Diallyl disulfide inhibits growth and metastatic potential of human triple-negative breast cancer cells through inactivation of the β-catenin signaling pathway *Mol. Nutr. Food Res.* **59** 1063–75

Hussain Y, Khan H, Alam W, Aschner M, Alsharif K F and Saso L 2022 Flavonoids targeting the mTOR signaling cascades in cancer: a potential crosstalk in anti-breast cancer therapy *Oxid. Med. Cell. Longev.* **2022** 4831833

Inoue-Yamauchi A *et al* 2017 Targeting the differential addiction to anti-apoptotic BCL-2 family for cancer therapy *Nat. Commun.* **8** 16078

Issinger O G and Guerra B 2021 Phytochemicals in cancer and their effect on the PI3K/AKT-mediated cellular signalling *Biomed. Pharmacother.* **139** 111650

Jain D *et al* 2021 Roles of therapeutic bioactive compounds in hepatocellular carcinoma *Oxidative Med. Cell. Longev.* **2021** 9068850

Jiang Q W, Chen M W, Cheng K J, Yu P Z, Wei X and Shi Z 2016 Therapeutic potential of steroidal alkaloids in cancer and other diseases *Med. Res. Rev.* **36** 119–43

Jiang X, Zhu X, Huang W, Xu H, Zhao Z, Li S, Li S, Cai J and Cao J 2017 Garlic-derived organosulfur compound exerts antitumor efficacy via activation of MAPK pathway and modulation of cytokines in SGC-7901 tumor-bearing mice *Int. Immunopharmacol.* **48** 135–45

Juaid N, Amin A, Abdalla A, Reese K, Alamri Z, Moulay M, Abdu S and Miled N 2021 Anti-hepatocellular carcinoma biomolecules: molecular targets insights *Int. J. Mol. Sci.* **22** 10774

Kamdje A H, Etet P F, Vecchio L, Muller J M, Krampera M and Lukong K E 2014 Signaling pathways in breast cancer: therapeutic targeting of the microenvironment *Cell. Signal.* **26** 2843–56

Kamga P T *et al* 2016 Notch signalling drives bone marrow stromal cell-mediated chemo-resistance in acute myeloid leukemia *Oncotarget* **7** 21713

Kang X, Lin Z, Xu M, Pan J and Wang Z W 2019 Deciphering role of FGFR signalling pathway in pancreatic cancer *Cell Prolif.* **52** e12605

Kanga K J, Mendonca P, Soliman K F, Ferguson D T and Darling-Reed S F 2021 Effect of diallyl trisulfide on TNF-α-induced CCL2/MCP-1 release in genetically different triple-negative breast cancer cells *Anticancer Res.* **41** 5919–33

Kashafi E, Moradzadeh M, Mohamadkhani A and Erfanian S 2017 Kaempferol increases apoptosis in human cervical cancer HeLa cells via PI3K/AKT and telomerase pathways *Biomed. Pharmacother.* **89** 573–7

Khan A Q *et al* 2020 Sanguinarine induces apoptosis in papillary thyroid cancer cells via generation of reactive oxygen species *Molecules.* **25** 1229

Khan H *et al* 2020 Targeting NF-κB signaling pathway in cancer by dietary polyphenols *Crit. Rev. Food Sci. Nutr.* **60** 2790–800

Khan I, Garikapati K R, Shaik A B, Makani V K, Rahim A, Shareef M A, Reddy V G, Pal-Bhadra M, Kamal A and Kumar C G 2018 Design, synthesis and biological evaluation of 1,4-dihydro indeno [1,2-c] pyrazole linked oxindole analogues as potential anticancer agents targeting tubulin and inducing p53 dependent apoptosis *Eur. J. Med. Chem.* **144** 104–15

Kim J H, Kang J W, Kim M S, Bak Y, Park Y S, Jung K Y, Lim Y H and Yoon D Y 2012 The apoptotic effects of the flavonoid N101-2 in human cervical cancer cells *Toxicol. In Vitro* **26** 67–73

Kim M S, Kang H J and Moon A 2001 Inhibition of invasion and induction of apoptosis by curcumin in H-ras-transformed MCF10A human breast epithelial cells *Arch. Pharmacal Res.* **24** 349–54

Lachej N, Jonušienė V, Mažeikė A, Sasnauskienė A, Dabkevičienė D, Šimienė J, Sužiedėlis K and Didžiapetrienė J 2019 Changes in the expression of notch and Wnt signalling molecules in human endometrial cancer *Acta Med. Litu.* **26** 181

Lamy M, Ferreira A, Dias J S, Braga S, Silva G and Barbas A 2017 Notch-out for breast cancer therapies *New Biotechnol.* **39** 215–21

Leverson J D *et al* 2015 Exploiting selective BCL-2 family inhibitors to dissect cell survival dependencies and define improved strategies for cancer therapy *Sci. Transl. Med.* **7** 279ra40

Li B, Gao Y, Rankin G O, Rojanasakul Y, Cutler S J, Tu Y and Chen Y C 2015 Chaetoglobosin K induces apoptosis and G2 cell cycle arrest through p53-dependent pathway in cisplatin-resistant ovarian cancer cells *Cancer Lett.* **356** 418–33

Li C, Li F, Zhao K, Yao J, Cheng Y, Zhao L, Li Z, Lu N and Guo Q 2014 LFG-500 inhibits the invasion of cancer cells via down-regulation of PI3K/AKT/NF-κB signaling pathway *PLoS One* **9** e91332

Li D D, Zhao C H, Ding H W, Wu Q, Ren T S, Wang J, Chen C Q and Zhao Q C 2018 A novel inhibitor of ADAM 17 sensitizes colorectal cancer cells to 5-fluorouracil by reversing Notch and epithelial-mesenchymal transition *in vitro* and *in vivo Cell Prolif.* **51** e12480

Li J M, Huang Y C, Kuo Y H, Cheng C C, Kuan F C, Chang S F, Lee Y R, Chin C C and Shi C S 2019 Flavopereirine suppresses the growth of colorectal cancer cells through P53 signaling dependence *Cancers* **11** 1034

Li X, Meng Y, Xie C, Zhu J, Wang X, Li Y, Geng S, Wu J, Zhong C and Li M 2018 Diallyl Trisulfide inhibits breast cancer stem cells via suppression of Wnt/β-catenin pathway *J. Cell. Biochem.* **119** 4134–41

Li X, Wu C, Chen N, Gu H, Yen A, Cao L, Wang E and Wang L 2016 PI3K/Akt/mTOR signaling pathway and targeted therapy for glioblastoma *Oncotarget* **7** 33440

Lim J S *et al* 2017 Intratumoural heterogeneity generated by Notch signalling promotes small-cell lung cancer *Nature* **545** 360–4

Lim W, Park S, Bazer F W and Song G 2016 Apigenin reduces survival of choriocarcinoma cells by inducing apoptosis via the PI3K/AKT and ERK1/2 MAPK pathways *J. Cell. Physiol.* **231** 2690–9

Liskova A, Kubatka P, Samec M, Zubor P, Mlyncek M, Bielik T, Samuel S M, Zulli A, Kwon T K and Büsselberg D 2019 Dietary phytochemicals targeting cancer stem cells *Molecules* **24** 899

Liu H T and Ho Y S 2018 Anticancer effect of curcumin on breast cancer and stem cells *Food Sci. Hum. Wellness* **7** 134–7

Liu J, Ma L, Chen X, Wang J, Yu T, Gong Y, Ma A, Zheng L and Liang H 2016 ERK inhibition sensitizes cancer cells to oleanolic acid-induced apoptosis through ERK/Nrf2/ROS pathway *Tumor Biol.* **37** 8181–7

Liu L J, Xie S X, Chen Y T, Xue J L, Zhang C J and Zhu F 2016 Aberrant regulation of Wnt signaling in hepatocellular carcinoma *World J. Gastroenterol.* **22** 7486

Long Q *et al* 2021 L20, a Calothrixin B analog, induces intrinsic apoptosis on HEL cells through ROS/γ-H2AX/p38 MAPK pathway *Biomed. Pharmacother.* **137** 111336

Lu J, Xia Y, Chen K, Zheng Y, Wang J, Lu W, Yin Q, Wang F, Zhou Y and Guo C 2016 Oncogenic role of the notch pathway in primary liver cancer (review) *Oncol Lett.* **12** 3–10 (Corrigendum)

Lv P C, Zhou C F, Chen J, Liu P G, Wang K R, Mao W J, Li H Q, Yang Y, Xiong J and Zhu H L 2010 Design, synthesis and biological evaluation of thiazolidinone derivatives as potential EGFR and HER-2 kinase inhibitors *Bioorg. Med. Chem.* **18** 314–9

McCarter A C, Wang Q and Chiang M 2018 Notch in leukemia *Molecular Mechanisms of Notch Signaling* (Cham: Springer) pp 355–94

Moloney J N and Cotter T G 2018 ROS signalling in the biology of cancer *Seminars in Cell and Developmental Biology* (New York: Academic)vol 80 pp 50–64

Mondal A, Gandhi A, Fimognari C, Atanasov A G and Bishayee A 2019 Alkaloids for cancer prevention and therapy: current progress and future perspectives *Eur. J. Pharmacol.* **858** 172472

Mu D W, Guo H Q, Zhou G B, Li J Y and Su B 2015 Oleanolic acid suppresses the proliferation of human bladder cancer by Akt/mTOR/S6K and ERK1/2 signaling *Int. J. Clin. Exp. Pathol.* **8** 13864

Murillo-Garzón V and Kypta R 2017 WNT signalling in prostate cancer *Nat. Rev. Urol.* **14** 683–96

O'Brien R and Marignol L 2017 The Notch-1 receptor in prostate tumorigenesis *Cancer Treat. Rev.* **56** 36–46

Pacini L, Jenks A D, Lima N C and Huang P H 2021 Targeting the fibroblast growth factor receptor (FGFR) family in lung cancer *Cells* **10** 1154

Pallichankandy S, Rahman A, Thayyullathil F and Galadari S 2015 ROS-dependent activation of autophagy is a critical mechanism for the induction of anti-glioma effect of sanguinarine *Free Radical Biol. Med.* **89** 708–20

Perez-Garcia J, Muñoz-Couselo E, Soberino J, Racca F and Cortes J 2018 Targeting FGFR pathway in breast cancer *Breast* **37** 126–33

Pham D C, Shibu M A, Mahalakshmi B and Velmurugan B K 2020 Effects of phytochemicals on cellular signaling: reviewing their recent usage approaches *Crit. Rev. Food Sci. Nutr.* **60** 3522–46

Phillips P A, Sangwan V, Borja-Cacho D, Dudeja V, Vickers S M and Saluja A K 2011 Myricetin induces pancreatic cancer cell death via the induction of apoptosis and inhibition of the phosphatidylinositol 3-kinase (PI3K) signaling pathway *Cancer Lett.* **308** 181–8

Pohl S G, Brook N, Agostino M, Arfuso F, Kumar A P and Dharmarajan A 2017 Wnt signaling in triple-negative breast cancer *Oncogenesis* **6** e310

Prabhu K S *et al* 2021 Sanguinarine mediated apoptosis in non-small cell lung cancer via generation of reactive oxygen species and suppression of JAK/STAT pathway *Biomed. Pharmacother.* **144** 112358

Pu Z, Yang F, Wang L, Diao Y and Chen D 2021 Advancements of compounds targeting Wnt and Notch signalling pathways in the treatment of inflammatory bowel disease and colon cancer *J. Drug Target.* **29** 507–19

Rahman M M *et al* 2022 Exploring the recent trends in perturbing the cellular signaling pathways in cancer by natural products *Front. Pharmacol.* **13** 950109

Raja K, Vignesh A, Lavanya P, Ravi M, Selvakumar S and Vasanth K 2023 Organosulfur compound identified from *Striga angustifolia* (D. Don) CJ saldanha inhibits lung cancer growth and induces apoptosis via p53/mtor signaling pathway *Appl. Biochem. Biotechnol.* 1–21 at press

Ravindran J, Prasad S and Aggarwal B B 2009 Curcumin and cancer cells: how many ways can curry kill tumor cells selectively? *AAPS J.* **11** 495–510

Rizwanullah M, Amin S, Mir S R, Fakhri K U and Rizvi M M 2018 Phytochemical based nanomedicines against cancer: current status and future prospects *J. Drug Target.* **26** 731–52

Rodriguez-Vida A *et al* 2015 Complexity of FGFR signalling in metastatic urothelial cancer *J. Hematol. Oncol.* **8** 1–8

Sanchez-Vega F *et al* 2018 Oncogenic signaling pathways in the cancer genome atlas *Cell* **173** 321–37

Sarkar B, Ullah M A, Islam S S, Rahman M H and Araf Y 2021 Analysis of plant-derived phytochemicals as anti-cancer agents targeting cyclin dependent kinase-2, human topoisomerase IIa and vascular endothelial growth factor receptor-2 *J. Recept. Signal Transduct. Res.* **41** 217–33

Seshadri V D 2021 Brucine promotes apoptosis in cervical cancer cells (ME-180) via suppression of inflammation and cell proliferation by regulating PI3K/AKT/mTOR signaling pathway *Environ. Toxicol.* **36** 1841–7

Shahi Thakuri P, Gupta M, Singh S, Joshi R, Glasgow E, Lekan A, Agarwal S, Luker G D and Tavana H 2020 Phytochemicals inhibit migration of triple negative breast cancer cells by targeting kinase signaling *BMC Cancer* **20** 1–4

Shang C, Lang B and Meng L R 2018 Blocking NOTCH pathway can enhance the effect of EGFR inhibitor through targeting CD133+ endometrial cancer cells *Cancer Biol. Therap.* **19** 113–9

Sharma P C, Bansal K K, Sharma A, Sharma D and Deep A 2020 Thiazole-containing compounds as therapeutic targets for cancer therapy *Eur. J. Med. Chem.* **188** 112016

Shi Q, Jiang Z, Yang J, Cheng Y, Pang Y, Zheng N, Chen J, Chen W and Jia L 2017 A flavonoid glycoside compound from Murraya paniculata (L.) interrupts metastatic characteristics of A549 cells by regulating STAT3/NF-κB/COX-2 and EGFR signaling pathways *AAPS J.* **19** 1779–90

Siddiqui A J *et al* 2022 Plants in anticancer drug discovery: from molecular mechanism to chemoprevention *BioMed Res. Int.* **2022** 5425485

Sohel M, Aktar S, Biswas P, Amin M A, Hossain M A, Ahmed N, Mim M I, Islam F and Mamun A A 2023 Exploring the anti-cancer potential of dietary phytochemicals for the patients with breast cancer: a comprehensive review *Cancer Med.* **12** 14556–83

Song X, Zhang M, Dai E and Luo Y 2019 Molecular targets of curcumin in breast cancer *Mol. Med. Rep.* **19** 23–9

Soylu H, Acar N, Ozbey O, Unal B, Koksal I T, Bassorgun I, Ciftcioglu A and Ustunel I 2016 Characterization of Notch signalling pathway members in normal prostate, prostatic intraepithelial neoplasia (PIN) and prostatic adenocarcinoma *Pathol. Oncol. Res.* **22** 87–94

Sun L R, Zhou W, Zhang H M, Guo Q S, Yang W, Li B J, Sun Z H, Gao S H and Cui R J 2019 Modulation of multiple signaling pathways of the plant-derived natural products in cancer *Front. Oncol.* **9** 1153

Sundaram M K, Khan M A, Alalami U, Somvanshi P, Bhardwaj T, Pramodh S, Raina R, Shekfeh Z, Haque S and Hussain A 2020 Phytochemicals induce apoptosis by modulation of nitric oxide signaling pathway in cervical cancer cells *Eur. Rev. Med. Pharmacol. Sci.* **24** 11827–44

Sung B, Kang Y J, Kim D H, Hwang S Y, Lee Y, Kim M, Yoon J H, Kim C M, Chung H Y and Kim N D 2014 Corosolic acid induces apoptotic cell death in HCT116 human colon cancer cells through a caspase-dependent pathway *Int. J. Mol. Med.* **33** 943–9

Tan H K, Moad A I and Tan M L 2014 The mTOR signalling pathway in cancer and the potential mTOR inhibitory activities of natural phytochemicals *Asian Pac. J. Cancer Prev.* **15** 6463–75

Tewari D, Patni P, Bishayee A, Sah A N and Bishayee A 2022 Natural products targeting the PI3K-Akt-mTOR signaling pathway in cancer: a novel therapeutic strategy *Seminars in Cancer Biology.* (New York: Academic)vol 80 pp 1–17

Tian Y *et al* 2012 Spirooxindole derivative SOID-8 induces apoptosis associated with inhibition of JAK2/STAT3 signaling in melanoma cells *PLoS One* **7** e49306

Tsai M H *et al* 2019 Correction: artocarpin, an isoprenyl flavonoid, induces p53-dependent or independent apoptosis via ROS-mediated MAPKs and Akt activation in non-small cell lung cancer cells *Oncotarget* **10** 3430

Tsuboi K *et al* 2014 Zerumbone inhibits tumor angiogenesis via NF-κB in gastric cancer *Oncol. Rep.* **31** 57–64

Venkatesh V, Nataraj R, Thangaraj G S, Karthikeyan M, Gnanasekaran A, Kaginelli S B, Kuppanna G, Kallappa C G and Basalingappa K M 2018 Targeting notch signalling pathway of cancer stem cells *Stem Cell Investig.* **5** 5

Wang J, Man G C, Chan T H, Kwong J and Wang C C 2018 A prodrug of green tea polyphenol (–)-epigallocatechin-3-gallate (Pro-EGCG) serves as a novel angiogenesis inhibitor in endometrial cancer *Cancer Lett.* **412** 10–20

Wang Y P, Pan F, Wang Y D, Khan A, Liu Y P, Yang M L, Cao J X, Zhao T R and Cheng G G 2022 Anti-leukemic effect and molecular mechanism of 11-methoxytabersonine from *Melodinus cochinchinensis* via network pharmacology, ROS-mediated mitochondrial dysfunction and PI3K/Akt signaling pathway *Bioorg. Chem.* **120** 105607

Wu G, Wilson G, George J and Qiao L 2015 Modulation of notch signaling as a therapeutic approach for liver cancer *Curr. Gene Therap.* **15** 171–81

Xie F, Su M, Qiu W, Zhang M, Guo Z, Su B, Liu J, Li X and Zhou L 2013 Kaempferol promotes apoptosis in human bladder cancer cells by inducing the tumor suppressor, PTEN *Int. J. Mol. Sci.* **14** 21215–26

Xie X, Wang Z, Chen F, Yuan Y, Wang J, Liu R and Chen Q 2016 Roles of FGFR in oral carcinogenesis *Cell Prolif.* **49** 261–9

Xiong T, Liu X W, Huang X L, Xu X F, Xie W Q, Zhang S J and Tu J 2018 Tristetraprolin: a novel target of diallyl disulfide that inhibits the progression of breast cancer *Oncol. Lett.* **15** 7817–27

Xu X, Rajamanickam V, Shu S, Liu Z, Yan T, He J, Liu Z, Guo G, Liang G and Wang Y 2019 Indole-2-carboxamide derivative LG25 inhibits triple-negative breast cancer growth by suppressing akt/mTOR/NF-κB signalling pathway *Drug Des. Devel. Ther.* **2019** 3539–50

Yang J, Chen J, He J, Li J, Shi J, Cho W C and Liu X 2016 Wnt signaling as potential therapeutic target in lung cancer *Expert Opin. Therap. Targets* **20** 999–1015

Yang Q, Fei Z and Huang C 2021 Betulin terpenoid targets OVCAR-3 human ovarian carcinoma cells by inducing mitochondrial mediated apoptosis, G2/M phase cell cycle arrest, inhibition of cell migration and invasion and modulating mTOR/PI3K/AKT signalling pathway *Cell. Mol. Biol.* **67** 14–9

Yang Y, Li X, Wang T, Guo Q, Xi T and Zheng L 2020 Emerging agents that target signaling pathways in cancer stem cells *J. Hematol. Oncol.* **13** 1–8

Yao Y, Ni Y, Zhang J, Wang H and Shao S 2017 The role of Notch signaling in gastric carcinoma: molecular pathogenesis and novel therapeutic targets *Oncotarget* **8** 53839

Yeh H T, Tsai Y S, Chen M S, Li Y Z, Lin W C, Lee Y R, Tseng Y S and Sheu S M 2019 Flavopereirine induces cell cycle arrest and apoptosis via the akt/p38 mapk/erk1/2 signaling pathway in human breast cancer cells *Eur. J. Pharmacol.* **863** 172658

Yip H Y and Papa A 2021 Signaling pathways in cancer: therapeutic targets, combinatorial treatments, and new developments *Cells* **10** 659

Yousefnia S, Seyed Forootan F, Seyed Forootan S, Nasr Esfahani M H, Gure A O and Ghaedi K 2020 Mechanistic pathways of malignancy in breast cancer stem cells *Front. Oncol.* **10** 452

Yuan X, Wu H, Xu H, Xiong H, Chu Q, Yu S, Wu G S and Wu K 2015 Notch signaling: an emerging therapeutic target for cancer treatment *Cancer Lett.* **369** 20–7

Zhang H W *et al* 2018 Flavonoids inhibit cell proliferation and induce apoptosis and autophagy through downregulation of PI3Kγ mediated PI3K/AKT/mTOR/p70S6K/ULK signaling pathway in human breast cancer cells *Sci. Rep.* **8** 1–3

Gu H F, Mao X Y and Du M 2020 Prevention of breast cancer by dietary polyphenols—role of cancer stem cells *Crit. Rev. Food Sci. Nutr.* **60** 810–25

Zhang X, Li T, Gong E S and Liu R H 2020 Antiproliferative activity of ursolic acid in MDA-MB-231 human breast cancer cells through Nrf2 pathway regulation *J. Agric. Food Chem.* **68** 7404–15

Zhang Y and Wang X 2020 Targeting the Wnt/β-catenin signaling pathway in cancer *J. Hematol. Oncol.* **13** 1–6

Zhao Y, Wang X, Sun Y, Zhou Y, Yin Y, Ding Y, Li Z, Guo Q and Lu N 2015 LYG-202 exerts antitumor effect on PI3K/Akt signaling pathway in human breast cancer cells *Apoptosis* **20** 1253–69

Zheng Z, Zhang L and Hou X 2022 Potential roles and molecular mechanisms of phytochemicals against cancer *Food Funct.* **13** 9208–25

Zhou Y, Ye Y, Zhu X, Jin T, Yi W, Gu L and Xiong X 2021 Meisoindigo inhibits cellular proliferation via down-regulation of the PI3K/Akt pathway and induces cellular apoptosis in glioblastoma U87 cells *Acta Biochim. Pol.* **68** 309–15

Zhu W, Wang H and Zhu D 2022 Wnt/β-catenin signaling pathway in lung cancer *Med. Drug Discov.* **13** 100113

IOP Publishing

Phytochemicals as an Epigenetic Modifier in Cancer Prevention

Nidhi Puranik, Deepa Yadav and Sangeeta Shukla

Chapter 9

Natural phytochemicals as anti-cancer agents: from past to present scenario

Divya Bisht, Deena Prakash and Arvind Kumar Shakya

Plants have long been known and utilized by humans for their medicinal properties with their therapeutic evidence in ancient literature. Plant phytochemicals exhibit antioxidants and ameliorative potential, and are known to treat various human diseases including cancer. Cancer is a major health concern accounting for about 10 million deaths annually, and is the second leading cause of global deaths. Numerous traditional remedies are known to treat cancer using herbal products. Approximately 70% of anti-cancer medicines in the market are derived from phytochemicals from medicinal plants. Phytochemicals like celastrol, curcumin, taxol, vincristine, topotecan, and irinotecan are some of the clinically used anti-cancer drugs. Nanotechnology is also employed to design green-synthesized anti-cancer nanodrugs from phytochemicals for better target specificity and higher efficacy. This chapter focuses on the evolution in the role of different phytochemicals as anti-cancer agents from the past as well as current contribution in the treatment of cancer.

Abbreviations

AD	Anno Domini
BBB	Blood–brain barrier
BC	Before Christ
BCE	Before Christian Era
CML	Chronic myelogenous leukaemia
CSCs	Cancer stem cells
DNA	Deoxyribonucleic acid
EVs	Extracellular vesicles
FTIR	Fourier transform infrared spectroscopy
HeLa	Henrietta Lacks
HPLC	High-performance liquid chromatography
NMR	Nuclear magnetic resonance

doi:10.1088/978-0-7503-5252-9ch9

NCI	National Cancer Institute
PBUH	Peace be upon him
TCM	Traditional Chinese medicine
TLC	Thin layer chromatography
UV	Ultraviolet
UVB	Ultraviolet B-rays
WHO	World Health Organization

9.1 Introduction

Cancer is a fatal metabolic disorder that can affect people of any age group and is the most talked about health topic in the world. It is one of the world's most prevalent causes of death globally, which accounts for over 7.6 million deaths every year, and an expected rise of 6 million by 2030 [1]. According to the World Health Organization (WHO), there are currently 22 million cancer patients living around the world, and the number is predicted to rise by nearly 50% during the next decade which ultimately shows the severity of this disease and impact on human life [2]. Cancer is a genetic disease resulting in uncontrolled proliferation of cells and formation of tumors, leading to disruption of various genetic and molecular mechanisms in the human body. These alterations disrupt the immunity mechanism of patients leaving them defenseless against many other infectious diseases that cause multidimensional damage to human health. Exponential cellular growth is caused by cancerous mutations in various genes responsible for cell growth metabolism, DNA repair, tumor suppression and oncogenes.

The most prevalent types of cancer include lung cancer followed by breast cancer, rectal cancer, colon cancer, pancreatic cancer, prostate cancer, and skin cancer which collectively accounts for maximum deaths worldwide after cardiac diseases [3, 4].

Cancer-causing factors, also known as carcinogens, are broadly classified as external factors and internal factors. External factors are various pollutants present around us in our environment (asbestos, benzene, benzidine, cadmium, nickel, arsenic, radon, vinyl chloride etc), high-energy radiations (UV radiations, x-rays, gamma rays etc), DNA damaging chemicals (such as polycyclic aromatic hydrocarbons, heterocyclic aromatic amines, aristolochic acid, nitrosamines), cancer causing metals (arsenic, cadmium, chromium, and nickel) and some infectious agents (hepatitis B and hepatitis C viruses, Epstein–Barr virus, human papillomavirus, human immunodeficiency virus type 1, *Helicobacter pylori* and *Streptococcus bovis*). Internal factors are mainly genetic mutations, weak immune system and various hormonal disorders that can cause cancer [5, 6].

Despite the advancement in medicinal science and technology with efficient techniques of diagnosis and treatment, cancer treatment remains a challenge to scientists across the world due to different reasons (social, economical, scientific, etc). Many cancer patients do not receive treatment due to a lack of appropriate diagnosis or non-availability of treatment options at their location or economic barriers to seeking specialized treatment facilities as cancer treatment is too expensive to be afforded by all. Even though the pharmaceutical industry offers different treatments to fight against cancer, it is hard to ignore the serious side effects associated with them. Methods of cancer treatment include anti-cancer drugs, surgical removal of tumor, stem cell transfer, vaccinations against cancer, cancer-controlling therapies like radiotherapy, immunotherapy, chemotherapy, photodynamic therapy, etc, which are mostly accompanied by severe side effects on patients causing more harm than good, even after numerous advancements being made to reduce the negative impact of these treatments and anti-cancer drugs [7].

The typical side effects of any of these cancer treatments vary in different patients depending on various factors like, their age, gender, type of cancer, stage of cancer, and immunity strength of individual patient. Major limitations of available anti-cancer treatments include nonspecificity of drug or therapy (making it toxic for the healthy cells in patients), limited bioavailability (less absorption offers less therapeutic potential), less efficiency, toxicity caused to other vital organs, non-ecofriendly and exorbitant cost (making it unaffordable to the common population) [8, 9]. The side effects of chemotherapy are sensory neuropathy, cardiovascular toxicity, nephrotoxicity, gastrointestinal toxicity, pulmonary and hematologic toxicity [10, 11].

All these shortcomings and side effects of available cancer treatment methods question the safety and effectivity of chemical anti-cancer drugs and promote the importance of medicinal plants in healthcare and to study their anti-cancer potential based on evidence in ancient medicinal literature worldwide. Traditional plant-based treatments of cancer are mentioned in ancient literature of many countries including India, China, Japan, Iran, Greece, etc [12–15]. These support the idea that plants have the properties to treat cancer as they were used as traditional remedies in past. Many phytochemical-derived anti-cancer drugs currently available in the market are extracted from plants that were used as traditional anti-cancer medicine through the ages. Medicinal plants can be considered as potential anti-cancer treatment options for treating cancerous cells in humans, because of the presence of numerous phytochemicals exhibiting antioxidant and anti-cancer properties. Using extensive knowledge of medicinal plants from ancient literature across the world, screening of their phytochemicals and anti-cancer potential is being done through various *in vitro* and *in vivo* methods for drug discovery with better efficacy, target specificity, and least harm to the normal cells in the human body for cancer treatment [16–19].

This chapter will focus on the limitations of cancer treatments currently available to mankind; the significance and efficiency of plants and their medicinal phytochemicals in healthcare, history of cancer treatment using plants; the current treatment approach that are been used in cancer treatment based on the knowledge from the past; and the future of phytochemicals as anti-cancer agents for development of better drugs with higher specificity and lower toxicity profile. It will be important to understand that past studies of cancer and traditional cancer treatment methods are used as evidence to validate the notion that plants have the potential to treat certain types of cancer, largely due to the presence of numerous phytochemicals well known for their antioxidant and therapeutic properties in the present. More recent studies have shown the possibilities of more effective and target-specific treatment of cancer by coupling phytochemicals with advanced approaches like nanotechnology and other methods.

9.2 Cancer treatment drugs and their limitations

There are numerous modalities that are used to treat cancer, which is a very complex problem for scientists. In the present time, there are many different ways to treat cancer which include surgery for the physical removal of the tumor from the patients, various therapies like radiotherapy (using ionizing radiation), immunotherapy (by stimulating the immune system), chemotherapy (using anti-cancer drugs), and cancer vaccines, among others. Even with all these methods and techniques of diagnosis and treatment of cancer, increasing deaths due to cancer are a serious concern which demand development of more efficient ways to fight cancer.

Cancer treatment is challenging because it is difficult to specifically target cancer stem cells (CSCs) among all the normal healthy cells in the body of a patient, as nonspecificity results in disastrous side effects, even the recurrence of the tumor following the cessation of drug use [20]. One such example is Gleevec (Imatinib), which is an anti-cancer drug used to treat chronic myelogenous leukaemia (CML) and has severe side effects.

Also, CSCs are resistant to anti-cancer drugs due to the drug resistance traits present in these cells. They exhibit specialized defences against any harmful xenobiotic agents, acquired after repeated processes of self-renewal and differentiation [21].

Another limitation is the absence of cancer epigenetic profiling as well as the lack of specificity in epidrugs presently available. As the traditional approach to cancer research was mainly concerned with identifying and figuring out the broad patterns of genetic anomalies that are caused by mutational or other chromosomal abnormality occurrences, there are only a small number of cancer-related genetic mutations found in patients, which is insufficient to explain the extensive genetic deviation that ultimately occurs in the malignant phenotype of cancer [22].

Chemotherapeutic medicines are chemical drugs used to stop the growth of or kill cancer cells. They work by inhibiting cellular growth processes or by causing cancer cell death. Chemotherapeutic medicines are either administered individually as a whole or in combination with surgery or radiation therapy. However, these chemotherapeutic agents also have numerous disadvantages. As they lack specificity and are thus toxic to all cells, including cancer and normal cells, causing normal cell death has adverse consequences, occasionally resulting in patient fatality. The side effects of chemotherapy can be appalling, and its effectiveness is never better than palliative. Doxorubicin causes cardiotoxicity as a side effect, while other chemotherapy drugs like oxaliplatin, melphalan, carboplatin, and cisplatin cause nephrotoxicity, gastrointestinal toxicity, cardiovascular toxicity, and pulmonary and hematologic toxicity in patients administered with chemotherapy, as shown in figure 9.1. Another chemotherapy drug, Irinotecan, also has side effects like neutropenia and sensory neuropathy [8, 10].

Cancer treatment has evolved significantly in recent years. Presently, there are a lot more treatment options available for a wide range of disease types.

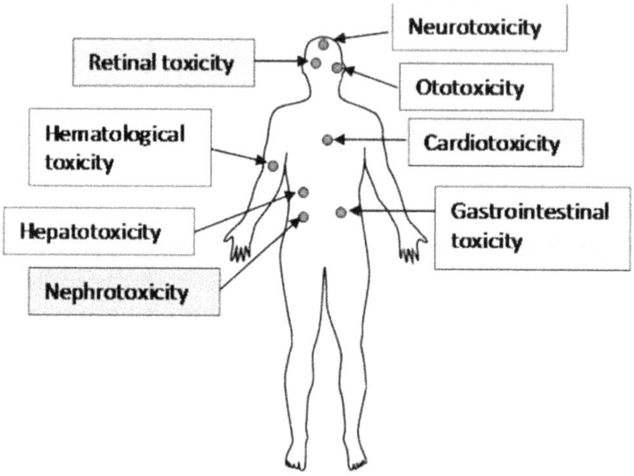

Figure 9.1. Adverse side effects of cancer treatment drugs on patients. Attribution-ShareAlike 4.0 International (CC BY-SA 4.0).

Unfortunately, the best method for treating cancer patients remains elusive. Alopecia, sensory neuropathy, nausea, vomiting, and other serious side effects are brought on by the use of these methods. We are still far from discovering a cure for many types of cancer, with cancer treatment drugs only acting as palliative rather than curative measures, despite enormous efforts and notable achievements in the field of cancer research [23, 24].

The most promising option for a more effective and less harmful cancer treatment, according to the existing ancient medical literature and thorough research findings, is phytochemicals and their derived analogs as they are considered safer to use with fewer side effects due to their natural origin and are more effective in treatment of numerous diseases in humans [19].

9.3 Plants and their medicinal properties

The plant kingdom is well known for its diversity in morphology, taxonomy, as well as phytochemical properties, having 374 000 plant species officially recognized and described so far with many more yet to be explored with continuous research. Though ancient civilizations across the world used plants in their medical practice, it was not until the 17th and 18th centuries that a unified nomenclature and cataloguing system was developed to classify plants on the basis of their morphological properties as well as therapeutic effects among humans that promoted the use of plants in therapeutic preparations to treat various ailments. Around 20 of the more than 450 plant families have a reputation for having medicinal qualities. Aristolochiaceae, Cucurbitaceae, Solanaceae, Piperaceae, Rubiaceae, Ranunculaceae, Zingiberaceae, Rutaceae and other families, are distinguished by the presence of specific classes of active molecules like monoterpene, phenolics, sesquiterpene, flavonoids, tannins, and alkaloids that are responsible for their medicinal properties [25, 26].

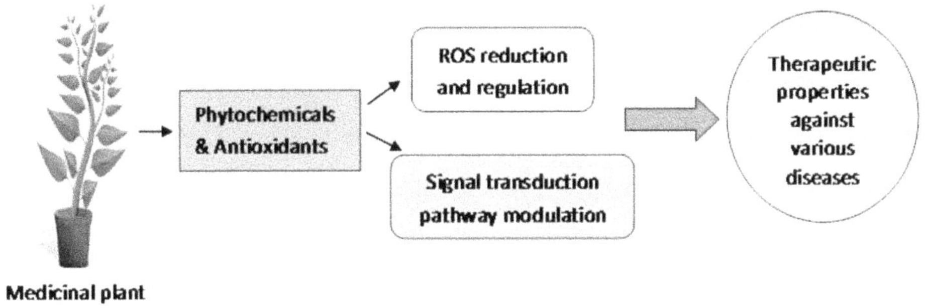

Figure 9.2. Therapeutic mechanism of medicinal plants. CC0 1.0 Universal (CC0 1.0) Public Domain Dedication.

More than 30 000 secondary metabolites are produced by plants and have important health effects that have been used in conventional medical procedures for ages. Many plant parts are known for their ability to prevent disease in addition to their direct therapeutic use against different human ailments. According to numerous studies, natural products have a diversity of biological effects, including stimulation of the immune system, antimicrobial, hepatoprotective, anti-ulcer, anti-inflammatory, antioxidant, and anti-cancer effects.

Numerous well-known pharmaceuticals are produced from natural products or their derivatives, and compounds derived from plants are used as medicines and their therapeutic mechanism is depicted in figure 9.2. More than 25% of the total drugs that are currently being used in medical industry come from plants [27].

Numerous studies have shown a connection between a high consumption of fruit like tomatoes, apples, and grapes as well as vegetables like broccoli and cauliflower and a lower risk of development of cancer [28–30]. It is noteworthy that 70% of the anti-cancer medications prescribed currently have their origins from plants. According to reports by WHO, about 80% of the world's population utilize plants for their primary healthcare requirements as plants have extensive potential to treat numerous diseases [31, 32].

9.3.1 History of plants as anti-cancer agents

From the earliest of civilizations, cancer was treated and recorded in medical history by humans. Medical and surgical care was the prime focus of cancer treatment in the past from what is mentioned in ancient records. The seven papyri that were found and understood in the latter part of the 19th century contain the oldest recorded characterizations of cancer with source materials that date back as far as 2500 BC reportedly. Vedic texts, which date back to around 600 BC, have descriptions of the fundamental concepts of cancer as an abnormal exponential growth and development of cells as well as its management. The literature from India and China's prehistoric periods both mention cancer as a curse to human population with various treatment methods to combat its effects. Many such major milestones in the history of cancer are mentioned in table 9.1 which gives you a brief tour of the development of knowledge about cancer and steps taken to treat this disease.

Table 9.1. This timeline provides a look at some of the key advances in cancer.

Year	Events/discoveries
3000 BC	First mention and description of breast cancer.
1500 BC	Description of soft tissue tumor.
	Introduction of herbal, mineral, and arsenic therapy.
375 BC	Introduction of cancer, carcinoma, scirrhus and condyloma.
	Identification of skin, mouth, stomach and breast cancers, cautery.
AD 50	Surgery as suggested cancer treatment.
	Identification of breast cancer in axilla, lymphedema of arm, cancer of liver, colon and spleen.
	Inoperable cancer treatment by honey, egg white, and cabbage mixture.
79	Book on drugs published.
	Internal remedies before and after surgery.
138	Classification of non-ulcerated and ulcerated uterine cancers.
200	Sarcoma introduced.
	Theory of humoral, yellow and black bile.
	Establishment of pharmacy in Rome.
403	Necrosis in cancer identified.
562	Mastectomy as treatment for breast cancer.
	Cancer of cervix, vulva and anus described.
690	Identification of intestinal cancer.
	Cancer stated to be painless.
932	Bile duct and intestinal obstructions.
1037	Polypectomy by wire loop.
1106	Bloodletting prior to surgery, no extensive surgery.
1162	Cancer of esophagus identified.
	Esophageal cannula for stricture and injection of nourishment, rectal obstruction, hysterectomy.
1215	Ban on surgery by the Pope.
1296	Rapid spread of cancer to other parts of the body found, treatment through surgery suggested.
	Identification of nasopharyngeal cancer.
	Livid tumors cannot be surgically removed.
	Opium administration as anesthesia.
1315	Clinical differentiation of benign and malignant breast tumors, surgeons learn regional anatomy.
1320	Identification of scirrhus and carcinoma as types of cancer.
	Cancer categorized according to size, placement, and depth.
	Cancer may be caused by external factors, suggested by research from England.
1368	Alternative cancer treatments such as diet and purgatives were suggested.
1390	No cure for anorectal cancers.

As cancer was a serious health issue in the past, various traditional healers and doctors around the world studied cancer and discovered treatments according to their cultural knowledge and medicinal plants available in their geographical area. In the Golden Age of Arab-Islamic civilization (7th to 14th century) many eminent Arab-Muslim doctors studied cancer and used various medications and surgical techniques to defeat cancer. In Islam, eating well is considered as the best way to prevent illness. Nutritional chemoprevention received immense attention and acceptance in the Arab-Islamic treatment of diseases because it plays a significant role in maintaining bodily health. The Prophet (PBUH) stated a variety of foods in the Holy Quran and Hadith, including grapes, citrus, melon, squash, figs, dates, honey, olive oil, and black seeds that are believed to cure all the ailments to maintain a healthy body.

Ibn Sina (980–1037), also called Avicenna in the west, was the most important Islamic philosopher-scientist. In his Canon, he listed four ways to treat cancer: (a) total elimination of cancer; (b) halting its progression; (c) avoiding ulceration; and (d) treatment of ulceration [33]. A pea flour poultice was effective in treating cancer, according to Khuzestani doctors. They also mentioned the possibility of gradual prevention as well as recovery from cancer with a poultice made from charred and melted cabbage (*Brassica oleracea*) roots. It was reported that a poultice made from common plantain (*Plantago major*) is effectual in treating a variety of cancers. For the cancerous wounds treatment, Aaron of Alexandria recommended applying a balm made from pulverized starch, sponge (*Spongia officinalis*), lead carbonate, black nightshade (*Solanum nigrum*), water, and rose oil. In the Roman Empire, Aelius Galenus, a Greek physician, surgeon, and philosopher cited Dioscorides as saying that non-ulcerative cancer can be treated by using a plaster made using hedge mustard (*Erysimum officinale*). The inner crust of walnuts (*Juglans regia*) applied to ulcerative melatonic swellings is a helpful treatment strategy, according to Greek physician Pedanius Dioscorides [14].

Worldwide cancer eradication efforts have recently incorporated a number of complementary and alternative medical approaches taken from the ancient medical literature. In China, traditional Chinese medicine (TCM) has gained widespread acceptance as a complementary and alternative treatment modality that has positive outcomes for people with cancer [34, 35]. The Chinese Materia Medica records the administration of 52 prescriptions from the Wu Shi Er Bing Fang as anti-cancer treatment, the first of which dates from at least 1100 BCE, 365 drugs from the Shennong Herbal (100 BCE), and 850 drugs from the Tang Herbal (659 BCE) [36, 37].

Cancer-like conditions are also referred to in Ayurveda as ‘granthi’ and ‘arbuda.’ Depending on the doshas involved, granthi and arbuda can either be inflammatory or non-inflammatory. The balance of three doshas in the body, mind, and consciousness is what Ayurveda defines as true health. Vata, pitta, and kapha are the three doshas that cause disease in the body. Tridoshicar budas are typically cancerous because the three main body humors become morbidly out of sync with one another which facilitates the origin and establishment of cancer in human body as per the Ayurveda [17].

In Indian Ayurveda, numerous medicinal plants have been mentioned for the treatment of cancer. These plants are categorized according to their properties and impact on human health. The properties taken in consideration include biophysical property, biopotency, and catabolic effects and taste, dryness, penetrating effect of plant. A list of a few such plants is given that were used as anti-cancer treatment in Ayurveda in table 9.2 [38]. Ayurveda promotes regular consumption of dietary medicinal plants such as ginger, garlic, pepper, cloves, tulsi and saffron along with seasonal antioxidants and detoxifiers like neem, and amla to take maximum advantage of their ability to prevent cancer [39–42].

The 1846 discovery of anesthesia facilitated surgeons Bilroth, Handley, and Halsted to perform surgery for complete tumor removals along with lymph node dissections during cancer operations. A surgeon named Paget reported afterward that the cancer cells show proliferation to other locations via the bloodstream (metastasis). During the last decades of the twentieth century, surgeons developed a novel cancer treatment method which is a combination of surgery with chemotherapy and/or radiation therapy. Later, researchers discovered that nitrogen mustard kills rapidly multiplying cancer cells [43]. This shows the continuous growth and improvement in the field of cancer studies in the past and also highlights the role of plants throughout this journey as a remedy to treat cancer.

9.3.2 Current contribution of phytochemicals in cancer treatment

In India, Ayurveda has been recognized as an effective medicinal system with a holistic approach of treatment. Ayurvedic herbal decoctions contain multiple herbs with anti-cancer properties; these compositions function precisely through a complex biochemical route and positively regulate different organs, along with providing nourishment to the whole body by strengthening its defence system. Medicinal plants speed up the curative process and decrease the adverse outcomes and complications linked with cancer, helping the patient to recover faster. Each medicinal plant comprises a range of active compounds that function synergistically to produce medicinal benefits while decreasing adverse effects, thereby eliminating the requirement of additional therapy to mitigate harsh symptoms of cancer [44]. It has made it critical to advocate for the utilization of natural Ayurvedic therapies in the treatment of a variety of cancers, as well as an integrated approach to tumor management and treatment [45].

Around half of all internationally approved anti-cancer drugs are originated from natural compounds. Nearly 30 plant-derived anti-cancer compounds have been shown positive anti-cancer properties in clinical trials against various types of tumors with some of them are mentioned in table 9.3 along with the type of cancer against which they showed anti-cancer property [46].

The therapeutic potential of medicinal plants is determined by various factors taken into consideration altogether, like the type of active phytochemicals found along with their specific quantity, which changes among different species based on their habitat (latitude, longitude, altitude, climate, and season). Further amount and effectivity of active phytochemicals change in different plant parts. To isolate

Table 9.2. Plants used in cancer treatment in past.

Scientific name	Hindi name	English name	Scientific name	Hindi name	English Name
Vinca rosea	Sadabahar	Periwinkle	*Bacopa monnieri*	Brahmi	Indian penny wort
Rubia cordifolia	Manjistha	Indian madder	*Curcuma longa*	Haridra	Turmeric
Saraca indica	Ashoka	Ashoka tree	*Boswellia serrata*	Shallaki	Indian olibanum
Allium sativum	Lasuna	Garlic	*Withania somnifera*	Ashwagandha	Indian ginseng
Aloe vera	Kumari	Aloe	*Jasminum auriculatum*	Juuhi	Jasmine
Alstonia scholaries	Sapta parni	Milky pine	*Datura metal*	Dhattura	Angel's trumpet
Cedrus deodara	Devadaru	Devdar	*Melia azadirachta*	Maha nimba	Neem tree
Holarrhena antidysenterica	Kutaja	Kurchi tree	*Moringa oleifera*	Shigru	Horseradish tree
Plumbago zeylanica	Chitraka	Leadwort	*Pisum sativum Kalaya*	Matar	Garden pea
Berberis aristata	Daru haridra	Indian ophthalmic barberry	*Centella asiatica*	Mandukaparni	Gotu kola
Piper betle	Nagavalli	Betel leaf pepper	*Occimum sanctum*	Tulasi	Holy basil
Paederia foetida	Gandha prasarani	Chinese fever vine	*Picrorrhiza kurroa*	Katuki	Kutki
Euphoria hirta	Dugdhika	Hairy spurge	*Azadiracta indica*	Nimba	Margosa tree
Nigella sativa	Krishna jeeraka	Black cumin	*Cymbopogon citrates*	Bhustrina	Lemongrass
Nerium indicum	Kara veera	Oleander	*Phyllantus fraternus*	Niruri	Leaf-flower
Anona squamosa	Sitaphala	Custard apple			

Table 9.3. Anti-cancer agent obtained from various dietary plants.

Plant name	Active compounds
Citrus aurantium	Hesperidin
Daucus carota sativus	Carotene
Glycyrrhiza sp.	Glycyrrhizin
Crocus sativus	Carotenoids
Ocimum sanctum	Ursolic acid
Camellia sinensis	Catechin and theaflavins
Lycopersicon esculentum	Lycopene, Lutein, Kaempferol
Azadirachata indica	Polyphenolics
Capsaicum annum	Capsaicinoids
Capsaicum frutens	Capsaicin
Piper nigrum	Purpurogallin
Glycine max	Genistein
Piper longum	Piperine
Pueraria lobata radix	Genistein
Betula alba	Betulinic acid
Prunus dulcis	Morin
Curcurbita moschata	Carotene
Rosmarinus officinalis	Carnosol
Silymarin marianum	Silymarin
Vitis vinifera	Resveratro
Zingiber officinale	Gingerol
Carica papaya	Cryptoxanthin
Prunus armeniaca	Carotenoids
Allium sativum	Allicin, *S*-allylcysteine

purified form of active phytomolecules methods like combinatorial chemistry along with different isolation tests, and bioassay coupled fractionation are performed. TLC, HPLC, FTIR, mass spectroscopy, NMR etc are a few well known methods used to access bioactivity of extracted active compounds to check their suitability as potential drug alternatives. Further evaluation and screening includes *in vitro* and *in vivo* methods to check anti-cancer activity of purified phytochemicals. If the molecule achieves a superior anti-cancer activity in all the previous tests, additional issues such as pharmacokinetics, pharmacodynamics, immunogenicity, metabolic fate, biosafety and side effects, drug interactions, dosage concentration, and so on must be explored for future anti-cancer drug design [47]. The cellular target and related anti-cancer mechanism of phytochemicals as anti-cancer drug are given in figure 9.3.

Active constituents isolated from numerous medicinal plants mentioned in ancient literature for their anti-cancer properties have been found to contain vital anti-cancer agents exhibiting significant pharmacological effects against cancer. Vinca alkaloids (vincristine, vinblastine, vindesine, vinorelbine), podophyllotoxin

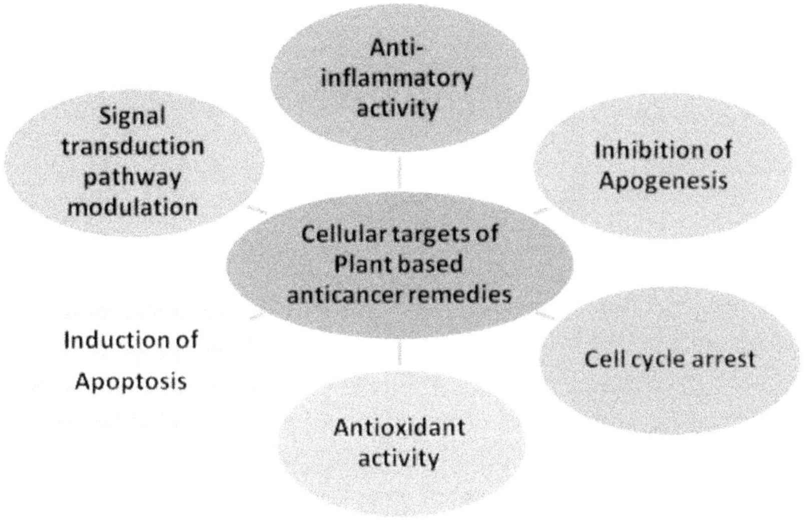

Figure 9.3. Cellular target and anti-cancer mechanism of plant-based remedies.

derivatives (etoposide, teniposide), taxanes (paclitaxel, docetaxel), camptothecin derivatives (irinotecan, topotecan) are some of the main natural drugs used as the primary approach in the battle against cancer. Vinca alkaloids, camptotectin quinolone alkaloid derivatives, epipodophyllotoxin lignans, and taxane diterpenoids are the major classes of cancer treatments from medicinal plants. The detailed effectivity and pharmacological utility of some of these anti-cancer agents are discussed in this section and their usage is depicted in figure 9.4.

Vinblastine and vincristine are two major anti-cancer vinca alkaloids extracted from the periwinkle plant (*Catharanthus roseus*). These two alkaloids along with some other chemotherapeutic drugs are used to treat Kaposi's sarcoma, breast cancer, leukemias, adenocarcinoma, lymphomas as well as advanced stage testicular cancer [29].

Paclitaxel (taxol) extracted from *Taxus brevifolia* (yew tree) had been approved as an anti-cancer agent in clinical trials by the US (1990s) for the treatment of cancer found in ovaries, breasts, and lungs [48].

Camptothecin is another such anti-cancer phytochemical obtained from *Camptotheca acuminate* that was approved in the 1970s for its anti-cancer properties by NCI. This along with two of its semi-synthetic derivatives are used in treatment of ovary cancer, oat cell cancer and colon cancers [49].

Celastrol found in *Tripterygium wilfordii* is a terpenoids, known for its anti-inflammatory activity. Research shows that it is an effective anti-cancer phytochemical due to its properties such as protein modification, angiogenesis suppression, proteasome repression, and apoptosis induction [50].

Elliptinium is another phytochemical that shows prominent anti-cancer activity against breast cancer and is extracted from *Bleekeria vitiensis* [29].

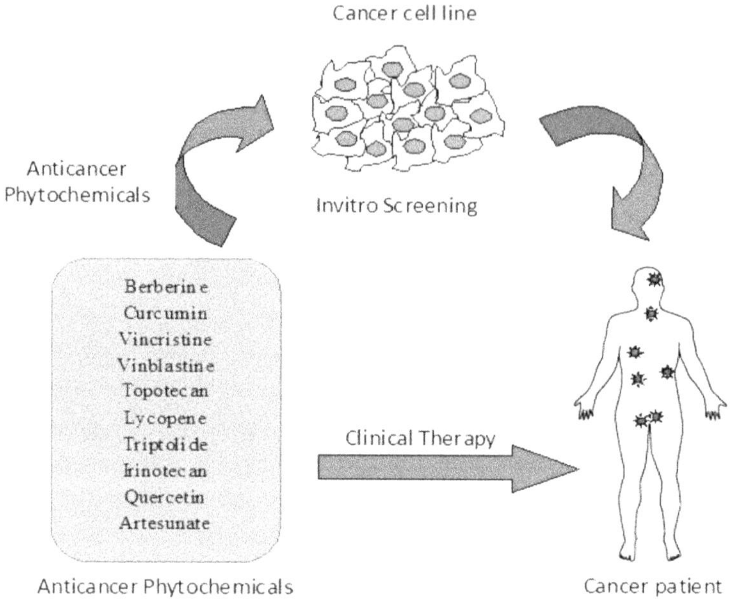

Figure 9.4. Anti-cancer phytochemicals actively used in treatment. Attribution-ShareAlike 4.0 International (CC BY-SA 4.0).

Human colon carcinoma is also found to be treated with two anti-cancer phytochemicals, schischkinnin and montamine, extracted from two different plant seeds, namely *Centaurea schischkinii* and *Centaurea montana* [51].

Curcumin is a dietary flavonoid extracted from *Curcuma longa* shows significant anti-carcinogenic activity in mouse and mice model to treat a skin cancer model [52–55].

Genistein is a dietary flavonoid isolated from *Glycine max* and *Ginkgo biloba* possessing anti-carcinogenic properties against skin carcinomas as per the *in vivo* studies performed on animal models [56–58].

Apigenin is another flavonoid sourced from vegetables, fruit and medicinal herbs that showed promising anti-cancer properties in the case of skin cancer in different animal models [59–61].

Proanthocyanidins found in grape seeds showed strong antitumor effects against UVB induced skin tumors in animal models [62–65].

There are various other phytochemicals that are actively present in our diet with sources in the form of fruit, vegetables, spices, beverages, pulses, nuts and cereals and are scientifically screened and proven to possess anti-cancer properties. A list of a few such anti-cancer agents from dietary phytochemicals is shown in table 9.4.

Some other phytochemicals with known and verified anti-carcinogenic activity are: Silymarin from *Silybum marianum* known for anti-carcinogenic effect against non-melanoma skin cancer in mice [66–71]. Taxanes (docetaxel and paclitaxel) that interfere in the cell division and thus inhibit tumor formation [72]. *Cephalotaxus* shows effects against lung cancer, HeLa, gastric cancer cell lines,

Table 9.4. Anti-cancer phytochemical in clinical practice.

Compound	Uses
Berberine	Colorectal cancer, prevention of recurrence
Curcumin	Advanced and metastatic breast cancer
Sulforaphane	Former smokers with a high risk of developing lung cancer
Vincristine	Leukemia, lymph tumor, adenocarcinoma, ductal carcinoma and childhood solid cancers
Epigallocatechin	Colorectal cancer
Vinblastine	Lymph tumor, breast germ-cell and renal cell carcinoma
Topotecan	Adenocarcinoma, ovarian and childhood cancers
Lycopene	Metastatic colorectal cancer
Triptolide	Pancreatic cancer
Irinotecan	Lung, and colorectal cancers
Quercetin	Prostate cancer
Homoharringtonine	Chronic myeloid leukemia and acute myeloid leukemia
Artesunate	Solid tumor, metastatic and locally advanced breast cancer, colorectal cancers
Tymoquinone	Oral potentially malignant lesion
Paclitaxel	Neck, head, ductal carcinoma, adenocarcinoma, bladder and ovarian cancer
Resveratrol	Low-grade GI neuroendocrine tumors
D-limonene	Pancreatic and breast cancer, submadullary and protid gland tumor
Docetaxel	Lung and breast cancers

etc by inhibiting protein formation and related biochemical pathways [73]. Berberine is another anti-cancer agent obtained from *Tinospora cordifolia* used to treat breast cancer, prostate cancer and colorectal cancer [74, 75]. Combretastatins extracted from *Combretum caffrum* has its mention in the Indian medicinal system as an anti-cancer plant as it suppresses tumor forming cells and inhibits cancer progression [76, 77]. Betulinic acid from *Ziziphus mauritiana* shows cytotoxicity towards human melanoma [78].

All these studies have shown that the extensive range of phytochemicals has anti-cancer properties that can be used for the treatment of cancer and may boost the effectivity of anti-cancer medicines with very few side effects.

9.3.3 Future possibilities of phytochemicals in cancer treatment

Plant-derived anti-cancer phytochemicals became popular in the field of science and medicine due to their significant protective and therapeutic properties proven in both animal studies as well as clinical trials. With elaborate knowledge and evidence (traditional medicinal literature and remedies) to support more such studies for the discovery of more effective and safer anti-cancer drug options there are several advanced methods and technologies being employed which show promising future for the treatment of cancer using phytochemicals. These treatment methods include the following.

Nanoparticles are innovative smart systems that include medicinal and imaging chemicals which show more precision and effectivity due to their highly compatible size, efficacy and surface topography. These systems are employed to administer drugs to specific target tissues and give sustained dose release treatment, improving bioavailability by adjusting concentration around tumor tissues [79]. Nanomedicines support successful administration of anti-cancer phytochemical by enhancing their solubility, improved bioavailability, better cellular uptake and increased specificity to avoid any damage to healthy cells and thus sustaining steady-state therapeutic quantities of phytochemicals through time with high blood stability, multifunctionality, minimal interaction with synthetic drugs, and increased anti--cancer activity [80].

Another technique involves extracellular vesicles (EVs) as efficient anti-cancer drug delivery vehicles as well as anti-cancer vaccines that also help in diagnosis and prognosis. These vesicles play a crucial role in cancer development as they regulate metastatic progression [81]. Exosomes generated from plants have exceptional biochemical properties including biocompatibility, non-toxicity and controlled immunogenicity, specificity, large-scale production and capability to permeate the blood–brain barrier (BBB) [82, 83]. Various dietary exosomes from grapefruit, blueberry, citrus and lemon possess antioxidant and antitumor properties [84–87].

Natural antioxidants have also received acceptance and appreciation among scientists, to be used as alternative anti-cancer treatment. Antioxidants are widely approved to treat cancer because of their anti-proliferative and pro-apoptotic properties. Examples of a few such natural antioxidants are phytochemicals like vitamins, alkaloids, flavonoids, carotenoids, curcumin, berberine, quercetin and many other compounds that are proposed as additional therapy to cancer [12, 88].

These approaches have entered a position of rapid development, and some of them have undergone successful clinical studies. However, numerous challenges still exist before these can be administered clinically. More research is essential to overcome such hurdles in the path of anti-cancer drug discovery. A combination of all these methods will be able to give the finest tailored medicines for cancer patients depending on the type of cancer they are suffering from along with its stage of severity, target molecules and pathways, emphasizing the need for merging several disciplines to get the greatest results.

9.4 Discussion

Cancer represents one of the major causes of death, with approximately 22 million patients with cancer worldwide. There are many different ways to treat cancer which includes surgery for the physical removal of the tumor. Nonspecificity of these methods results in disastrous side effects, at times as severe as the recurrence of the tumor. The side effects of treatment methods can be appalling, and their effectiveness is never better than palliative. In ancient literature healthy eating was noted as one of the methods to combat all diseases including cancer. Ayurveda has been considered as an efficient medicinal system with a comprehensive therapy approach. Plants and herbs with medicinal properties hasten the recovery and mitigate the negative consequences of cancer. In clinical studies also, plant-derived anti-cancer agents have shown anti-cancer activity. Plant-derived phytochemicals may include important anti-cancer agents with considerable anti-cancer pharmacological effects. Plant-based anti-cancer medicines mainly include phytochemicals like vinca alkaloids, camptotectin quinolone alkaloid derivatives, epipodophyllotoxin lignans, and taxane diterpenoids, that gained popularity in research and medicine due to considerable preventive and therapeutic effects demonstrated in both animal studies and clinical trials. Several innovative approaches and technologies are being used, indicating a potential future for the treatment of cancer with phytochemicals. Plant-derived exosomes exhibit extraordinary biological characteristics. To produce next-generation cancer therapies, further study is needed to understand and enhance the design, complexity, manufacturing, and biological interaction of phytonanomedicine. Furthermore, clever methods must be developed to provide phytonamomedicine to as many patients as feasible through the collaborative efforts of academics/researchers, doctors, pharmaceutical corporations, and regulatory agencies. A substantial amount of research has been carried out to evaluate the anti-cancer potential of different phytochemicals in *in vitro* studies on different cancer cell lines, and it is established that medicinal plants and their phytochemicals are key players in the creation of novel anti-cancer medications. Many phytochemicals have been emphasized in this chapter, that have been investigated for anti-cancer ability to decrease carcinogenesis, which includes variables such as proliferation, growth, metastasis, angiogenesis, and invasion. However, these potential phytochemicals must yet be tested in preclinical and clinical trials to evaluate their safety, effectiveness, and pharmacokinetic characteristics. Increased investment in the growing use of current cancer prevention methods, as well as fundamental and clinical research to improve understanding and treatment alternatives, will likely accelerate cancer treatment progress and bridge the racial and socioeconomic differences. We must look into whether the anti-cancer phytochemicals will disperse throughout the body after being absorbed post intake to confirm their bioavailability and thus their effectivity. It is the role of scientists (as well as doctors) to investigate the effectiveness, biochemical activity, and cellular target of those plant extracts and active components.

9.5 Conclusion

Medical science has made tremendous progress in the field of cancer treatment, making certain forms of cancer completely curable (pediatric lymphoblastic leukaemia, lymph tumor and testis cancer) with prolonged survival in others in the past few decades. A huge part of this success is a result of rigorous research on the identification and application of natural compounds against cancer. Plants make a great contribution to human healthcare and further research is being performed continuously to utilize the maximum benefits of their miraculous healing and curing properties. Medicinal plants have always been used to treat various diseases in humans since ancient times with cancer being no exception. Even in the past, various plants were believed to treat cancer by different tribes and communities globally. A number of popular plant-derived anti-cancer drugs presently available in the market have their links to the plants mentioned in the ancient medicinal literature across the globe and many such plants which contain phytochemicals with anti-cancer properties are yet to be screened for potential drug discovery at preclinical and clinical level to evaluate the safety, efficacy and pharmacokinetic profiles. In this chapter, many plants as well as phytochemicals have been highlighted that either have their mention in history as a treatment to cancer or are being used presently for their anti-cancer activity to obstruct carcinogenesis, including procreation, growth, expansion, angiogenesis, and invasion factors. New technologies are further adding to the efficiency of drug discovery against cancer. The use of metallic nanoparticles in combination with medicinal plants is being considered as one of the promising methods to aid cancer with improved tumor specificity, promising anti-cancer activity, and minimal toxicity to healthy cells using metallic nanoparticles. Only intensive preclinical and clinical research as well as a thorough understanding of the pharmacology of new compounds, can ensure the selection of active and safe anti-cancer and chemopreventive drugs, such as natural compounds. The challenges of cancer disease necessitate a scientific battle to combat cancer on any and all fronts.

References

[1] American Cancer Society 2016 *Cancer Facts & Figures 2016* (Atlanta, GA: American Cancer Society)

[2] Siegel R L, Miller K D and Jemal A 2016 Cancer statistics, 2016 *CA: Cancer J. Clin.* **66** 7–30

[3] Horn L, Pao W and Johnson D H 2012 Neoplasms of the lung. Chapter89 ed D L Longo, D L Kasper, J L Jamson, A S Fauci, S L Hauser and J Loscalzo *Harrisons Principles of Internal Medicine* 18th edn (New York: McGraw-Hill)

[4] Zhou Z, Tang M, Liu Y, Zhang Z, Lu R and Lu J 2017 Apigenin inhibits cell proliferation, migration, and invasion by targeting Akt in the A549 human lung cancer cell line *Anti-Cancer Drugs* **28** 446–56

[5] Ames B N, Gold L S and Willett W C 1995 The causes and prevention of cancer *Proc. Natl Acad. Sci. USA* **92** 5258–65

[6] Anand P, Kunnumakkara A B, Kunnumakara A B, Sundaram C, Harikumar K B, Tharakan S T, Lai O S, Sung B and Aggarwal B B 2008 Cancer is a preventable disease that requires major lifestyle changes *Pharm. Res.* **25** 2097–116

[7] Vinogradov S and Wei X 2012 Cancer stem cells and drug resistance: the potential of nanomedicine *Nanomedicine* **7** 597–615

[8] Patra C R, Mukherjee S and Kotcherlakota R 2014 Biosynthesized silver nanoparticles: a step forward for cancer theranostics *Nanomedicine* **9** 1445–8

[9] Mukherjee S and Patra C R 2016 Therapeutic application of anti-angiogenic nanomaterials in cancers *Nanoscale* **8** 12444–70

[10] Weaver B A 2014 How taxol/paclitaxel kills cancer cells *Mol. Biol. Cell.* **25** 2677–81

[11] Caruso M, Colombo A L, Fedeli L L, Pavesi A, Quaroni S D, Saracchi M and Ventrella G 2000 Isolation of endophytic fungi and actinomycetes taxane producers *Ann. Microbiol.* **50** 3–13

[12] Singh S, Sharma B, Kanwar S S and Kumar A 2016 Lead phytochemicals for anticancer drug development *Front. Plant Sci.* **7** 1667

[13] Kharb M, Jat R K and Gupta A 2012 A review on medicinal plants used as a source of anticancer agents *Int. J. Drug Res. Tec.* **2** 177–83

[14] Emami S A, Sahebkar A, Tayarani-Najaran N and Tayarani-Najaran Z 2012 Cancer and its treatment in main ancient books of Islamic Iranian traditional medicine (7th to 14th century AD) *Iran. Red Crescent Med. J.* **14** 747–57

[15] Hajdu S I 2011 A note from history: landmarks in history of cancer, part 1 *Cancer* **117** 1097–102

[16] Saxe T G 1987 Toxicity of medicinal herbal preparations *Am. Fam. Phys.* **35** 135–42

[17] Shukla S and Mehta A 2015 Anticancer potential of medicinal plants and their phytochemicals: a review *Braz. J. Bot.* **38** 199–210

[18] Belayachi L, Aceves-Luquero C, Merghoub N, Bakri Y, de Mattos S F, Amzazi S and Villalonga P 2013 Screening of North African medicinal plant extracts for cytotoxic activity against tumor cell lines *Eur. J. Med.Plants* **3** 310–32

[19] Saklani A and Kutty S K 2008 Plant-derived compounds in clinical trials *Drug Discov. Today* **13** 161–71

[20] Copland M, Jørgensen H G and Holyoake T L 2005 Evolving molecular therapy for chronic myeloid leukaemia—are we on target? *Hematology* **10** 349–59

[21] Raaijmakers M H, de Grouw E P, Heuver L H, van der Reijden B A, Jansen J H, Scheper R J, Scheffer G L, de Witte T J and Raymakers R A 2005 Breast cancer resistance protein in drug resistance of primitive CD34+38- cells in acute myeloid leukemia *Clin. Cancer Res.* **11** 2436–44

[22] Chen W *et al* 2004 Epigenetic and genetic loss of Hic1 function accentuates the role of p53 in tumorigenesis *Cancer Cell* **6** 387–98

[23] Chakraborty S and Rahman T 2012 The difficulties in cancer treatment *Ecancermedicalscience* **6** ed16

[24] Pucci C, Martinelli C and Ciofani G 2019 Innovative approaches for cancer treatment: current perspectives and new challenges *Ecancermedicalscience* **13** 961

[25] Reddy J 2017 Important medicinal plant families and plant based drugs: a review *Proc. of 5th Int. Conf. on Civil, Architecture, Environment and Waste Management (CAEWM-17) (Singapore)*

[26] Macêdo M J F, Ribeiro D A, Santos M O, de Macêdo D G, Macedo J G F, de Almeida B V, Saraiva M E, de Lacerda M S L and Souza M M A 2018 Fabaceae medicinal flora with therapeutic potential in Savanna areas in the Chapada do Araripe, Northeastern Brazil *Rev. Bras. Farmacogn.* **28** 738–50

[27] Priya S and Satheesh kumar P K 2020 Natural products from plants: recent developments in phytochemicals, phytopharmaceuticals, and plant-based neutraceuticals as anticancer agents *Functional and Preservative Properties of Phytochemicals* (New York: Academic) ch 5 pp 145–63

[28] Chan J M, Wang F and Holly E A 2005 Vegetable and fruit intake and pancreatic cancer in a population-based case-control study in the San Francisco bay area *Cancer Epidemiol., Biomarkers Prev.* **14** 2093–7

[29] Cragg G M and Newman D J 2005 Plants as a source of anti-cancer agents *J. Ethnopharmacol.* **100** 72–9

[30] Vainio H and Weiderpass E 2006 Fruit and vegetables in cancer prevention *Nutr. Cancer* **54** 111–42

[31] Heinrich M B J, Gibbons S and Williamson E M 2004 *Fundamentals of Pharmacognosy and Phytotherapy* 1st edn (Edinburgh: Churchill Livingstone)
[32] Tag H, Kalita P, Dwivedi P, Das A K and Namsa N D 2012 Herbal medicines used in the treatment of diabetes mellitus in Arunachal Himalaya, northeast, India *J. Ethnopharmacol.* **141** 786–95
[33] Avi Senna A H 1993 *AlKanoon Fi Altib (The Rules of Medicine). Four Volumes, 1993* (Beirut, Lebanon: Iz Aldin Publications) p 1037 (in Arabic)
[34] Cui Y, Shu X O, Gao Y, Wen W, Ruan Z X, Jin F and Zheng W 2004 Use of complementary and alternative medicine by chinese women with breast cancer *Breast Cancer Res. Treat.* **85** 263–70
[35] Chen Z, Gu K, Zheng Y, Zheng W, Lu W and Shu X O 2008 The use of complementary and alternative medicine among Chinese women with breast cancer *J. Altern. Complement. Med.* **14** 1049–55
[36] Yuan W 1988 [The formation and development of basic theories as an independent discipline in Chinese traditional medicine] (Chi) *Zhonghua yi shi za zhi (Beijing, China : 1980)* **18** 154–8
[37] Li B 2008 [On interest-oriented teaching method for the basic theories of traditional Chinese medicine] *Zhong xi yi jie he xue bao (J. Chin. Integr. Med.)* **6** 643–4
[38] Garodia P, Ichikawa H, Malani N, Sethi G and Aggarwal B B 2007 From ancient medicine to modern medicine: ayurvedic concepts of health and their role in inflammation and cancer *J. Soc. Integr. Oncol.* **5** 25–37
[39] Shan B, Cai Y Z, Sun M and Corke H 2005 Antioxidant capacity of 26 spice extracts and characterization of their phenolic constituents *J. Agric. Food Chem.* **53** 7749–59
[40] Lai P K and Roy J 2004 Antimicrobial and chemopreventive properties of herbs and spices *Curr. Med. Chem.* **11** 1451–60
[41] Shobana S and Naidu K A 2000 Antioxidant activity of selected Indian spices *Prostaglandins Leukot. Essent. Fatty Acids* **62** 107–10
[42] Abdullaev F I 2002 Cancer chemopreventive and tumoricidal properties of saffron (*Crocus sativus* L.) *Exp. Biol.d Med. (Maywood, N.J.)* **227** 20–5
[43] Sudhakar A 2009 History of cancer, ancient and modern treatment methods *J. Cancer Sci. Therap.* **1** 1–4
[44] Ganguly S 2014 Ayurveda for cancer therapy *World J. Pharm. Res.* **3** 1476–9
[45] Patel B, Das S, Prakash R and Yasir M 2010 Natural bioactive compound with anticancer potential *Int. J. Adv. Pharm.* **1** 32–41
[46] Nirmala J M, Samundeeswari A A and Sankar D P 2011 Natural plant resources in anti-cancer therapy—a review *Res. Plant Biol.* **1** 1–14
[47] Iqbal J, Abbasi B A, Mahmood T, Kanwal S, Ali B, Shah S A and Khalil A T 2017 Plant-derived anticancer agents: a green anticancer approach *Asian Pac J Trop. Biomed.* **7** 1129–50
[48] Rowinsky E K, Onetto N, Canetta R M and Arbuck S G 1992 Taxol: the first of the taxanes, an important new class of antitumor agents *Semin. Oncol.* **19** 646–62
[49] Potmeisel M and Pinedo H 1995 *Camptothecins: New Anticancer Agents* (Boca Raton, FL: CRC Press) pp 149–50
[50] Safe S and Kasiappan R 2016 Natural products as mechanism-based anticancer agents: Sp transcription factors as targets *Phytother. Res : PTR* **30** 1723–32
[51] Shoeb M, MacManus S M, Jaspars M, Trevidadu J, Nahar L, Thoo-Lin P K and Sarker S D 2006 Montamine, a unique dimeric indole alkaloid, from the seeds of *Centaurea montana* (Asteraceae), and its *in vitro* cytotoxic activity against the CaCo2 colon cancer cells *Tetrahedron* **62** 11172–7

[52] Perrone D, Ardito F, Giannatempo G, Dioguardi M, Troiano G, Lo Russo L, Lillo A D E, Laino L and Lo Muzio L 2015 Biological and therapeutic activities, and anticancer properties of curcumin *Exp. Ther. Med.* **10** 1615–23

[53] Huang M T, Ma W, Yen P, Xie J G, Han J, Frenkel K, Grunberger D and Conney A H 1997 Inhibitory effects of topical application of low doses of curcumin on 12-O-tetradecanoylphorbol-13-acetate-induced tumor promotion and oxidized DNA bases in mouse epidermis *Carcinogenesis* **18** 83–8

[54] Huang M T, Ma W, Lu Y P, Chang R L, Fisher C, Manchand P S, Newmark H L and Conney A H 1995 Effects of curcumin, demethoxycurcumin, bisdemethoxycurcumin and tetrahydrocurcumin on 12-O-tetradecanoylphorbol-13-acetate-induced tumor promotion *Carcinogenesis* **16** 2493–7

[55] Sonavane K *et al* 2012 Topical curcumin-based cream is equivalent to dietary curcumin in a skin cancer model *J. Skin Cancer* **147863** 2012

[56] Kim S H, Kim C W, Jeon S Y, Go R E, Hwang K A and Choi K C 2014 Chemopreventive and chemotherapeutic effects of genistein, a soy isoflavone, upon cancer development and progression in preclinical animal models *Lab. Anim. Res.* **30** 143–50

[57] Wei H, Saladi R, Lu Y, Wang Y, Palep S R, Moore J, Phelps R, Shyong E and Lebwohl M G 2003 Isoflavone genistein: photoprotection and clinical implications in dermatology *J. Nutr.* **133** 3811S–9S

[58] Wei H, Bowen R, Zhang X and Lebwohl M 1998 Isoflavone genistein inhibits the initiation and promotion of two-stage skin carcinogenesis in mice *Carcinogenesis* **19** 1509–14

[59] Yan X, Qi M, Li P, Zhan Y and Shao H 2017 Apigenin in cancer therapy: anti-cancer effects and mechanisms of action *Cell Biosci.* **7** 50

[60] Wei H, Tye L, Bresnick E and Birt D F 1990 Inhibitory effect of apigenin, a plant flavonoid, on epidermal ornithine decarboxylase and skin tumor promotion in mice *Cancer Res.* **50** 499–502

[61] Birt D F, Mitchell D, Gold B, Pour P and Pinch H C 1997 Inhibition of ultraviolet light induced skin carcinogenesis in SKH-1 mice by apigenin, a plant flavonoid *Anticancer Res.* **17** 85–91

[62] Jing S, Zhang X and Yan L J 2015 Antioxidant activity, antitumor effect, and antiaging property of proanthocyanidins extracted from Kunlun *Chrysanthemum* flowers *Oxid. Med. Cell. Longev.* **2015** 983484

[63] Zhu Y, Shi Z, Yao Y, Hao Y and Ren G 2017 Antioxidant and anti-cancer activities of proanthocyanidins-rich extracts from three varieties of sorghum (*Sorghum bicolor*) bran *Food Agric. Immunol.* **28** 1530–43

[64] Zhao J, Wang J, Chen Y and Agarwal R 1999 Anti-tumor-promoting activity of a polyphenolic fraction isolated from grape seeds in the mouse skin two-stage initiation-promotion protocol and identification of procyanidin B5-3′-gallate as the most effective antioxidant constituent *Carcinogenesis* **20** 1737–45

[65] Mittal A, Elmets C A and Katiyar S K 2003 Dietary feeding of proanthocyanidins from grape seeds prevents photocarcinogenesis in SKH-1 hairless mice: relationship to decreased fat and lipid peroxidation *Carcinogenesis* **24** 1379–88

[66] Kaur M and Agarwal R 2007 Silymarin and epithelial cancer chemoprevention: how close we are to bedside *Toxicol. Appl. Pharmacol.* **224** 350–9

[67] Ramasamy K and Agarwal R 2008 Multitargeted therapy of cancer by silymarin *Cancer Lett.* **269** 352–62

[68] Anthony K P and Saleh M A 2013 Free radical scavenging and antioxidant activities of silymarin components *Antioxidants (Basel, Switzerland)* **2** 398–407
[69] Lani R *et al* 2015 Antiviral activity of silymarin against chikungunya virus *Sci. Rep.* **5** 11421
[70] Montgomery A, Adeyeni T, San K, Heuertz R M and Ezekiel U R 2016 Curcumin sensitizes silymarin to exert synergistic anticancer activity in colon cancer cells *J. Cancer* **7** 1250–7
[71] Katiyar S K, Korman N J, Mukhtar H and Agarwal R 1997 Protective effects of silymarin against photocarcinogenesis in a mouse skin model *J. Natl. Cancer Inst.* **89** 556–66
[72] Heiblig M, Sobh M and Nicolini F E 2014 Subcutaneous omacetaxine mepesuccinate in patients with chronic myeloid leukemia in tyrosine kinase inhibitor-resistant patients: review and perspectives *Leuk. Res.* **38** 1145–53
[73] Mantena S K, Sharma S D and Katiyar S K 2006 Berberine, a natural product, induces G1-phase cell cycle arrest and caspase-3-dependent apoptosis in human prostate carcinoma cells *Mol. Cancer Ther.* **5** 296–308
[74] Barzegar E, Fouladdel S, Movahhed T K, Atashpour S, Ghahremani M H, Ostad S N and Azizi E 2015 Effects of berberine on proliferation, cell cycle distribution and apoptosis of human breast cancer T47D and MCF7 cell lines *Iran. J. Basic Med. Sci.* **18** 334–42
[75] Cragg G M, Newman D J and Yang S S 2006 Natural product extracts of plant and marine origin having antileukemia potential. The NCI experience *J. Nat. Prod.* **69** 488–98
[76] Lauritano C, Andersen J H, Hansen E, Albrigtsen M, Escalera L, Esposit F, Helland K, Hanssen K Ø, Romano G and Ianora A 2016 Bioactivity screening of microalgae for antioxidant, anti-inflammatory, anticancer, anti-diabetes, and antibacterial activities *Front. Marine Sci.* **3** 68
[77] Prakash O, Kumar A and Kumar P 2013 Anticancer potential of plants and natural products: a review *Am. J. Pharmacol.* **1** 104–15
[78] Martinelli C, Pucci C and Ciofani G 2019 Nanostructured carriers as innovative tools for cancer diagnosis and therapy *APL Bioeng.* **3** 011502
[79] Kumar P *et al* 2022 Promises of phytochemical based nano drug delivery systems in the management of cancer *Chem. Biol. Interact.* **351** 109745
[80] Cai Y, Zhang L, Zhang Y and Lu R 2022 Plant-derived exosomes as a drug-delivery approach for the treatment of inflammatory bowel disease and colitis-associated cancer *Pharmaceutics* **14** 822
[81] Yang C, Zhang M and Merlin D 2018 Advances in plant-derived edible nanoparticle-based lipid nano-drug delivery systems as therapeutic nanomedicines *J. Mater. Chem.* B **6** 1312–21
[82] Sarvarian P, Samadi P, Gholipour E, Shams Asenjan K, Hojjat-Farsangi M, Motavalli R, Motavalli Khiavi F and Yousefi M 2022 Application of emerging plant-derived nanoparticles as a novel approach for nano-drug delivery systems *Immunol. Invest.* **51** 1039–59
[83] Xiao J *et al* 2018 Identification of exosome-like nanoparticle-derived microRNAs from 11 edible fruits and vegetables *Peer J.* **6** e5186
[84] Hua S 2014 Orally administered liposomal formulations for colon targeted drug delivery *Front. Pharmacol.* **5** 138
[85] Pérez-Bermúdez P, Blesa J, Soriano J M and Marcilla A 2017 Extracellular vesicles in food: experimental evidence of their secretion in grape fruits *Eur. J. Pharm. Sci.* **98** 40–50
[86] De Robertis M, Sarra A, D'Oria V, Mura F, Bordi F, Postorino P and Fratantonio D 2020 Blueberry-derived exosome-like nanoparticles counter the response to TNF-α-induced change on gene expression in EA.hy926 cells *Biomolecules* **10** E742

[87] Chikara S, Nagaprashantha L D, Singhal J, Horne D, Awasthi S and Singhal S S 2018 Oxidative stress and dietary phytochemicals: role in cancer chemoprevention and treatment *Cancer Lett.* **413** 122–34

[88] González-Vallinas M, González-Castejón M, Rodríguez-Casado A and Ramírez de Molina A 2013 Dietary phytochemicals in cancer prevention and therapy: a complementary approach with promising perspectives *Nutr. Rev.* **71** 585–99

Chapter 10

An overview of phytochemicals under clinical trials for various cancers

Sumana Pal and Rohit Kumar Singh

Cancer refers to an ailment where certain cells in the body experience uncontrolled growth and can subsequently invade other body parts. These cells can give rise to tumors, which can be either malignant (cancerous) or benign (non-cancerous). Worldwide, cancer is a significant contributor to mortality, with approximately 10 million deaths recorded in 2020. The increased understanding of molecular mechanisms involved in cancer development has resulted in the creation of numerous drugs to fight against cancer. In the last few decades, it was seen that the efficacy of chemically synthesized drugs is not greatly significant for cancer treatment and also shows notable side effects. Phytochemicals or naturally occurring plant-derived molecules are important sources for cancer treatment and are also important for the development of innovative drugs. Preclinical and clinical research is accumulating evidence that phytochemicals can influence the formation and progression of cancer by favorably modulating many signaling pathways. The utilization of combinations of phytochemicals in cancer treatment is highly effective due to their ability to induce cell death, inhibit cell growth and invasion, enhance the sensitivity of cancer cells, and consequently boost the body's immune system. Allicin, curcumin, epigallocatechin and resveratrol are some phytochemicals that affect cancer cell lines by working synergistically to suppress cell proliferation, lessen cellular migration and invasion, and trigger cell cycle arrest and apoptosis.

10.1 Introduction

A growing number of cancer cases are being reported in both developed and developing countries [1]. The findings show that more than 19.3 million new cancer cases have lately been identified and recorded, with an estimated 10 million deaths from cancer by 2020 [2]. Chemotherapy, radiation, and surgery are the primary cancer treatments currently available. Chemotherapy can lead to various unwanted

doi:10.1088/978-0-7503-5252-9ch10

effects, including but not limited to hair loss, suppression of bone marrow function, development of drug resistance, gastrointestinal damage, neurological impairments, and toxicity to the heart [3, 4]. There is an urgent need for novel ways of cancer control because cancer incidences are continuously rising globally and are responsible for millions of deaths annually. Instead of seeking to treat cancer in its advanced stages, an alternative strategy for this issue would be to concentrate on carcinogenesis control [4]. Chemoprevention involves the utilization of natural, synthetic, or biological substances to hinder, prevent, or reverse the early stages of cancer development, or to inhibit the invasive potential of precancerous cells [5]. Natural substances are excellent sources for the creation of novel treatments for many diseases. Numerous medicinal plants and herbal compounds have been shown in studies to have anti-cancer properties [7–9].

Phytochemicals have been demonstrated experimentally to be useful in the treatment and prevention of cancer and the outcomes are highly encouraging. It has been shown that phytochemicals derived from medicinal herbs can suppress angiogenesis, slow metastasis, and trigger apoptosis in cells [10, 11]. Phytochemicals, found in plants, impact the taste and appearance of plants and beverages. They can be classified into phenolics, carotenoids, organosulfur compounds, nitrogen-containing compounds, and alkaloids. These biologically active phytochemicals have the ability to hinder cancer development at various stages [6]. Medicinal plants are the most abundant natural resource of substances found in traditional medicine, modern drugs, health supplements, traditional remedies, intermediate compounds for pharmaceuticals, and synthetic drugs [98]. Phytochemicals, present in commonly consumed foods like fruit, vegetables, and nuts, hold great potential for treating various diseases. These nutraceutical phytochemicals play a significant role in promoting human health by offering protection against a wide range of conditions, including cancer, heart disease, diabetes, high blood pressure, inflammation, infections, mental illness, spasmodic conditions, ulcers, osteoporosis, and related disorders [7]. In modern times, phytochemicals and their derivatives have been widely employed in the pharmaceutical and nutraceutical sectors for various purposes, including serving as substrates, enzymatic cofactors, modulators, inhibitors, antioxidants, and even as primary compounds for drug advancement [8]. Leaves, out of all parts of a plant, have the highest capacity to gather bioactive substances, including secondary metabolites [9].

Phytochemicals have traditionally been classified into primary and secondary metabolites, depending on their role in plant metabolism. Primary metabolites include vital compounds like sugars, amino acids, proteins, nucleic acid components, and chlorophylls. Secondary metabolites, on the other hand, encompass a wide range of plant substances such as alkaloids, terpenes, flavonoids, lignans, plant steroids, curcuminoids, saponins, phenolics, and glucosides [10].

Certain phytochemicals possess toxic properties for humans [11]. Aristolochic acid, for instance, is a carcinogen even at low levels [12]. Some phytochemicals act as antinutrients, hindering nutrient absorption [13]. Additionally, specific polyphenols and flavonoids, when consumed in excessive quantities, can exhibit pro-oxidant effects.

The phytochemicals involved in treatment of cancers (figure 10.1) are as follows.

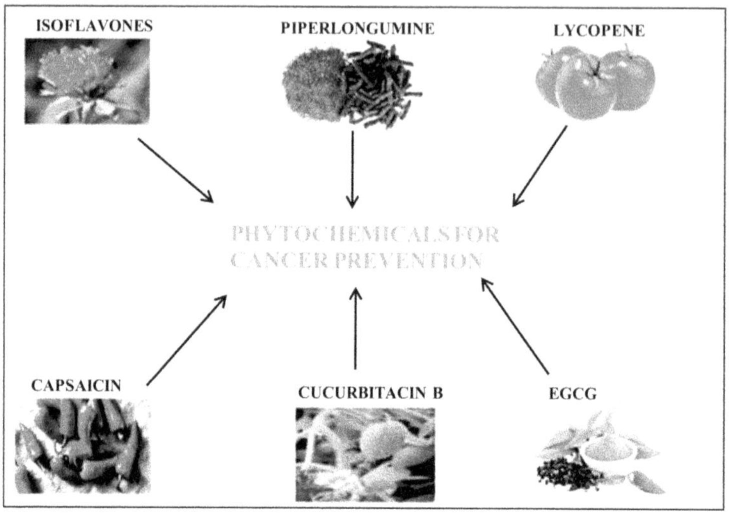

Figure 10.1. Phytochemicals involved in treatment of cancer.

Phytochemicals can impact the important ERK and MAPK pathway that is crucial for cell growth and survival. They regulate cancer progression through various mechanisms. Specifically, resveratrol, genistein, and isothiocyanates (ITCs) induce apoptosis by targeting the MAPK and ERK pathways.

The Akt/PI3 signaling pathway is crucial for controlling and advancing cancer, regulating factors like NF-κB, caspases, Bcl-2, GSK3β, and mTOR. EGF levels influence this pathway, leading to resistance to apoptosis and uncontrolled cell growth. Alkaloids and phenolics significantly affect these factors. Substances such as resveratrol, flavone, and curcumin have anti-cancer properties by impacting the cell cycle, promoting apoptosis, inhibiting Akt/PI3K signaling, activating FOXO3a, and displaying characteristics that hinder proliferation and invasion.

The tumor suppressor protein p53 triggers cell apoptosis, playing a role in anti-cancer activities. Phytochemicals such as resveratrol and EGCG raise p53 levels, reduce Akt levels, induce apoptosis, and pause the cell cycle. There is a notable connection between p53 and the MAPK and JNK pathways. JAKs activate the JAK/STAT signaling pathways, regulating essential genes linked to cell death, proliferation, and apoptosis. Phytochemicals inhibit JAK/STAT signaling, initiating apoptotic cascades and causing cell death in diverse cancer types.

The Wnt/β-Catenin signaling pathways are activated by Wnt-protein binding to frizzled family transmembrane receptors. This results in β-catenin accumulation in the nucleus, regulating transcriptional factors related to cell proliferation, survival, and migration. Phytochemicals like curcumin, resveratrol, and EGCG inhibit β-catenin movement and build-up in the nucleus by activating glycogen synthase kinase 3 (GSK3).

Curcumin induces autophagy, controlling abnormal cell growth and progression. Dietary phytochemicals also regulate various anti-tumor functions, including inflammation control, angiogenesis inhibition, and prevention of invasion and

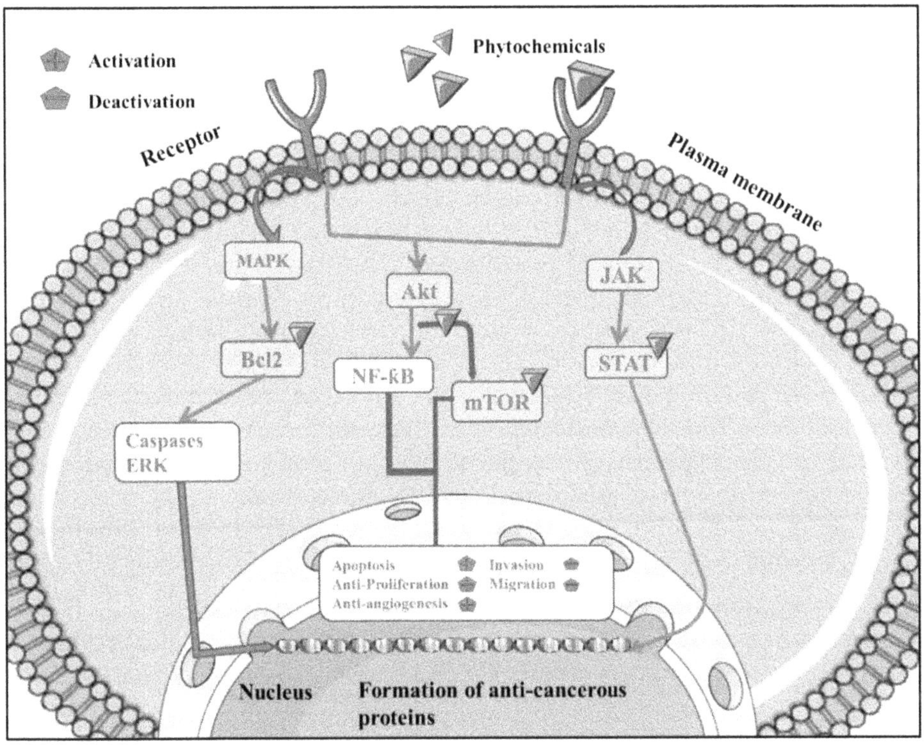

Figure 10.2. Mechanism of phytochemicals.

metastasis. Phytochemicals effectively aid in cancer development through these signaling pathways [14] (figure 10.2).

10.2 Herbal plants and their role in cancer prevention

10.2.1 Garlic (*Allium sativum*)

Garlic (*Allium sativum*) has been an integral part of culinary and medicinal practices across multiple countries for centuries. Its widespread utilization, both in cooking and as a topical remedy, in diverse cultures has solidified its reputation for providing a diverse array of health benefits [15]. According to reports, garlic has a variety of health benefits, such as anti-diabetic, hypolipidemic, antimicrobial, anti-hypertensive, and anti-cancer effects [16]. Furthermore, a double-blind placebo-controlled study conducted on patients with advanced digestive system cancer demonstrated that administering garlic led to an increase in the quantity and effectiveness of natural killer cells [17]. Garlic may reduce the risk of cancer-related death because it increases natural-killer cell production, which is linked to a favorable tumor outcome [18]. The growth of the Hep-2 human laryngeal cancer cell line is also inhibited by garlic [19].

Primarily, it is known for its efficacy in reducing cholesterol levels. Allicin, a sulfur-containing compound found in garlic, is believed to play a crucial role in this property, as suggested by several *in vivo* studies [20]. Allicin, the primary component of garlic, is converted to allicin by the enzyme alliinase. Allicin further breaks down into ajoene and polysulfides, which give garlic its distinctive aroma.

10.2.2 *Camptotheca acuminata*

Camptothecin, a natural alkaloid, can be derived from several plant species such as *Camptotheca acuminata* and *Nothapodytes nimmoniana* [21]. The topoisomerase I enzyme, which is involved in the relaxation of DNA supercoils, is the target of this strong anti-cancer phytochemical [22]. According to reports, there is evidence suggesting that CPT-11, a novel compound derived from camptothecin, shows promise in treating metastatic colorectal cancer. Two FDA-approved semi-synthetic derivatives of camptothecin, irinotecan and topotecan, have proven effective in cancer treatment and are considered safer than the original drug. Topotecan is approved for the treatment of recurrent ovarian, small cell lung, and cervical cancers, while irinotecan is used for advanced colorectal cancer [23].

10.2.3 Curcumin

The rhizome of the turmeric plant yields curcumin, a yellow polyphenol. The anti-inflammatory, antioxidant, and cytoprotective characteristics of curcumin are responsible for its therapeutic effects [24]. Curcumin's potential as an anti-cancer agent stems from its various effects on mutagenesis, cell cycle control, apoptosis, oncogene expression, and metastasis. Curcumin can influence cancer at different stages, including initiation, progression, and metastasis [25]. Curcumin possesses favorable chemopreventive qualities, including minimal toxicity, cost-effectiveness, and easy availability. It targets important molecules like COX-2, NF-kB, TNF-a, and cyclin D1, contributing to cancer cell death [26]. In both clinical and preclinical studies, these molecular targets have exhibited substantial anti-inflammatory and anti-tumor properties. Treatment with curcumin has been observed to significantly reduce the levels of cyclin D1 and CDK-4 in breast and skin cancers [27]. Recent research has uncovered that curcumin has anti-cancer properties as it influences various biological pathways associated with mutagenesis, oncogene expression, regulation of the cell cycle, apoptosis, tumorigenesis, and metastasis [26].

10.2.4 *Hibiscus sabdariffa*

Research utilizing human cell and xenograft models has demonstrated the inhibitory effects of *Hibiscus sabdariffa* leaf extract on the growth of LNCaPtumors. Moreover, the extract has exhibited the capacity to induce apoptosis in leukemia and gastric carcinoma cells, as well as initiate autophagic cell death in melanoma cells [28]. The potential of Hibiscus anthocyanins (HAs) to trigger apoptosis has been observed in gastric cancer and leukemia cells. Conversely, PCA has been shown to hinder the carcinogenic effects of various substances in different tissues of rat models *in vivo*. In healthy men, the intake of *H. sabdariffa* has resulted in notable declines in the urinary concentrations of creatinine, uric acid, citrate, tartrate, calcium, sodium, potassium, and phosphate, with the exception of oxalate [29].

10.2.5 *Viola tricolor*

Viola tricolor, belonging to the Violaceae plant family, is a widely found ornamental plant in Iran. During a study conducted on a human cell line, it was observed that the ethyl acetate and n-butanol fractions derived from *Viola tricolor* effectively suppressed the growth of neuroblastoma N2a cells. The ethyl acetate component of *Viola tricolor* showed promising cytotoxic effects, potentially attributed to its ability to induce apoptosis, inhibit angiogenesis, and decrease the proliferation of tumor cells in thechorioallantoic membrane (CAM) [30]. It is known for its various medicinal properties, including anti-inflammatory, antimicrobial, antioxidant, sedative, and diuretic activities [30].

10.2.6 Resveratrol

Extensive research has been conducted on resveratrol, which is a polyphenolic phytoalexin known as a stilbenoid. The aim of this research has been to investigate its potential to hinder the proliferation of different types of tumor cells, including those found in the breast, colon, prostate, liver, and lung. The results of these studies have shown that resveratrol effectively reduces the growth of tumors and prevents the spread of cancer to the lungs in mice with highly metastatic Lewis lung carcinoma tumors [23].

The skin of various fruits and vegetables, such as grapes, peanuts, berries, and certain other fruits, contains a phytoalexin called resveratrol, specifically known as trans-3, 4', 5-tri-hydroxystilbene. Resveratrol is found in grape powder and exhibits notable anti-inflammatory and antioxidant properties. Moreover, it possesses the capability to hinder the growth of diverse cancer cell types [31]. While it may not directly block the Wnt pathway in colon cancer, it has the potential to decrease the expression of Wnt target genes in the healthy mucosal tissue of individuals with colorectal cancer [32]. Resveratrol has the potential to prevent the initiation and metastasis of colon cancer by targeting the processes controlled by Wnts and their downstream effectors, which include tumor initiation, growth, cell death, and metastasis [33].

10.2.7 Green tea

Green tea is a widely popular drink that enjoys significant consumption, especially in Asia, Europe, and North America. Extensive research has shed light on the diverse health benefits it offers. Green tea consists of proteins, amino acids, carbohydrates, minerals, lipids, vitamins, and volatile components [34]. Recent research has shown that the majority of the biological effects of green tea are caused by catechins, a type of polyphenol [35]. Green tea catechins were proven to be both safe and beneficial for treating premalignant prostate cancer in a double-blind, placebo-controlled research [34]. Additionally, case-control studies confirm green tea's protective effect against pancreatic, prostate, esophageal, colon, and rectum cancers.

It demonstrates anti-proliferative effects on hepatoma cells and reduces lipid levels in rats with hepatoma. It also prevents hepatoxicity and acts as a preventive agent for mammary cancer. The consumption of green tea has been associated with a lower risk of various cancers, such as lung, colon, esophagus, mouth, stomach, small intestine, kidney, pancreas, and mammary glands. Epidemiological studies and trials offer supporting evidence that green tea, along with black and Oolong teas to a lesser extent, can contribute to reducing the likelihood of developing chronic diseases. These effects are attributed to the abundant polyphenols in green tea, which possess strong antioxidant properties. Green tea has the potential to lower blood pressure, reducing the likelihood of stroke and coronary heart disease. Its components offer protection against environmental cancer risk through their antioxidant, antimutagenic, and anticarcinogenic effects [36].

10.2.8 *Panax ginseng*

In Asia, ginseng roots have been used medicinally for thousands of years. The three most often utilized ginsengs in the world are *Panax quinquefolius* (American ginseng), *Panax japonicus* (Japanese ginseng), and *Panax ginseng* (Korean or Chinese ginseng) [37]. Clinical research has shown that P. ginseng both lowers cancer incidence and has positive effects on cancer patients. According to case-control studies, drinking ginseng tea, juice, or fresh slices lowers the incidence of most cancers, including those of the pharynx, larynx, esophagus, stomach, colon, pancreatic, liver, lung, and ovary [41, 42]. It was learned that ginseng use before cancer diagnosis was associated with a higher overall survival rate in a group of 1455 breast cancer patients [38]. Pharmacological effects of ginseng have been seen in cardiovascular, diabetic, and cancer cases. It is utilized to boost immune system health, improve central nervous system (CNS) performance, lessen stress, and display antioxidant properties [39]. Ginsenoside has anti-proliferative, anti-angiogenic, anti-inflammatory, and antioxidant characteristics that are thought to be responsible for its chemotherapeutic effects. Numerous cancers, including breast, lung, liver, colon, and skin cancer, have been shown to be resistant to ginseng's anti-cancer properties [40].

10.2.9 *Rhus verniciflua*

East Asia is the native home of *Rhus verniciflua*, also known as *Toxicodendron vernicifluum*, which is grown in some parts of China, Japan, and Korea. Due to its antioxidant, antibacterial, anti-inflammatory, and anti-cancer characteristics, this plant is also known as the 'lacquer tree' and has long been employed in traditional Korean medicine [44–46]. Patients with advanced non-small cell lung cancer have experienced notable enhancements in survival rates and disease progression durations. These findings indicate that *R. verniciflua* demonstrates synergistic effects and may offer potential benefits to individuals who are ineligible for chemotherapy treatment [47, 48]. By inhibiting a number of transcription factors, raising the expression of p53, caspases, and Bax, and decreasing the levels of survivin, cyclins, and Bcl-2, resveratrol has an anti-proliferative impact. Apoptosis is influenced by the upregulation of caspases and the Bax/Bcl-2 ratio. Resveratrol has been proven to possess protective properties that are effective throughout all stages of carcinogenesis, including initiation, promotion, and progression [1].

10.2.10 *Viscum album*

The mistletoe species known as 'European mistletoe' is called the *Viscum album* and belongs to the Santalaceae family. One of the most popular complementary and alternative cancer treatments in Europe is mistletoe phytochemical preparations [41]. Recent studies have shown that a standardized aqueous extract of *V. album* can mitigate the adverse effects of chemotherapy and improve the quality of life for individuals undergoing cancer treatment. [50, 51]. In patients with various types of cancer, Iscador extends survival duration, enhances self-control, and reduces the suppression of natural killer cell activity [52, 53]. The pharmacological activities of *V. album* have been substantiated through clinical research and experimental models. These activities encompass immunomodulatory, anti-hypertensive, antioxidant, cytotoxic, anti-tumor, anti-inflammatory, anti-diabetic, anti-microbial, and sedative actions [42].

10.2.11 Isoflavones

Flavonoids, which are synthesized by plants, play a vital role in the light-dependent stage of photosynthesis by aiding in electron transportation. These compounds originate from phenylalanine, tyrosine, and acetate components [43] (figure 10.3). Flavonoids, which make up the majority of polyphenolic secondary plant metabolites consumed by humans, are present in a wide range of sources including citrus fruit, nuts, and herbal trees [44]. Due to their various pharmacological attributes, such as their anti-cancer action, flavonoids have drawn a lot of interest. Flavonoids exert their main anti-cancer effects through their role as anti-inflammatory and antioxidant agents [56, 57]. They can suppress the activity of fatty acid synthase, and flavonoids have also been associated with the triggering of apoptosis [45]. Women who consume a lot of phytoestrogens, especially isoflavones, equol, lignans,and enterolactone, have a significantly lower risk of developing breast cancer [46]. The scavenging effect of soy isoflavones on free radicals provides cellular protection within the CNS. Furthermore, they aid in preventing the oxidative modification of low-density lipoprotein (LDL), ensuring its preservation. A relationship between phytoestrogen intake and the incidence of breast cancer was investigated in a case-control research by Ingram *et al.* According to the study, women who consumed a lot of enterolactone, a lignan, and the isoflavone phytoestrogen equol had a significantly lower risk of developing breast cancer. Urinary excretion was used to measure phytoestrogen consumption. The researchers suggested that these findings have the potential to contribute to breast cancer prevention [47].

10.2.12 Isothiocyanates

Fruit and vegetables contain beneficial compounds that go beyond basic nutrition and offer potential health benefits. Glucosinolates, which are found in many plants of the Brassicaceae family, are secondary metabolites. When these plants come into contact with water, a plantenzyme called myrosinase breaks down the glucose group in glucosinolates, resulting in the rapid formation of thiocyanates, ITCs, or nitriles.

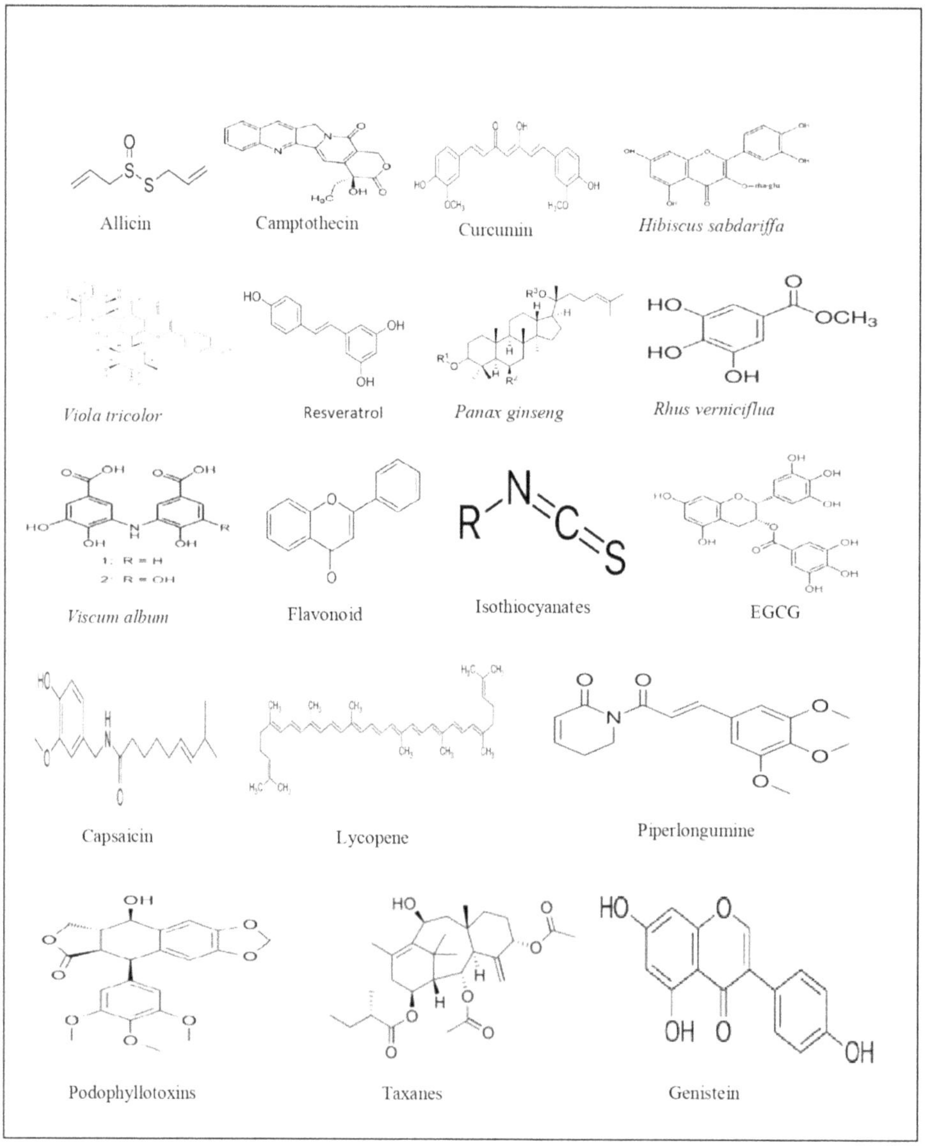

Figure 10.3. Chemical structures of different phytochemicals.

These active compounds are used by plants to defend against parasites. Although heat may deactivate the plant myrosinase, the myrosinase activity of bacteria in the human intestines enables the production and absorption of ITCs [48]. ITCs can prevent the development of cancer (pre-initiation) [49]. Nevertheless, administering excessive amounts of phenethylisothiocyanate (PEITC) or benzyl isothiocyanate (BITC) to rats after exposure to a chemical carcinogen has been observed to encourage bladder cancer [50]. ITCs have proven to be successful in preventing cancer [51]. In this context, their main function is to activate detoxifying enzymes, preventing the start of cancer development [52]. A recent study showed that orally administering a synthetic isothiocyanate called PHI (phenylhexylisothiocyanate) toimmuno-deficient mice with human leukemia HL-60 cell xenografts, at a dosage of 12 μmol/day, significantly reduced the formation of tumors. Importantly, there were no indications of harm to normal tissue cells [53].

10.2.13 (−)-Epigallocatechin-3-gallate (EGCG)

Tea, derived from *Camellia sinensis* leaves, is a highly popular beverage globally and a natural source of polyphenols, particularly catechins. Among these catechins, (−)-Epigallocatechin-3-gallate (EGCG) stands out as the most biologically active compound found in green tea. This fact has been supported by numerous cell culture studies [54], animal models, and epidemiological evidence [55]. A significant body of research has focused on investigating EGCG's anti-cancer properties, primarily its ability to prevent cancer (chemopreventive effects). Similar to other plant-based chemicals, EGCG regulates various signaling pathways that contribute to its cancer-preventing and potential cancer-treating effects. It exhibits antioxidant properties that safeguard against oxidative damage to DNA, lipids, and proteins, which are believed to be associated with cancer development [54]. The compound EGCG triggers programmed cell death and stops the cell cycle in different cancer cell lines originating from solid tumors and human leukemia. Importantly, this effect is exclusive to cancer cells and has no impact on normal cells. Cutting-edge scientific techniques, such as surface plasmon resonance assay and cold spray ionization-mass spectrometry, have provided evidence of the direct interaction between EGCG and nucleic acids [55]. Researchers have discovered that the 67 kDa laminin receptor (67LR) acts as a cell surface receptor for EGCG, mediating its anti-cancer properties. Tumor cells expressing 67LR respond to EGCG, while normal cells like fibroblasts or PBMC are not affected. EGCG has also been found to enhance the efficacy of various anti-cancer drugs, including retinoids [56]. When AM80, a synthetic retinoid used in relapsed and difficult acute promyelocyticleukemia cases, was combined with EGCG in lung cancer, it was discovered that the two substances synergistically triggered apoptosis and increased the expression of DNA damage-inducible genes like GADD153, death receptor 5 (DR5), and p21waf1.

10.2.14 Capsaicin

Capsaicin, a potent alkaloid found in chili peppers from the Capsicum plant genus, has been identified as an effective compound with multiple properties in fighting cancer [68, 69]. It has been documented to have chemopreventive, tumor-suppressing, radio-sensitizing, and anti-cancer effects in different cancer models [57]. The activation of activator protein 1 (AP-1), nuclear factor kappa B (NF-B), and signal transducer and activator of transcription 3 (STAT3) signaling pathways is impeded by capsaicin treatment. These pathways have a significant impact on the advancement of tumors, and capsaicin treatment is responsible for their inhibition [71, 72]. The inhibition of catenin signaling was found to be linked to the induction of apoptosis in pancreatic cancer cells caused by capsaicin. Administering capsaicin orally at a dosage of 5 mg kg^{-1} effectively suppressed the growth of pancreatic tumors implanted in mice [58]. Capsaicin demonstrates its ability to inhibit carcinogens and induce apoptosis in various cancer cell lines *in vitro* as well as inrodents, utilizing multiple pathways [59].

10.2.15 Lycopene

Lycopene, belonging to the carotenoid group, is predominantly present in tomatoes and other foods like watermelons [60]. Its potent antioxidant properties are linked to its protective effects against a range of conditions, including cardiovascular diseases, neurodegenerative disorders, hypertension, osteoporosis, diabetes, and cancer, as it effectively counteracts oxidation [61]. There have been approximately 250 articles published thus far discussing the anti-cancer properties of lycopene. From a chemical perspective, lycopene is a highly lipophilic tetraterpene hydrocarbon that is synthesized by plants and certain microorganisms [62]. Naturally, lycopene exists predominantly in the all-trans-isomer form. Zu *et al* conducted a study showing that higher consumption of lycopene was linked to a reduced occurrence of prostate cancer. Furthermore, individuals with increased lycopene intake exhibited decreased expression of tumor tissue biomarkers associated with angiogenesis, apoptosis, cell proliferation, and differentiation. This suggests that lycopene inhibits tumor growth by preventing the formation of new blood vessels in the tumor [60]. According to reports, lycopene tends to accumulate more in prostate tissue compared to other tissues. This specific accumulation may contribute to its anti-prostate cancer properties [63].

Lycopene hinders the growth of prostate and breast cancer cells by obstructing NF-kB signaling [64]. Furthermore, it boosts the efficacy of quinacrine in combating breast cancer cells by blocking Wnt-TCF signaling [65]. In an experiment using BALB/c nude mice with DU145 prostate cancer cells, lycopene was administered at doses of 100 and 300 mg kg^{-1}. The results showed a 55.6% reduction in tumor growth with the 100 mg kg^{-1} dose and a 75.8% reduction with the 300 mg kg^{-1} dose [66]. In a recent study, it was discovered that lycopene prevents the proliferation of human hepatoma SK-Hep-1 cells in athymic nude mice [66]. Chen *et al* demonstrated the anti-angiogenic effects of lycopene in diverse laboratory and animal models, indicating its potential involvement in regulating PI3K-Akt and ERK/p38 signaling pathways [67]. Multiple studies have provided evidence that the combined use of lycopene and melatonin exhibits powerful chemopreventive effects through their antioxidant and anti-inflammatory actions [68]. The oral administration of 16 mg kg^{-1} of lycopene over a period of 7 weeks resulted in a significant 67% suppression of prostate tumor growth in athymic nude mice, in comparison to the control group. Moreover, the study found that lycopene reduced the levels of proliferating cell nuclear antigen (PCNA) in tumor tissues and vascular endothelial growth factor (VEGF) in plasma [69].

10.2.16 Piperlongumine

Piperlongumine also known as Piplartine, is a chemical compound extracted from the roots of the long pepper plant, *Piper longum* L., from the Piperaceae family.

Long peppers have significant importance in Indian Ayurvedic medicine and Latin American folk medicine [70], and they are utilized for treating cancer [71]. In general, piperlongumine demonstrates considerable potential as both a chemotherapy and chemoprevention agent, offering a viable choice for treating cancer. More specifically, when applied to pancreatic cancer cells, piperlongumine induces the production of reactive oxygen species (ROS), leading to DNA damage linked to oxidative stress [72]. A study demonstrates that piperlongumine triggers autophagy-mediated apoptosis by inhibiting the PI3K/Akt/mTOR pathway in lung cancer [73]. By blocking the activation of STAT3, piperlongumine successfully impedes the metastatic capabilities of pancreatic cancer and melanoma. This inhibition also suppresses the resistance to anoikis, a process involved in detachment-induced cell death [74]. Cucurbitacins, which are tetracyclic triterpenoids derived from traditional Chinese medicinal plants of the Cucurbitaceae family, include Cucurbitacin B (CuB) as the most powerful anti-cancer compound. CuB demonstrates promising effects in various cancer models [75]. Recent studies have validated the anti-angiogenic properties of CuB, indicating its ability to inhibit the formation of new blood vessels. This effect is associated with the suppression of VEGF/FAK/MMP-9 signaling in highly metastatic breast cancer cells [76]. In the case of pancreatic cancer, CuB has been found to enhance the ability of gemcitabine, a chemotherapy drug, to inhibit cell proliferation by blocking the JAK-STAT pathway [77]. To compare the way CuB behaves in the body with CuB that is encapsulated in solid lipid nanoparticles, scientists conducted studies on its pharmacokinetic profile. They discovered that the CuB-loaded nanoparticles were taken up by tumor cells 3.4 times more effectively than regular CuB, resulting in improved suppression of tumor growth [78]. In another investigation, researchers demonstrated that modifying phospholipid complexes with CuB led to better therapeutic effectiveness, increased bioavailability, and targeted delivery of the drug for cholangiocarcinoma treatment [79].

10.2.17 Podophyllotoxins

Podophyllotoxin, obtained from *Podophyllum peltatum* and *Podophyllum emodi* (Berberidaceae), is a natural compound. It can reversibly bind to tubulin. On the other hand, its derivatives, etoposide, and teniposide, can inhibit topoisomerase II and cause DNA cleavage through the action of this enzyme. Additionally, Podophyllotoxin shows promise in combating drug-resistant tumor cells of various types, indicating its potential as an anti-multidrug-resistant agent [80].

10.2.18 Cabazitaxel

Taxanes, powerful drugs used to combat cancer, were originally extracted from the Yew tree's bark. Their mechanism of action involves stabilizing microtubules, resulting in the interruption of the cell cycle and abnormal cell division. Cabazitaxel, a more recent derivative of docetaxel, exhibits cytotoxic effects on various tumor types that have developed resistance to docetaxel. Moreover, it offers the advantage of fewer side effects [81]. Taxanes play a crucial role in treating type II endometrial cancers, which are not influenced by estrogen and encompass grade 3 endometrioid, serous, and clear-cell histotypes [82].

10.2.19 Genistein

Isoflavones, a type of flavonoid, are naturally occurring compounds that are present in limited quantities. Soyfoods, primarily consumed by the Asian population, are the main dietary source of these beneficial plant chemicals. Soyfoods contribute to about 10% of the total protein intake for individuals in this population [83]. Scientific studies conducted in laboratories have demonstrated that genistein, a specific compound found in isoflavones, possesses the capability to impede the growth of different types of cancer cells, including both hormone-dependent and hormone-independent ones. The impact of genistein on cellular signaling, however, is dependent on the dosage administered [84]. During binding assays, genistein competes with 17-β-estradiol (E2) for estrogen receptors (ERs) binding. ERs, specifically ERβ, have a critical role in the functions of estrogens and selective ER modulators in breast cancer. Notably, approximately 70% of breast cancer cases express the ERβ variant. ERs mediate hormone effects in estrogen-dependent tissues such as the uterus, ovary, and breast, where the levels and proportions of these receptors can significantly vary. When genistein is present at a concentration of 300 nM, it activates both ERs. The final impact on gene expression and cell fate depends on the ligand dosage and the varying ability of ligand-ER complexes to recruit modulators at binding sites of hormone-regulated genes [85]. It is reasonable to infer that the ability of genistein to inhibit tyrosine kinase (PTK) plays a significant role in its anti-proliferative activity at concentrations exceeding 10 μM. Notably, genistein demonstrates substantial *in vitro* inhibitory effects on PTKs, particularly EGF-R (tables 10.1 and 10.2).

10.3 Conclusion

When it comes to the various combinations of genetic and epigenetic events that take place in a single cell to produce a neoplastic distortion, the process of carcinogenesis is complex and heterogeneous. Finding novel cancer treatments is crucial because it is a leading cause of death worldwide and is on the rise. Natural products are becoming more popular since they are more dependable and affordable than present pharmaceuticals, which have negative effects. For the discovery of new treatments for human ailments, medicinal plants have traditionally been a significant source. Hence, the vital source for the identification and advancement of new pharmacological approaches continues to be medicinal plants. Utilizing plant-based chemicals for cancer chemoprevention has become a popular strategy in cancer care. Chemoprevention involves various classes of phytochemicals, including phenolics, carotenoids, alkaloids, organosulfur compounds, and nitrogen-containing compounds. Limiting proliferation, inducing cell cycle arrest and apoptosis, raising antioxidant status, neutralizing carcinogens, limiting growth, and immune system control are all ways that phytochemicals prevent cancer. A major objective of anticancer research is the quest for new chemopreventive phyto-compounds, which also

Table 10.1. Different phytochemicals and their molecular targets against cancer.

Phytochemicals (compound class)	Botanical name (family)	Molecular targets	References
Allicin	*Allium sativum* (Amaryllidaceae)	STAT3 signaling pathway	[86]
Curcumin	*Curcuma longa* (Zingiberaceae)	Modulates cell signaling and gene expression regulatory pathways	[87]
Epigallocatechin	*Camellia sinensis* (Theaceae)	Prevent cell proliferation and apoptosis	[55]
Genistein	*Glycine max* (legumes)	wnt/b-catenin and Akt signaling pathway	[85]
Resveratrol	*Polygonumcuspidatum* (Polygonaceae)	Regulating cell cycle and apoptosis pathways	[88]
Camptothecin (alkaloid)	*Camptotheca acuminate* (Nyssaceae)	Inhibition of type I topoisomerase	[89]
Viola tricolor	*Violaceae*	Induces apoptosis and also causes angiogenesis	[30]
EGCG	*Camellia sinensis* (Theaceae)	reducing the growth and triggering apoptosis in pancreatic cancer cells that had PTEN expression	[90]
Piperlongumine	Amide alkaloid	Causes redox imbalance in cancer cells by increasing ROS level	[91]
Podophyllotoxin	Cupressaceae	Hampers cell growth via polymerization of tubulin	[92]
Capsaicin	Vanilloid	Changes expression of different genes that cause cancer cell growth and metastasis	[93]
Taxanes	Diterpenes	Stops mitosis and also interacts with microtubules	[94]
Lycopene	Carotenoid	Inhibits tumor cell-cycle progression, IGF-1 signaling transduction	[95]
Isothiocyanates	Brassicaceae	Generate apoptosis through a caspase-3-dependent mechanism	[96]

aid in the identification of new targets for therapy. A number of the dietary chemicals discussed in this study may be effective cancer chemopreventive agents, and it has been demonstrated that eating foods containing these bioactive compounds provides protective and curative effects on many cancer types. The anti-cancer and chemopreventive properties of phytochemicals have gained growing interest among oncology researchers due to their low toxicity in healthy cells and notable impact on malignant cells. Further clinical trials must be conducted to examine the efficacy and toxicity documentation of the anti-cancer phytochemicals presented in this chapter.

Table 10.2. Phytochemicals clinically tested in cancerous patients.

Phytochemicals	Type of cancer	Effects	References
Allicin	Liver, pancreatic cancer	Increase in the number and activity of natural killer cells.	[95]
Curcumin	Advanced and metastatic breast cancer	Preventing carcinogenicity.	[96]
Epigallocatechin	Colorectal cancer	Compared to the baseline, the methylation pattern has changed.	[97]
Resveratrol	GI neuro endocrine tumors with a low grade	Activation of Notch1 and toxicity.	[1]
Camptotheca acuminata	Gastric cancer, intestinal cancer, head and neck tumors, and bladder carcinoma	Response rates ranging from 20% to 30% were observed in single-agent trials for multiple cancer types, such as non-small cell lung, cervical, ovarian, colorectal, and breast cancers. In patients with non-small cell lung cancer and acute T-cell leukemia or lymphoma, the response rates varied between 30% and 40%. Importantly, Phase I trials that combined a CPT analog with cisplatinum achieved impressive response rates of up to 40%–50% in non-small cell lung cancer patients.	[23]
Green tea	Adenocarcinoma of the prostate	Greater consumption of green tea over longer durations is associated with a reduced risk of prostate cancer. Furthermore, consuming green tea is linked to a lower chance of developing esophageal cancer.	[97]
Panax ginseng	Cancer of uterine,ovary, rectum, stomach	Case-control studies have indicated that the consumption of various ginseng products, such as fresh sliced ginseng, ginseng juice, and tea, is associated with enhanced mental and physical performance. Additionally, ginseng products have been linked to a reduced risk of cancers affecting the pharynx, larynx, esophagus, stomach, colon, pancreas, liver, lung, and ovary.	[97]
Rhus verniciflua	Metastatic colorectal or pancreatic cancer	Enhancement of the overall survival rate.	[1]

References

[1] Hosseini A and Ghorbani A 2015 Cancer therapy with phytochemicals: evidence from clinical studies *Avicenna J. Phytomed.* **5** 84–97

[2] Global Cancer Statistics 2022: The Trends Projection Analysis. https://researchgate.net/publication/364185741_Global_Cancer_Statistics_2022_the_trends_projection_analysis (accessed 23 May 2023)

[3] Monsuez J J, Charniot J C, Vignat N and Artigou J Y 2010 Cardiac side-effects of cancer chemotherapy *Int. J. Cardiol.* **144** 3–15

[4] Tsao A S, Kim E S and Hong W K 2004 Chemoprevention of cancer *CA: Cancer J Clin.* **54** 150–80

[5] Sharma H, Parihar L and Parihar P 2011 Review on cancer and anticancerous properties of some medicinal plants *J. Med. Plants Res.* **5** 1818–35

[6] Ghorbani A 2013 Phytotherapy for diabetic dyslipidemia: evidence from clinical trials *Clin. Lipidol.* **8** 311–9

[7] Thakur M, Singh K and Khedkar R 2020 *Phytochemicals* (Amsterdam: Elsevier) pp 341–61

[8] Singh M K, Singh S K, Singh A V, Verma H, Singh P P and Kumar A 2020 Phytochemicals: Intellectual property rights *Functional and Preservative Properties of Phytochemicals* ed B Prakash (New York: Academic) pp 363–75

[9] Kumar M *et al* 2021 Mango (*Mangifera indica* L.) leaves: nutritional composition, phytochemical profile, and health-promoting bioactivities *Antioxid Basel Switz* **10** 299

[10] Koche D, Shirsat R and Kawale M 2016 An overview of mahor classes of phytochemicals: their types and role in disease prevention *Hislopia J.* **9** 1–11

[11] Chinese herbology. In: *Wikipedia.* 2023 https://en.wikipedia.org/w/index.php?title=Chinese_herbology&oldid=1150374563 (accessed 23 May 2023)

[12] Smith A 2000 *Oxford Dictionary of Biochemistry and Molecular Biology* (Oxford: Oxford University Press) 2nd edn

[13] Halliwell B 2007 Dietary polyphenols: good, bad, or indifferent for your health? *Cardiovasc. Res.* **73** 341–7

[14] George B P, Chandran R and Abrahamse H 2021 Role of phytochemicals in cancer chemoprevention: insights *Antioxidants* **10** 1455

[15] Blumenthal M, Goldberg A and Brinckmann J 2023 *Herbal Medicine* (CAB International)

[16] Ishikawa H, Saeki T, Otani T, Suzuki T, Shimozuma K and Nishino H *et al* 2006 Aged garlic extract prevents a decline of NK cell number and activity in patients with advanced cancer *J. Nutr.* **136** 816S–20S

[17] Coca S, Perez-Piqueras J, Martinez D, Colmenarejo A, Saez M A and Vallejo C *et al* 1997 The prognostic significance of intratumoral natural killer cells in patients with colorectal carcinoma *Cancer* **79** 2320–8

[18] de Jonge M J A, Kaye S, Verweij J, Brock C, Reade S and Scurr M *et al* 2004 Phase I and pharmacokinetic study of XR11576, an oral topoisomerase I and II inhibitor, administered on days 1–5 of a 3-weekly cycle in patients with advanced solid tumours *Br. J. Cancer* **91** 1459–65

[19] Mortazavian S M, Ghorbani A and Ghorbani Hesari T 2012 Effect of hydro-alcoholic extracts of *Viola tricolor* and its fractions on proliferation of cervix carcinoma cells *Iran. J. Obstet Gynecol. Infertil.* **15** 9–16

[20] *American Botanical Council.* https://herbalgram.org/resources/herbalgram/issues/37/table-of-contents/article1013/ (accessed 3 June 2023); Foster S 1996 Garlic: the science and

therapeutic application of Allium sativum L. and related species (book review) *HerbalGram* **1996** 64

[21] Li Q Y, Zu Y G, Shi R Z and Yao L P 2006 Review camptothecin: current perspectives *Curr. Med. Chem.* **13** 2021–39

[22] Shimada Y, Yoshino M, Wakui A, Nakao I, Futatsuki K and Sakata Y *et al* 1993 Phase II study of CPT-11, a new camptothecin derivative, in metastatic colorectal cancer. CPT-11 gastrointestinal cancer study group *J. Clin. Oncol. Off J. Am. Soc. Clin. Oncol.* **11** 909–13

[23] Choudhari A S, Mandave P C, Deshpande M, Ranjekar P and Prakash O 2020 Phytochemicals in cancer treatment: from preclinical studies to clinical practice *Front. Pharmacol.* **10** 1614

[24] Alinejad B, Ghorbani A and Sadeghnia H R 2013 Effects of combinations of curcumin, linalool, rutin, safranal, and thymoquinone on glucose/serum deprivation-induced cell death *Avicenna. J. Phytomed.* **3** 321–8

[25] Cheng A L, Hsu C H, Lin J K, Hsu M M, Ho Y F and Shen T S *et al* 2001 Phase I clinical trial of curcumin, a chemopreventive agent, in patients with high-risk or pre-malignant lesions *Anticancer Res.* **21** 2895–900

[26] Wilken R, Veena M S, Wang M B and Srivatsan E S 2011 Curcumin: a review of anti-cancer properties and therapeutic activity in head and neck squamous cell carcinoma *Mol. Cancer* **10** 12

[27] Mukhopadhyay A, Banerjee S, Stafford L J, Xia C, Liu M and Aggarwal B B 2002 Curcumin-induced suppression of cell proliferation correlates with down-regulation of cyclin D1 expression and CDK4-mediated retinoblastoma protein phosphorylation *Oncogene* **21** 8852–61

[28] Chiu C T, Hsuan S W, Lin H H, Hsu C C, Chou F P and Chen J H 2015 *Hibiscus sabdariffa* leaf polyphenolic extract induces human melanoma cell death, apoptosis, and autophagy *J. Food Sci.* **80** H649–658

[29] Ali B H, Wabel N A and Blunden G 2005 Phytochemical, pharmacological and toxicological aspects of *Hibiscus sabdariffa* L.: a review *Phytother Res.* **19** 369–75

[30] Sadeghnia H R, Ghorbani Hesari T, Mortazavian S M, Mousavi S H, Tayarani-Najaran Z and Ghorbani A 2014 *Viola tricolor* induces apoptosis in cancer cells and exhibits antiangiogenic activity on chicken chorioallantoic membrane *BioMed. Res. Int.* **2014** 625792

[31] Athar M, Back J H, Tang X, Kim K H, Kopelovich L and Bickers D R *et al* 2007 Resveratrol: a review of preclinical studies for human cancer prevention *Toxicol. Appl. Pharmacol.* **224** 274–83

[32] Nguyen A V, Martinez M, Stamos M J, Moyer M P, Planutis K and Hope C *et al* 2009 Results of a phase I pilot clinical trial examining the effect of plant-derived resveratrol and grape powder on Wnt pathway target gene expression in colonic mucosa and colon cancer *Cancer Manag. Res.* **1** 25–37

[33] Anastas J N and Moon R T 2013 WNT signalling pathways as therapeutic targets in cancer *Nat. Rev. Cancer* **13** 11–26

[34] Gao Y T, McLaughlin J K, Blot W J, Ji B T, Dai Q and Fraumeni J F 1994 Reduced risk of esophageal cancer associated with green tea consumption *J. Natl. Cancer Inst.* **86** 855–8

[35] Bettuzzi S, Brausi M, Rizzi F, Castagnetti G, Peracchia G and Corti A 2006 Chemoprevention of human prostate cancer by oral administration of green tea catechins in volunteers with high-grade prostate intraepithelial neoplasia: a preliminary report from a one-year proof-of-principle study *Cancer Res.* **66** 1234–40

[36] Chacko S M, Thambi P T, Kuttan R and Nishigaki I 2010 Beneficial effects of green tea: a literature review *Chin. Med.* **5** 13

[37] Yun T K and Choi S Y 1990 A case-control study of ginseng intake and cancer *Int. J. Epidemiol.* **19** 871–6

[38] Cui Y, Shu X O, Gao Y T, Cai H, Tao M H and Zheng W 2006 Association of ginseng use with survival and quality of life among breast cancer patients *Am. J. Epidemiol.* **163** 645–53

[39] Park B J, Lee Y J, Lee H R, Jung D H, Na H Y and Kim H B *et al* 2012 Effects of Korean red ginseng on cardiovascular risks in subjects with metabolic syndrome: a double-blind randomized controlled study *Korean. J. Fam. Med.* **33** 190–6

[40] Majeed F, Malik F Z, Ahmed Z, Afreen A, Afzal M N and Khalid N 2018 Ginseng phytochemicals as therapeutics in oncology: recent perspectives *Biomed. Pharmacother.* **100** 52–63

[41] Kienle G S, Berrino F, Büssing A, Portalupi E, Rosenzweig S and Kiene H 2003 Mistletoe in cancer—a systematic review on controlled clinical trials *Eur. J. Med. Res.* **8** 109–19

[42] Singh B N, Saha C, Galun D, Upreti D K, Bayry J and Kaveri S V 2016 European *Viscum album*: a potent phytotherapeutic agent with multifarious phytochemicals, pharmacological properties and clinical evidence *RSC Adv.* **6** 23837–57

[43] Batra P and Sharma A K 2013 Anti-cancer potential of flavonoids: recent trends and future perspectives *3 Biotech.* **3** 439–59

[44] Pallauf K, Duckstein N and Rimbach G 2017 A literature review of flavonoids and lifespan in model organisms *Proc. Nutr. Soc.* **76** 145–62

[45] Brusselmans K, Vrolix R, Verhoeven G and Swinnen J V 2005 Induction of cancer cell apoptosis by flavonoids is associated with their ability to inhibit fatty acid synthase activity *J. Biol. Chem.* **280** 5636–45

[46] Ingram D, Sanders K, Kolybaba M and Lopez D 1997 Case-control study of phyto-oestrogens and breast cancer *Lancet Lond Engl.* **350** 990–4

[47] Rudzińska A, Juchaniuk P, Oberda J, Wiśniewska J, Wojdan W and Szklener K *et al* 2023 Phytochemicals in cancer treatment and cancer prevention—review on epidemiological data and clinical trials *Nutrients* **15** 1896

[48] Shapiro T A, Fahey J W, Wade K L, Stephenson K K and Talalay P 1998 Human metabolism and excretion of cancer chemoprotective glucosinolates and isothiocyanates of cruciferous vegetables *Cancer Epidemiol. Biomark Prev.* **7** 1091–100

[49] Kuroiwa Y, Nishikawa A, Kitamura Y, Kanki K, Ishii Y and Umemura T *et al* 2006 Protective effects of benzyl isothiocyanate and sulforaphane but not resveratrol against initiation of pancreatic carcinogenesis in hamsters *Cancer Lett.* **241** 275–80

[50] Okazaki K, Umemura T, Imazawa T, Nishikawa A, Masegi T and Hirose M 2003 Enhancement of urinary bladder carcinogenesis by combined treatment with benzyl isothiocyanate and N-butyl-N-(4-hydroxybutyl)nitrosamine in rats after initiation *Cancer Sci.* **94** 948–52

[51] Hecht S S 1995 Chemoprevention by isothiocyanates *J. Cell. Biochem. Suppl.* **22** 195–209

[52] Zhang Y and Talalay P 1994 Anticarcinogenic activities of organic isothiocyanates: chemistry and mechanisms *Cancer Res.* **54** 1976s–81s

[53] Rao C V, Wang C X, Simi B, Lubet R, Kelloff G and Steele V *et al* 1997 Enhancement of experimental colon cancer by genistein *Cancer Res.* **57** 3717–22

[54] Khan N, Afaq F, Saleem M, Ahmad N and Mukhtar H 2006 Targeting multiple signaling pathways by green tea polyphenol (−)-epigallocatechin-3-gallate *Cancer Res.* **66** 2500–5

[55] Carlson J R, Bauer B A, Vincent A, Limburg P J and Wilson T 2007 Reading the tea leaves: anticarcinogenic properties of (−)-epigallocatechin-3-gallate *Mayo Clin. Proc.* **82** 725–32
[56] Shammas M A, Neri P, Koley H, Batchu R B, Bertheau R C and Munshi V *et al* 2006 Specific killing of multiple myeloma cells by (−)-epigallocatechin-3-gallate extracted from green tea: biologic activity and therapeutic implications *Blood* **108** 2804–10
[57] Venier N A, Colquhoun A J, Sasaki H, Kiss A, Sugar L and Adomat H *et al* 2015 Capsaicin: a novel radio-sensitizing agent for prostate cancer *Prostate* **75** 113–25
[58] Suresh D and Srinivasan K 2010 Tissue distribution and elimination of capsaicin, piperine and curcumin following oral intake in rats *Indian J. Med. Res.* **131** 682–91
[59] Bley K, Boorman G, Mohammad B, McKenzie D and Babbar S 2012 A comprehensive review of the carcinogenic and anticarcinogenic potential of capsaicin *Toxicol. Pathol.* **40** 847–73
[60] Chen J, O'Donoghue A, Deng Y F, Zhang B, Kent F and O'Hare T 2014 The effect of lycopene on the PI3K/Akt signalling pathway in prostate cancer *Anticancer Agents Med. Chem.* **14** 800–5
[61] Agarwal S and Rao A V 2000 Tomato lycopene and its role in human health and chronic diseases *CMAJ Can. Med. Assoc. J. J. Assoc. Medicale Can.* **163** 739–44
[62] Zu K, Mucci L, Rosner B A, Clinton S K, Loda M and Stampfer M J *et al* 2014 Dietary lycopene, angiogenesis, and prostate cancer: a prospective study in the prostate-specific antigen era *J. Natl. Cancer Inst.* **106** djt430
[63] Assar E A, Vidalle M C, Chopra M and Hafizi S 2016 Lycopene acts through inhibition of IκB kinase to suppress NF-κB signaling in human prostate and breast cancer cells *Tumour. Biol.* **37** 9375–85
[64] Preet R, Mohapatra P, Das D, Satapathy S R, Choudhuri T and Wyatt M D *et al* 2013 Lycopene synergistically enhances quinacrine action to inhibit Wnt-TCF signaling in breast cancer cells through APC *Carcinogenesis* **34** 277–86
[65] Tang L, Jin T, Zeng X and Wang J S 2005 Lycopene inhibits the growth of human androgen-independent prostate cancer cells *in vitro* and in BALB/c nude mice *J. Nutr.* **135** 287–90
[66] Huang C S, Liao J W and Hu M L 2008 Lycopene inhibits experimental metastasis of human hepatoma SK-Hep-1 cells in athymic nude mice *J. Nutr.* **138** 538–43
[67] Oguz E, Kocarslan S, Tabur S, Sezen H, Yilmaz Z and Aksoy N 2015 Effects of lycopene alone or combined with melatonin on methotrexate-induced nephrotoxicity in rats *Asian Pac. J. Cancer Prev. APJCP* **16** 6061–6
[68] Moselhy S S 2008 Al mslmani MAB. Chemopreventive effect of lycopene alone or with melatonin against the genesis of oxidative stress and mammary tumors induced by 7,12 dimethyl(a)benzanthracene in sprague dawely female rats *Mol. Cell. Biochem.* **319** 175–80
[69] Bezerra D P, Pessoa C, de Moraes M O, Saker-Neto N, Silveira E R and Costa-Lotufo L V 2013 Overview of the therapeutic potential of piplartine (piperlongumine) *Eur. J. Pharm. Sci. Off. J. Eur. Fed. Pharm. Sci.* **48** 453–63
[70] Prasad S and Tyagi A K 2016 Historical spice as a future drug: therapeutic potential of piperlongumine *Curr. Pharm. Des.* **22** 4151–9
[71] Dhillon H, Chikara S and Reindl K M 2014 Piperlongumine induces pancreatic cancer cell death by enhancing reactive oxygen species and DNA damage *Toxicol. Rep.* **1** 309–18
[72] Wang F, Mao Y, You Q, Hua D and Cai D 2015 Piperlongumine induces apoptosis and autophagy in human lung cancer cells through inhibition of PI3K/Akt/mTOR pathway *Int. J. Immunopathol. Pharmacol.* **28** 362–73

[73] Fofaria N M and Srivastava S K 2014 Critical role of STAT3 in melanoma metastasis through anoikis resistance *Oncotarget.* **5** 7051–64
[74] Fofaria N M and Srivastava S K 2015 STAT3 induces anoikis resistance, promotes cell invasion and metastatic potential in pancreatic cancer cells *Carcinogenesis* **36** 142–50
[75] Sinha S, Khan S, Shukla S, Lakra A D, Kumar S and Das G *et al* 2016 Cucurbitacin B inhibits breast cancer metastasis and angiogenesis through VEGF-mediated suppression of FAK/MMP-9 signaling axis *Int. J. Biochem. Cell Biol.* **77** 41–56
[76] Thoennissen N H, Iwanski G B, Doan N B, Okamoto R, Lin P and Abbassi S *et al* 2009 Cucurbitacin B induces apoptosis by inhibition of the JAK/STAT pathway and potentiates antiproliferative effects of gemcitabine on pancreatic cancer cells *Cancer Res.* **69** 5876–84
[77] Hu H, Liu D, Zhao X, Qiao M and Chen D 2013 Preparation, characterization, cellular uptake and evaluation *in vivo* of solid lipid nanoparticles loaded with cucurbitacin B *Drug Dev. Ind. Pharm.* **39** 770–9
[78] Cheng L, Xu P H, Shen B-D, Shen G, Li J-J and Qiu L *et al* 2015 Improve bile duct-targeted drug delivery and therapeutic efficacy for cholangiocarcinoma by cucurbitacin B loaded phospholipid complex modified with berberine hydrochloride *Int. J. Pharm.* **489** 148–57
[79] Cao B, Chen H, Gao Y, Niu C, Zhang Y and Li L 2015 CIP-36, a novel topoisomerase II-targeting agent, induces the apoptosis of multidrug-resistant cancer cells *in vitro Int. J. Mol. Med.* **35** 771–6
[80] Kotsakis A, Matikas A, Koinis F, Kentepozidis N, Varthalitis I I and Karavassilis V *et al* 2016 A multicentre phase II trial of cabazitaxel in patients with advanced non-small-cell lung cancer progressing after docetaxel-based chemotherapy *Br. J. Cancer* **115** 784–8
[81] Lampe J W, Nishino Y, Ray R M, Wu C, Li W and Lin M G *et al* 2007 Plasma isoflavones and fibrocystic breast conditions and breast cancer among women in shanghai, China *Cancer Epidemiol Biomark Prev.* **16** 2579–86
[82] Schwab C L, English D P, Roque D M and Santin A D 2014 Taxanes: their impact on gynecologic malignancy *Anticancer Drugs* **25** 522–35
[83] Kurahashi N, Iwasaki M, Sasazuki S, Otani T, Inoue M and Tsugane S *et al* 2007 Soy product and isoflavone consumption in relation to prostate cancer in Japanese men *Cancer Epidemiol Biomark Prev.* **16** 538–45
[84] Kuiper G G, Lemmen J G, Carlsson B, Corton J C, Safe S H and van der Saag P T *et al* 1998 Interaction of estrogenic chemicals and phytoestrogens with estrogen receptor beta *Endocrinology* **139** 4252–63
[85] Akiyama T, Ishida J, Nakagawa S, Ogawara H, Watanabe S and Itoh N *et al* 1987 Genistein, a specific inhibitor of tyrosine-specific protein kinases *J. Biol. Chem.* **262** 5592–5
[86] Huang L, Jia S, Wu R, Chen Y, Ding S and Dai C *et al* 2022 The structure, antioxidant and antibacterial properties of thiol-modified soy protein isolate induced by allicin *Food Chem.* **396** 133713
[87] Kunnumakkara A B, Bordoloi D, Padmavathi G, Monisha J, Roy N K and Prasad S *et al* 2017 Curcumin, the golden nutraceutical: multitargeting for multiple chronic diseases *Br. J. Pharmacol.* **174** 1325–48
[88] Banerjee S, Bueso-Ramos C and Aggarwal B B 2002 Suppression of 7,12-dimethylbenz(a)anthracene-induced mammary carcinogenesis in rats by resveratrol *Cancer Res.* **62** 4945–54
[89] Avemann K, Knippers R, Koller T and Sogo J M 1988 Camptothecin, a specific inhibitor of type I DNA topoisomerase, induces DNA breakage at replication forks *Mol. Cell. Biol.* **8** 3026–34

[90] Almatroodi S A, Almatroudi A, Khan A A, Alhumaydhi F A, Alsahli M A and Rahmani A H 2020 Potential therapeutic targets of epigallocatechin gallate (EGCG), the most abundant catechin in green tea, and its role in the therapy of various types of cancer *Molecules* **25** 3146

[91] Tripathi S K and Biswal B K 2020 Piperlongumine, a potent anticancer phytotherapeutic: Perspectives on contemporary status and future possibilities as an anticancer agent *Pharmacol. Res.* **156** 104772

[92] Ardalani H, Avan A and Ghayour-Mobarhan M 2017 Podophyllotoxin: a novel potential natural anticancer agent *Avicenna J. Phytomed.* **7** 285–94

[93] Clark R and Lee S H 2016 Anticancer properties of capsaicin against human cancer *Anticancer Res.* **36** 837–43

[94] Cortes J and Vidal M 2012 Beyond taxanes: the next generation of microtubule-targeting agents *Breast Cancer Res. Treat.* **133** 821–30

[95] Qi W J, Sheng W S, Peng C, Xiaodong M and Yao T Z 2021 Investigating into anti-cancer potential of lycopene: molecular targets *Biomed. Pharmacother.* **138** 111546

[96] Wu X, Zhou Q H and Xu K 2009 Are isothiocyanates potential anti-cancer drugs? *Acta Pharmacol. Sin.* **30** 501–12

[97] Hosseini A and Ghorbani A 2015 Cancer therapy with phytochemicals: evidence from clinical studies *Avicenna J. Phytomed.* **5** 84–97

[98] Ncube N S, Afolayan A J and Okoh A I 2008 Assessment techniques of antimicrobial properties of natural compounds of plant origin: current methods and future trends *Afri. J. Biotechnol.* 71797e1806

Chapter 11

Screening of possible anti-cancer phytochemicals against cancer by structure-based docking studies

Deena Prakash, Divya Bisht and Arvind Kumar Shakya

In recent years, cancer has been the leading cause of death world-wide. It is identified as the uncontrolled growth and abnormal spread of the cells in the human body. Major cancer causing factors are environmental influence, aging, diet, infectious agents, hormonal imbalance and chronic inflammation. Although there are various synthetic drugs available in the market, plant derivatives are known to have better efficacy and reduced side effects in the treatment of various cancer. Various molecular docking studies have been performed on the phytochemicals to evaluate their anti-cancer potency and are useful in providing the insights to molecular identification. Molecular docking study is an important tool in the process of drug discovery for searching potential hits. This chapter aims to focus on the finding of the molecular docking study performed on various phytochemicals and different cancerous proteins and their future drug discovery potential.

11.1 Introduction

Cancer is the genetic disorder related to the dysfunction of various important proteins which are essential for cell survival, cell division and cell death. Due to the lack of proper functioning of these proteins and their further communicating pathways, normal cells behave aberrantly causing unlimited cell division and proliferation of the cancerous cells in the body followed by the spread of these cells to other body parts, making it incurable. After cardiovascular illnesses, cancer is currently the second biggest cause of death. A WHO report suggests that cancer is responsible for nearly 10 million deaths worldwide in which breast cancer is the commonest one accounting for 2.26 million cases, followed by lung cancer (2.21 million cases), colon cancer, prostate cancer, skin cancer and stomach cancer [1]. By 2030, it is expected that cancer will be the primary cause of mortality and an

doi:10.1088/978-0-7503-5252-9ch11

estimated 23.6 million new cases are likely to be recorded annually [2, 3]. This rise in cases can be due to the numerous factors like environment, food, pathogens, hormonal imbalance, and long-term inflammation etc [4]. Another major cause of increase in cancer cases is the incompetence of current treatment such as synthetic medicines, chemotherapy, radiation therapy, and surgery which is expensive and has more severe side effects. Moreover, another reason for the failure of the conventional treatment is the acquired resistance by the cancerous cells and this necessitates the discovery of new anti-cancer drugs in the market with better efficacy, fewer side effects and that are cost effective. The use of plants and their active phytochemicals in the treatment of various ailments, such as cancer, hypertension, heart disease, liver diseases has been noteworthy [5]. The fact that 25%–28% of all current drugs are either directly or indirectly derived from higher plants highlights their tremendous therapeutic potential and lengthy history of use. Additionally, almost 60% of anti-cancer medications come from the plant kingdom. Nowadays, phytochemicals are frequently studied for new drug discovery [6]. About 35% cancer cases can be reduced by consuming plant-based foods including vegetables, fruit and different types of grains that have carotenoids, flavonoids, coumarins, terpenoids, monoterpenes, etc. These phytochemicals exhibit a wide range of therapeutic properties, such as anti-cancerous, antiviral, antimicrobial, central nervous system (CNS) stimulants, blood thinner and anti-inflammatory [7–9]. In order to find new potent and effective therapeutic drugs for cancer, molecular docking is the crucial tool where the identification of phytochemicals and the interaction between phytochemicals and cascade proteins which are directly or indirectly involved in the cancer causing mechanism can easily be discovered and studied. This chapter uncovers the various reported findings of a molecular docking study conducted on numerous phytochemicals and cancer causing proteins, as well as the possibility for new drugs to be developed using these findings.

11.2 Mechanism of cancer

11.2.1 Classification of cancer

The primary and fundamental flaw in cancer development is the unrestrained and continuing expansion of cancerous cells. Cancer cells multiply and divide uncontrollably instead of effectively reacting to the signals that control normal cell activity, infecting healthy tissues and organs and eventually dispersing throughout the body. There are two types of cancer as per their spread—benign which remains limited to its origin, neither invading adjacent tissues nor spreading to distant tissues, for example, normal skin warts which can be easily removed surgically; whereas malignant cancer has the potential to spread throughout the body by invading neighboring healthy tissue and doing so via the lymphatic or circulatory systems (metastasis).

On the basis of the origin of the cancer, there are three types of cancers: leukemias/lymphomas, sarcomas and carcinomas. Carcinomas are originated from the epithelial cells and account for 90% of human epithelial cancers, primarily being malignant in nature. Sarcomas are rarely found and are basically originated from connective tissues such as fibrous tissues, cartilage, muscle and bone. 8% of human malignancies are caused by leukemias and lymphomas, which are, respectively, produced by immune cells and blood producing cells. Leukaemia and lymphomas are common in young age groups. Furthermore, tissues are classified according to the origin tissues such as lung cancer, prostate cancer, colon cancer, breast carcinomas, fibrosarcomas (fibroblasts) and erythroid (erythrocytes). Lung cancer is the most lethal one by far, and is responsible for approximately 30% of cancer deaths worldwide.

11.2.2 Causes of cancer

Carcinogens like chemicals, viruses and radiation are reported to have the ability to mutate or damage the DNA which is the basic reason for the development of cancer. Cancer is the multistep process started via mainly carcinogens followed by activation of oncogenic cascades to the development of cancer. Carcinogens like aflatoxin, tobacco smoke, and sunlight are the major contributor to skin cancer [10]. Nicotine smoke contains nickel compounds, dimethylnitrosamine, and benzo(a) pyrene, which are the main recognized causes of lung cancer. 80%–90% of lung cancer cases are caused by active or passive smoking [11]. Some carcinogens promote cell proliferation instead of causing mutations which leads to the cancer development, phorbol esters is the classical example of this kind of carcinogen, it promotes cell proliferations by activation of protein kinase C [12]. Since they enhance uncontrolled cell division, which is necessary for the expansion of a tumor in its initial stage, these substances are called tumor promoters. As the name suggests, they stimulate the growth of tumor cells in the healthy tissue. For example, estrogen is required in the normal menstruating cycle, stimulating the proliferation of uterine endometrium wall, but women who have excessive levels of estrogen have high chances of endometrial cancer.

Hence, postmenopausal estrogen replacement therapy increases the risk of endometrial cancer. To counteract the stimulatory effect of estrogen, progesterone is administered. Unfortunately, long-term use of estrogen and progesterone combo therapies may increase the risk of breast cancer [13, 14]. There are many other ways to activate oncogenes, including infections with retroviruses or DNA viruses, which either insert oncogenes into the human genome or they insert sequences that are similar to those of proto-oncogene in order to cause cancer. For instance, when a host is infected by a retrovirus harboring SRC oncogenes, the viral chromosome is integrated into the host chromosome, the viral progeny is multiplied, and the surrounding cells are then infected [15]. This results in the overexpression of the surrounding cells abnormal genes and uncontrolled cell proliferation.

Oncogenes development is carried out by numerous mechanisms like gene addition, deletion, duplication, chromosomal translocation or rearrangement. Oncogenes/proto-oncogenes are divided into five categories—growth factors (TGF/NGF/EGF), growth hormone/factor receptors (VEGFRa), serine/threonine kinases (AKT), GTPase molecules and transcription factors. Cancers like fibrosarcoma, glioma (brain cancer), osteosarcoma, etc, result from mutations in the growth factors. Some tumors have deletions in the epidermal growth factor receptor that cause the subsequent activation of receptors even in the absence of the ligand carrying the tyrosine kinase activity [16]. This activation leads to the deregulation of multiple signaling pathways and interactions with other cytoplasmic proteins including SRC domain [17]. GFR mutations typically appear in gastrointestinal, breast, and lung malignancies. Similar to this, excessive Raf-1 kinase and cyclin-dependent kinase expression brought on by unchecked phosphorylation can result in a variety of malignancies, including thyroid and ovarian cancer.

Activation of oncogene via point mutation, insertion, deletions, amplification or chromosomal translocation is a primary cause in cancer formation, for example, point mutation in the RAS gene in colon cancer. ERB gene deletion in breast cancer, N-myc multiplication in neuroblastoma and BCR and ABL genes translocation in blood cancer. These biomarkers can facilitate the correct and timely diagnosis of cancer and also can ease the treatment [18].

11.2.3 P53 gene and protein

It is reported that 60% of cancer occurs due to the formation of unusual formation of protein which is because of mutation in the p53 gene, a tumor protein. P53 gene is critical for angiogenesis, differentiation, cell death, senescence, cell division, and DNA metabolism under normal circumstances and has been called 'the guardian of the genome'. In normal circumstances, p53 plays an essential role in apoptosis and cell cycle control and is found in very low levels. The concentration of p53 in cells is tightly regulated by Mdm2, a protein made for the degradation of p53 by ubiquination. During apoptosis, p53 activates the expression of apoptotic protease activating factor-1 (Apaf1) and apoptotic regulator proteins (Bax1) which will bind to caspase 9 and activate the apoptotic pathway. It also stimulates the release of cytochrome c from mitochondria [19–21].

P53 gene keeps cells in check in the G1 and G2 checkpoints with the help of cyclin-dependent kinase (CDK) CDK2 and CDC 2, respectively. Actually, it acts as an inhibitor as well as a promoter of cancerous cells. DNA damage leads to the stimulation of the WAF 1 genes which further leads to binding of p53 with CDK2 inhibiting the p21 effect for the next cycle. P53 also repairs proteins, induces apoptosis and arrests cell cycles in G1/S phase [21]. Another important process in cell growth is methylation which can be hypermethylated or hypomethylated in the case of cancer progress. Hypermethylation of promoter causes inactivation of the repair genes like Hmlh1, WRN, BRCA1, CRB1, RARB2 inducing cancer [22].

11.2.4 EGFR

The epidermal growth factor receptor (EGFR), a member of the tyrosine kinase receptor (RTK) family, plays a crucial role in the physiology of epithelial cells. Since it is frequently mutated and/or overexpressed in a variety of human malignancies, it is used as a target for several cancer medicines. EGFR's role in the regulation of autophagy and metabolism has given rise to the idea that simultaneous targeting of the EGFR and stress pathways may present a window of opportunity for the treatment of cancer [23]. EGFR activates various signaling pathways like the PI3K/AKT pathway, Ras/MAPK pathway and the phospholipase C (PLC)/protein kinase C (PKC) signaling cascade [24]. Numerous cellular processes, including survival, proliferation, differentiation, and motility, depend on these EGFR signaling pathways. Large genomic rearrangements and oncogenic EGFR mutations, as seen in glioblastoma, brain, lung, breast, and ovarian malignancies, frequently result in altered receptor endocytosis, which enhances signaling pathways. Some mutations, such as those in the EGFRvIV and EGFRvV mutants, directly impact the E3 ligase, Cbl, recruitment site in the intracellular domain of the receptor, influencing receptor ubiquitination and lysosomal degradation. In NSCLC patients, some mutations are seen in the extracellular domain (EGFRvIII), activating the receptor even in the absence of a ligand [25]. EGFR ligand activation elicits a classic signaling pathway via PI3K recruitment leading to the full activation of PIP3-AKT complex via phosphorylation AKT on Thr 308 and Ser 473. This activated AKT complex inhibits autophagy and blocks GLUT 1 endocytosis. This pathway is one of the best characterizations of cancer cells, increased uptake and metabolism of intracellular glucose into pyruvate to lactate is seen in cancerous cells [26]. Various EGFR-targeted medicines have been created due to EGFR's crucial role in cancer, including monoclonal humanized antibodies (mAbs) that target the receptor's extracellular domain. EGFR inhibitors like gefitinib, erlotinib, and afatinib are chosen for the first line of therapy in lung cancer treatment [27].

11.2.5 COX proteins

One of the most noticeable characteristics of cancer is inflammation, which plays a crucial part in the pathophysiology of the disease. The function of cyclooxygenase (COX) enzymes has been related to cancer and inflammation throughout the course of several decades of intensive research [28]. COX enzymes are involved in the process of production of prostaglandin (PG) from arachidonic acid. The catalysis of PGH2 (a kind of PG) is aided by the two COX isoforms, COX-1 and COX-2, which are homo-dimeric proteins. COX-2 catalyse is the first step in the prostaglandin production which later stimulates tumor invasion, cancer development and resistance of cell death. Substantially increased COX-2 expression is the characterization for the carcinogenesis with increased enzymatic product, i.e., PGE2. Hence, inhibition of PGE2 synthesis with COX-2 inhibitors can decrease the various types of cancer like prostate cancer, pancreatic cancer, osteosarcoma and breast cancer. In the cancer cells, the inhibition of COX-2 can also reduce the effect of upstream mediator of EGFR, mitogen activated kinases (MAK), nuclear factor-κβ (NF-κβ). Therefore, inhibiting the COX-2 can potentially decrease the cancer possibility [29].

11.2.6 JAK/STATs signaling pathways

JAK/STAT signaling pathway is activated by cytokines and growth factors, which is in charge of cellular transcription activation. It controls a wide range of biological reactions, including proliferation, division, migration and cell death. Numerous developmental and homeostatic processes including as immunity cell formation, maintenance of stem cells, hematopoiesis, mammary gland development and maturation of organism are controlled by JAK/STATs signaling. It includes three major proteins—cell surface receptor (gp 130), Janus Kinase (JAK), and signaling transducer and activator of transcription proteins (STATs). This pathway starts with the activation of the receptors by cytokines like IL-6 resulting in the phosphorylation activation of JAK further phosphorylation of tyrosine residue turning into activation loops for STATs possession, leading to the dissociation of STAT from the receptor. The dimerization of loosened STATs helps them enter the nucleus, activating their target genes. Any change in this pathway leads to the cancer development. It is seen that increased activation of the JAK/STATs signaling pathway is accountable for the uncontrolled growth of the cells in any body part leading to cancer. This process also stimulates the transcription of cell division genes like BCL2 and c-Myc. Therefore, by targeting this pathway protein can inhibit the cancer [30].

11.3 Methodology

After the completion of the Human Genome Project, there has been an increase in the finding of new therapeutic targets for drug discovery [31]. Numerous types of techniques like nuclear magnetic resonance spectroscopy, crystallography, and high-throughput protein purification have been developed for the better understanding of structural features of protein and protein–ligand complexes. Virtual screening and high-throughput screening offer the advantage of low cost and efficient screening of potential leads and hits (figure 11.1).

11.3.1 Ligand preparation

In this chapter, those phytochemicals which are known to have medicinal properties are taken as ligands. Ligand structures were first determined by any structural techniques like LCMS, GCMS, NMR etc. The chemical structure of shortlisted phytochemicals was accessed from the Pubchem database (https://pubchem.ncbi.nlm.nih.gov/) and drawn in Advanced Chemistry Development's Chemsketch, which were converted into 3D structure using the Open Babel software[32] or Lig

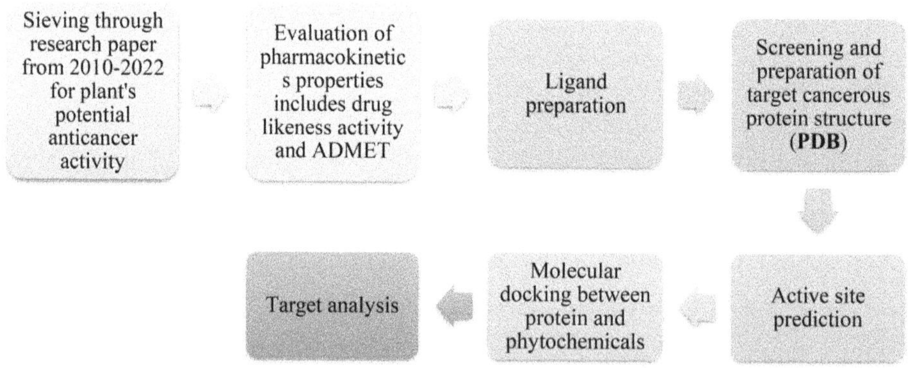

Figure 11.1. Schematic representation of *in silico* studies.

prep 2.2 application. Now these ligands are further used for molecular docking analysis [33].

11.3.2 Preparation of protein structure

The structure of the cancer target proteins (HER2/ERBB2, HER3/ERBB3, VEGFR2 [33], GLUT 4 [32], CDK2, human topoisomerase IIa etc) were retrieved from the protein data bank. The proteins were then cleaned by removing the bound inhibitor, non-essential molecule like heteroatoms and hydrogen atoms. Finally, optimization of protein structure was done by Weblab Viewer, Argus Lab 4.0, Dockprep or Swiss PDB Viewer. Now these proteins had stable structure and were ready to be docked with their respective ligand.

11.3.3 Active site prediction

Active site prediction is used to identify the potential ligand binding site. The active binding sites of the proteins were identified via DoGSiteScorer.24, Castp or online server Metapocket2.0 [68].

11.3.4 Docking studies

Molecular docking is a computer simulation tool used to predict the interaction of a receptor–ligand complex, where the receptor is often a protein or a nucleic acid molecule and the ligand is either a small molecule or another protein. The most important application of docking software is the virtual screening, in which the most promising molecules are selected from an existing database for further research. Various tools were used for the docking analysis in this chapter such as Auto Dock Variants [32], Patchdock Server, Argus Lab Docking Software, Dock, Gold, UCSF etc [34]. It is the most reliable automated tool used to understand the protein–ligand interactions and protein–protein interactions.

11.4 Pharmacological potential of phytochemicals

There are more than 11 000 extracts screened out for the anti-cancer activity. These phytochemicals samples were extracted from 35 000 plant samples collected from 20 different countries. In 1983, approximately 60% synthetic anti-cancer drug were of plant origin.

There are few plants which have been reported to have anti-cancer properties, like Madagascar periwinkle, *Catharanthus roseus*, Pacific yew, *Murraya koenigii*, *Taxus brevifolia* nutt., *Lupinus luteus*, *Taxus canadensis* marshall, *Taxus baccata* [35–37]. For example, Paclitaxel from bark of the Pacific Yew has notable activity against breast cancer, ovarian cancer and lung cancer. Topotecan, irinotecan from the plant *Camptotheca* acuminate was found to have anti-ovarian cancer effect. Homoharringtonine, the plant derived molecule from *Cephalotaxus harringtonia* was found effective against leukaemia. Many more compounds have been isolated and investigated for their anti-cancerous properties. Some of the reported pharmacological potential of phytochemicals is reported in table 11.1.

Table 11.1. Pharmacological properties of phytochemicals.

S. No.	Phytochemcials	Plant	Pharmacological effect	References
1.	Girinimbine murrayanine, murrastinine-b, mukolidine	*Murraya koenigii*	Anti-inflammatory activity via COX inhibition	[38]
3.	Glabranin, anthocyanin, eriosemation	*Glycyrrhiza glabra* *Lupinus luteus*	Anti-angiogenic, anti-inflammatory, blood thinner, anti-allergic, antimicrobial anti-cancer activity	[39, 40]
4.	Chlorogenic acid	Coffee, sunflowers	Anti-cancer, antioxidant	[33]
5.	Theaflavin	Tea	Antioxidant	[33]
6.	Silibinin	*Silybum marianum* (milk thistle)	Antioxidant	[33]
7.	Genistein	Soy and soy products	Tyrosine kinase Inhibitor, anti-tumor	[33]
8.	Yuanhuanin	*Daphne sericea* *Diuris pedunculata*	Anti-tumor	[33]
9.	Apigenin, caffiec acid, esculin, lupeol, scopoletein, solasodine, stigmasterol	*Solanum xanthocarpum*	Anti-cancer	[32]

10.	Xanthotoxol, bergapten, angelicin, psoralen, isoimperatorin	Carrot, legumes and citrus families	Anti-cancer, antimicrobial, blood thinner, anti-inflammatory, CNS stimulants	[41]
11	Ursolic acid, cleomiscosin-A rhamnetin, berberastine, berberine,	Apples, berries, mango, goldenseal, barberry and Oregon grape	Anti-inflammatory, antioxidant, antiviral, serum lipid-lowering, anti-cancer	[42]
12	7-hydroxy-4′-methoxy-3,11-dehydrohomoiso-flavanone, luteolin, quercetin, kaempferol, 4,4′-dihydroxy-2’-methoxychalcone, 7,4′-dihydroxy-3,11-dehydrohomoisoflavanone,	*Guilandina bonduc*	Antiplasmodial, anti-cancer	[43]
13	Schinilenol	*Zanthoxylum* species	Antithrombotic	[44]
14	Epigallocatechin gallate, nordihydroguaiaretic acid	Green tea extract, *Larrea tridentata*	Antioxidant, anti-inflammatory, anti-cancer neurological disorders	[45]
15.	daidzein quercetin	Soybeans and soy kale cherry tomatoes broccoli blueberries apples	Antioxidant anti-inflammatory effects anti-cancer	[46]

(*Continued*)

Table 11.1. (*Continued*)

S. No.	Phytochemcials	Plant	Pharmacological effect	References
16	9,19-cyclolanost-24-en-3-ol,acetate, campesterol, stigmasterol, desmosterol, ergosterol	*Calotropis gigantea*	Anti-cancer anti-atherogenic cardiovascular treatment	[47]
17	Mussaenosidic acid, betulinic acid	*Picrorhiza kurroa*, *Aegle marmelos*	Hepatoprotective, antioxidant, anti-cancerous activity, radioprotective, antiproliferative, analgesic, anti-inflammatory, antimicrobial	[48]
18	Boswellic acid, ursolic acid	*Fagonia indica* *Boswellia*	Anti-inflammatory, antioxidant, anti-cancer, hepatoprotective	[49]
19	Tricetinidin, myricetin, camellianin, myricetin 3-glucoside	*Camelia sinensis*	Anti-cancer, antioxidant, anti-coagulant, blood pressure and cholesterol lowering activity, antimicrobial	[50]
21	Casticin, isoorientin, p-hydroxybenzoic acid, chrysophanol	*Vitex negundo*	Treatment of eye disease, toothache, anti-inflammatory, leukoderma, to treat enlargement of the spleen, skin ulcers	[51]
22	Ajmalicidine, rawolscine, yohimbine ajmaline papaverine	*Rauwolfia serpentina*	Antihypertensive, antibacterial, antifungal, anti-inflammatory, anti-cancer	[52]

23	Cubenene muurolene pinene aucalyptol	*Ficus carica*	Metabolic disorders, cardiovascular diseases, respiratory diseases anti-cancer anti-inflammatory antispasmodic remedy	[53]
24	Ponicidin	*Isodon* and *Rabdosia* genus	Antiviral, immunoregulatory, anti-inflammatory, anti-tumor	[54]
25	Thymol	*Euphrasia rostkoviana*, *Nigella sativa*, *Origanum Compactum*, *Thymus glandulosus*	Antioxidant anti-inflammatory antimicrobial, anti-diabetic, antiobesity antihyperglycemic, hypolipidemic effects	[55]
26	5α,7α,8ξ,13α,17α)–17-(3-furyl)–4,4,8-trimethyl-3,16-dioxoandrosta-1,14-dien-7-yl acetate isomargosinolide 17-epiazadiradione	*Azadirachta indica*	Antimicrobial, antioxidant, anti-inflammatory activities	[56]
27	Fanchinoline	*Fangji Huangqi*	Anti-inflammatory	[57]
28	Coumarin, kaempferol	*Fagonia indica*	Anti-inflammatory, anti-diabetic, anti-cancer, antimicrobial, antipyretic, laxative, hepatoprotective effects	[58]
29	p-hydroxycinnamic acid	*Clitoria ternatea*	Antioxidant, anti-tumor, Anti-inflammatory, antimicrobial anti-diabetic activity	[59]
30	isorhamnetin-3-o-glucoside, 3,7-di-o-α-l-rhamnoside	*Zygophyllum coccineum*	Anti-diabetes, hypertension, wound-healing, burns and infections, gout, rheumatoid antipyretic, anthelmintic	[60]

(Continued)

Table 11.1. (*Continued*)

S. No.	Phytochemcials	Plant	Pharmacological effect	References
31	Gallic acid, vanillic acid, 4-hydroxy-3-methoxy benzoic acid, coumaric acid syringic acid	*Moringa oleifera*	Antipyretic anti-allergic decreased blood pressure, anti-diabetic, to treat skin infection, sores, tumors, weakness, wound	[61]
32	4-methyl-5-oxo-tetrahydrofuran-3-yl acetate) methyl-4-hydroxy-3-methoxybenzoate	*Polygonum hydropiper*	Anti-angiogenic anti-tumor	[62]
33	24-methylene cycloartanol	*Amaranthus*	Anti-cancer	[63]
34	azelaic acid	*Bruguiera gymnorhiza*	Anti-inflammatory	[64]
35	acetyleugenol	*Cyanthillium cinereum*	Anti-asthma, anti-cancer, against diarrhea, dysentery, impotency night-blindness	[65]
36	Apiol, asarone, taraxasterol, hopa-22(29)-ene-3alpha-ol	*Pleurospermum candollei*	Cures abdominal problems, hypolipidemic effects, decreased blood pressure	[66]

11.5 Physicochemical/pharmacokinetics properties of phytochemicals

In recent years, it has become crucial to incorporate drug property research into the initial phases of drug discovery. To lessen the clinical trials failure, virtual characterization physicochemical/pharmacokinetics aspects like bioavailability of phytochemicals are explored on the basis of molecular structure of the molecule. According to certain structural investigation essentially operated according to Lipinski's Rule of Five, a molecular structure is more likely to succeed as a medicine. Lipinski's Rule of Five is conducted using online tools (Molinspiration) or software such as Instant JChem, the Discovery Studio software, etc. A general guideline is to consider drug resemblance qualities as compared to large molecular weight molecules, low molecular weight compounds are more easily absorbed, dispersed, and transported. The log *P* value is used to assess the lipophilic efficiency that determines the potency and oral bioavailability of the drug. Log P value was found out to be in the acceptable range (less than 5) for the drugs to penetrate the cellular membranes. Topological polar surface area (TPSA)/PSA has shown to be a very good parameter characterizing drug absorption. The surface areas occupied by the oxygen, nitrogen, and hydrogen atoms that are bound to them were used to determine the TPSA. Thus, the TPSA is closely related to the hydrogen bonding potential of a compound. Good bioavailability of a compound is more likely with $\leqslant$10 rotatable bonds and TPSA of $\leqslant$140 Å. As the number of rotatable bonds increases, the molecule becomes more flexible and more adaptable for efficient interaction with a particular binding pocket. It predicts high probability of success or failure [67, 68] (table 11.2).

The following are the rules for the evaluation of drug likeness for molecules:

1. Molecular mass less than 500 Dalton;
2. High lipophilicity (expressed as log *P* less than 5);
3. Less than 5 hydrogen bond donors;
4. Less than 10 hydrogen bond acceptors;
5. Molar refractivity should be between 40 and 130.

11.6 Docking analysis

Table 11.3 shows the docking result of various phytochemicals and target cancer protein with binding score and interacting amino acid.

11.7 Docking results and discussion

11.7.1 EGFR-HER2/3 and VEGFR

EFGR AND VEGFR are the most characteristic proteins increased in breast cancer and colorectal cancer. Identifying phytochemicals from plants with potential ability to bind these proteins can decrease its overexpression which can be therapeutically beneficial for the treatment of breast and colorectal cancer. Studies suggest that VEGF is the main angiogenic factor in colorectal cancer and is expressed in about 50% of colorectal patients. Several anti-cancer drugs like 5-fluorouracil (5-FU),

Table 11.2. Drug-likeness properties of phytochemicals.

Phytochemicals	Molecular weight <500	H-bond donors ⩽5	H-bond acceptors ⩽10	log P ⩽5	References
4-methoxycoumesterol	282.2	2	2	−3.03	[69]
Apigenin	270.24	3	3	−2.83	
Biochanin	284.27	1	1	−1.92	
Coumesterol	282.25	2	2	−3.03	
Crocetin	328.41	5	5	3.78	
Curcumin	368.39	1	1	−1.26	
Daidzein	254.24	2	2	−0.95	
Diosgenin	414.63	0	0	5.17	
Formononetin	268.27	2	2	−0.84	
Gabridin	324.38	0	0	−1.26	
Genestein	284.27	1	1	−1.92	
Hesperatin	302.28	4	4	−3.12	
Indole-3-carbinol	147.18	5	3	−0.74	
Kaempferol	286.24	2	2	−3.46	
Lignan	302.37	0	0	0.01	
Luteolin	286.24	1	1	−3.46	
Lycopene	536.89	5	5	11.11	
Naringenin	272.26	1	1	−2.15	
Quercetin	302.24	4	4	−4.54	
Resveratrol	228.25	3	2	−0.62	
Berberin	336.4	0	4	3.6	[70]
Choline	104.17	1	1	3.6	
Magnoflorine	342.4	2	4	2.7	
Tinosporin	406.4	2	8	1.1	
Palmatine	352.4	0	4	3.7	
Isocolumbin	358.4	1	6	2.2	
Aporphine	235.32	0	1	3	
Jatrorrhizine	338.4	1	4	3.4	
Tetrahydropalmatine	355.4	0	5	3.2	
Palmarin	374.4	1	7	1.3	
Tembetarine	344.4	2	4	3	
Eugenol	164.2	1	2	2	
Methyl eugenol	178.23	0	2	2.5	
Cirsilineol	344.3	2	7	2.9	
Cirsimartin	314.29	2	6	2	
Isothymusin	330.29	3	7	2.6	
Apigenin	270.24	3	5	1.7	
Rosemeric acid	360.31	5	8	2.36	
Luteolin	286.24	4	6	2.53	
Bornyl acetate	196.29	0	2	4.3	
Myrtenal	150.22	0	1	2.98	
Neral	152.23	0	1	3.03	

Alpha elemene	204.35	0	0	5	
Podophyllotixin	414.41	1	8	2.01	
4-dimethylpodophylloto xin	400.38	2	8	1.68	
Quercetin	302.24	5	7	1.54	
Kaempferol	286.24	4	6	1.9	
Andrographolide	350.45	3	5	2.16	
Isopropylideneandrog rapholide	390.51	1	5	3.17	
14-deoxy-11,12-didehydroandrograph olide	332.43	2	4	3.23	
Dehydroandrographolide	332.43	2	4	3.38	
Moslosooflavone	298.29	1	5	3.32	
19-O-acetyl-14-deoxy-11,12-didehydroandrograph olide	374.47	1	5	3.26	
(8S,12R)-Isoandrographolide	350.45	2	5	2.34	
14-acetylandrographolide	392.49	2	6	2.74	
Azatoxin	380.39	2	5	2.94	
Betaine	117.15	0	2	0	
Ferulic acid	194.18	2	4	1.51	
Caffeic acid	180.16	3	4	1.15	
p-Coumaric acid	164.16	2	3	1.46	
Syringic acid	198.17	2	5	1.04	
Rhamnetin	316.26	4	7	1.87	
Rhamnocitirin	300.26	3	6	2.22	
Betaxanthin	358.35	2	7	1.38	
Orientin	448.38	8	11	0	
Vicenin-2	594.52	11	15	−2.26	
Ursolic acid	456.7	2	3	7.34	
Podophyllotoxinglucoside	576.55	4	13	0.42	
Etoposide	588.56	3	13	0.6	
Teniposide	656.65	3	13	1.24	
NK611	652.09	2	13	2.12	
GL331	520.49	2	9	3.88	
TOP-53	512.59	1	9	3.02	
Etoposide phosphate	668.54	4	16	0	
Tafluposide	1116.71	2	30	4.84	
Beta-Sitosterol	414.71	1	1	9.34	
Stigmasterol	412.69	1	1	8.56	
Rutin	610.52	10	16	0	
Astragalin	448.38	7	11	0.72	
Oleanolic acid	456.7	2	3	7.49	
Beta-carotene	536.87	0	0	13.54	
Lutein	568.87	2	2	11.01	
Apigenin	270.00	3	5	2.41	[32]
Caffeic acid	170.00	2	4	−0.13	

(Continued)

Table 11.2. (*Continued*)

Phytochemicals	Molecular weight <500	H-bond donors ⩽5	H-bond acceptors ⩽10	log *P* ⩽5	References
Esculin	340.00	5	9	−1.49	
Lupeol	426.00	1	1	8.02	
Scopoletin	192.00	1	4	1.33	
Solasodine	414.00	3	2	4.26	
Stigmasterol glucoside	574.00	4	6	5.62	
Pristimerin	464.64	1	4	4.28	
Ixocarpalactone A	504.60	8	4	3.29	
Viscosalactone B	488.61	7	3	2.84	
Zhankuic acid A	468.62	5	1	3.25	
Xanthotoxol	202.16	4	1	2.00	[41]
Bergapten	216.19	4	0	2.28	
Angelicin	186.17	3	0	2.29	
Psoralen	186.17	3	0	2.29	
Isoimperatorin	270.28	4	0	3.95	
Cudraxanthone 1	326.35	2	5	3.87	[71]
Atalantoflavone	336.34	2	5	4.06	
Ursolic acid	456.71	2	2	7.09	
Akummidine	352.432	1	5	3.2	[72]
Gallic acid	170	5	4	0.55	[60]
p-Coumaric acid	164	3	2	2.07	
4-Hydroxy-3-methoxycinnamic acid	194	4	2	2.04	
Isobavachin	324.38	4	2	4.45	[73]
Glabranin	324.38	4	2	4.85	
Anthocyanin	207.25	1	0	1.31	
Erioemation	314.38	4	2	4.85	

irinotecan, and oxaliplatin block specifically the EGFR and VEGFR. Therefore, the use of targeted anti-VEGF treatment for colorectal cancer can be useful in the treating CRC treatment. Whereas, EGFR, is cell surface protein, it activates the tyrosine kinase phosphorylation, which is crucial in the cell proliferation pathway. Therefore, by inhibiting EGFR, we can directly halt the cell proliferation of cancerous cells. The inhibitors of EGFR are being used to treat CRC along with chemotherapy. Qawoogha *et al* docked phytochemical with respective CRC target protein and found out that these molecules are forming hydrogen bonding in the active site of proteins and hence can block these proteins, which can further hinder other related pathways of cell cycle, cell progression and cell division. In table 11.4, the docking of various phytochemicals was done with EGFR, HER2, and vascular endothelial growth factor receptor (VEGFR2) [52, 53, 62, 74, 79]. In this paper, these three flavonoids were found to have minimum binding score (–10.2 kcal mol^{-1}–9.8 kcal mol^{-1}) [33].

Table 11.3. The docking result of various phytochemicals and target cancer protein with binding score and interacting amino acid.

Target protein	Phytochemicals	Binding amino residue	Binding score (kcal mol^{-1})	Reference
Androgen receptor (1E3G)	Isobavachin	L873, G708, R752, M745,	−13.73	[73]
	Glabranin	G708, Q711, R752, M745, M749	−13.26	
	Anthocyanin	D879, L880, M780, W741, L873, M787, M895, R752, Q711	−13.01	
	Eriosemation	T877, L873	−12.78	
EGFR-HER2 receptors (3PP0)	Theaflavin	—	−10.2	[33]
EGFR-HER3 receptors (3lMG)	Genistein	—	−9.8	
VEGF receptor (4AG8)	Yuanhuanin	—	−10.2	
Glucose transporter (GLUT) (4PYP)	Apigenin	I42, Y308, F307	−163.48	[32]
	Caffeic acid	R225, E162, T166, P165, A256	−106.04	
	Esculin	Q298, F395, I42, Q299, N333	−60.32	
	Scopoletin	E259, E162 T166, A256	−98.43	
	Lupeol	V85, V89, N304, I42, I180, I184, F307, F395, Y 308	−211.25	
	Solasodine	N304, Y308, F307, I42, I184, I303, F395, Y308	−257.41	
	Stigmasterol ecoside	Q439, A86, I184, N431, F88, I42, Y308, V85, A86, I184	−289.94	
Epidermal growth factor receptor	Pristimerin	C773, M769, L820	−13.6	[74]
HER2	Pristimerin ixocarpactone a viscosactone b zhankuic acid a	L860, A751, L852, F864	−14.1–14.4–1.9–12.8	
Estrogen receptor	Viscosactone b	M528	−11.8	
Nf-κβ	Ixocarpactone a zhankuic acid a	T23, D166	−13.9–13.6	
Epidermal growth factor receptor (2J6M)	Xanthotoxol	T854, A743, F723, L844, V726.	−19.2199	[41]

(Continued)

Table 11.3. (*Continued*)

Target protein	Phytochemicals	Binding amino residue	Binding score (kcal mol^{-1})	Reference
Estrogen receptor α (3ERT)		A350, L384, L391, L387, L346	−34.43	
Progesterone receptor (4OAR)		M759, L763, L718, F778	−21.1074	
Mammalian target of rapamycin (mTOR) (4DRH)		L121, H71, Y2038, T2098, W2101, F2039	−12.4596	
P53R2	Berberastine	S99, D100, E131, N132	−9.7	[75]
Cytotoxic T-lymphocyte protein 4 (CTAL-4)	Ursolic acid	T57, G68, T69, F70, V75, N76	−7.6	
VEGF(1VPF)	7-hydroxy-4′-mhoxy-3,11-dehydrohomoisoflavanone	I29, G58, G59, L32, T31, E30, C57	−6.7	[76]
	4,4′-dihydroxy-2′-mhoxy-chalcone	I29, G58, G59, L32, T31, E30, C57, R56	−5.9	
	7,4′-dihydroxy-3,11-dehydrohomoisoflavanone	G59, C60, C61, E64, E67, S50, D63, F47,F36, L66	−6.6	
	Luteolin	F36, F47, L107, E67, L66, C60, G59 N62, D63	−7.0	
	Quercetin-3-mhyl	G59, C68, C61, C51, E67, L107, L66, F36, I46, N62, D34	−6.3	
Tyrosine kinase (1FMK)	7-hydroxy-4′-mhoxy-3,11-dehydrohomoisoflavanone	G344, Y340, M341, V323, F405, I336, S345, D348	−8.6	
	4,4′-dihydroxy-2′-mhoxy-chalcone	F405, I336, V323, Y340, L393, S345, S342, M341, G344, G274, D348	−7.7	
	7,4′-dihydroxy-3,11-dehydrohomoisoflavanone	G 344, Y 340, M 341, V 323, V 281, I 336, S 345	−8.8	
	Luteolin	Y 340, V 323, I 336	−8.7	
	Quercetin-3-mhyl	M 341, A 293, T 338, D 404,R 388, C 277, Q 275, S 345, G 274, G 344	−7.7	

Matrix metalloproteinases (2OXU)	7-hydroxy-4′-mhoxy-3,11-dehydrohomoisoflavanone	P 232, A 234, F 237, Y 240, T 215, L 181, F 248, L 214, P 238, ZN 264	−10.7	
	4,4′-dihydroxy-2′-mhoxy-chalcone	P 232, A 234, F 237, Y 240, T 215, L 181, F 248,L 214, P 238, E 219,	−9.3	
	7,4′-dihydroxy-3,11-dehydrohomoisoflavanone	P 232, A 234, F 237, Y 240, T 215, L 181, F 248, L 214, P 238, L 241	−10.4	
	Luteolin	F 248, V 243, A 234, F 237, A 182, T 215, L 214, ZN 264	−8.8	
	Quercetin-3-mhyl	H 183, A 184, H 222, A 182, E 219, V 235, L 241, L 214, Y 240, L 181, P 238, ZN 264	−7.8	
CDK2	Schininol	T14, N132, D86, Q131, L129, L33	-8.10	[77]
Mdm2 protein	Epigallocatechin Gallate	W23, L26, L24, E28, Q59, G58, L51, M62	— 17.40	[78]
	Alvaradoin m	W23, L26, L54, E28, L51, L24, F55	— 14.22	
	Alvaradoin e	W23, L26, L54, L24, L51, E28, F55	— 12.19	
	Nordihydroguaiaretic acid	W23, Q59, L51, L24, F55, E28, L54, M62	— 11.54	
Cyclin-dependent kinase-2 (3EZV)	Remangiflavano ne b	L 55, V 64, L 134, A 144, F 80, F 146, A 31, D 135, L 33, V 18	−8.531	[79]
	Epigallocatechin gallate	L 89, L 289, H 84, E 08, I 10, L 134, Q 131	−8.616	
Human topoisomerase (1ZXM)	Daidzein	N 120, T 215, I 125, N 91, A 167, F 142, T 147, L 168, I 141	−8.152	
	Camptothecin	I 125, S 149, G 164, S 148, N 150, A 167, G 166	−8.871	
	Salvicine	A 32, N 91, I 88, I 217	−9.064	
Vascular endothelial growth factor 2 (2OH4)	Decursinol	L 838, V 846, A 864, L 866, F 916, C 917, V 914, L 1033, V 897, L 887, E 883	−9.829	
	Plumbagin	V 846, L 838, L 1033, C 917, F 916, E 915, A 864	−8.602	
	Quercitin	E 883, LINE 866, V 846, A 864, L 838, V 914, E 915, F1045, F 916, D 1044, C 1043, L 1033, C 917	−12.030	

(Continued)

Table 11.3. (*Continued*)

Target protein	Phytochemicals	Binding amino residue	Binding score (kcal mol^{-1})	Reference
Anaplastic lymphoma kinase (ALK) protein (4ANL)	62 –p hydroxybenoyl mussaenosidic acid	R1120 D1203 G1202 E1210 S1206	−127.723	[52, 80]
	Betulinic acid	G1269 D1270 L1122	−95.598	
	Viridiflorol	M1199	−75.1202	
	Ptocatechuic acid	D 1160 D1163 E1167 T1151 L1152 F1164	−63.0854	
	Ajmalicidine	A864, L866, V912, L838, V846, V865, E883, V897, I913,	−10.08	[52]
	1, 2-Dihydrovominine	E915, F916, C917, L1033, C1043, D1044, F1045	−10.6	
	Rauwolscine	L866, E883, L838, A864, V897, V912, V914, E915, F1045	−10.4	
	Yohimbine	L838, R1049, A864, V897, V914, E915, F916, F1045	−9.7	
	Ajmaline	E915, L838, V846, A864, L866, E883, V914, C917, L1033, C1043,D1044	−9.44	

Abbreviations for amino acid used in the table: L (leucine), G (glycine), R (arginine), M (methionine), D (aspartic acid), W (tryptophan), Q (glutamine), T (threonine), I (isoleucine), Y (tyrosine), F (phenylalanine), E (glutamic acid), P (proline), A (alanine), N (asparagine), V (valine), C (cysteine), H (histidine), S (serine).

Table 11.4. 2D and 3D docking representation of phytochemicals with HER2, VEGFR2 and EGFR.

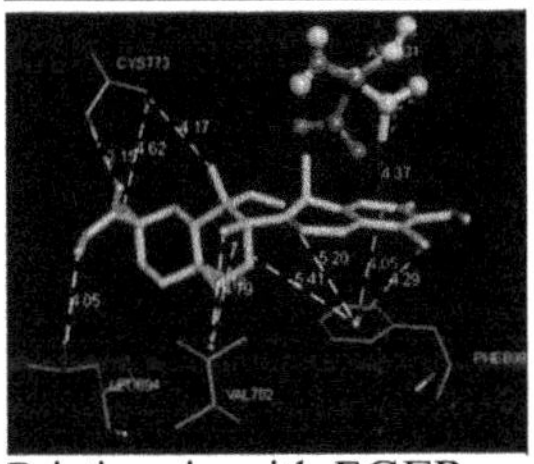

Pristimerin with EGFR protein. Reproduced from [74] with permission from Taylor & Francis.

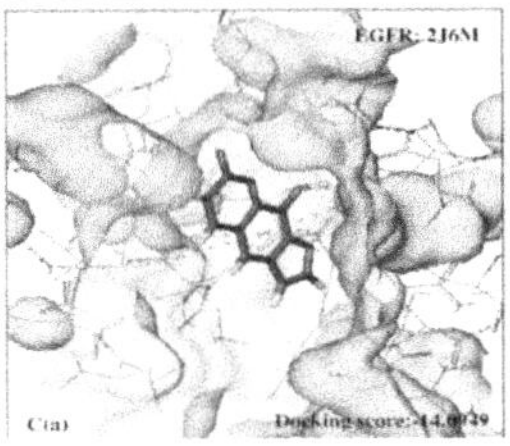

Xanthotoxol with EGFR. Reproduced from [62] with BMC permission.

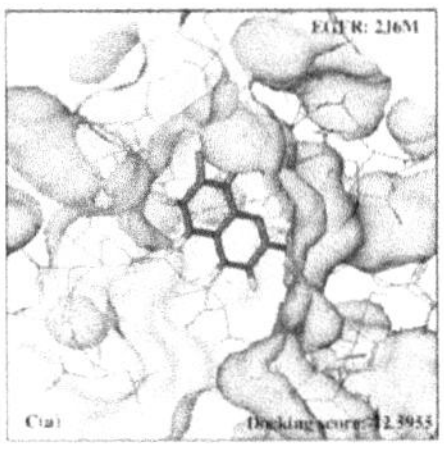

Angelicin with EGFR. Reproduced from [62] with BMC permission.

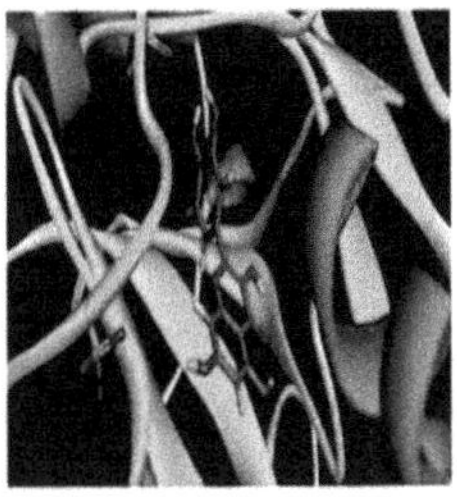

Quercitin with EGFR2. Reproduced from [79] with permission from Taylor & Francis.

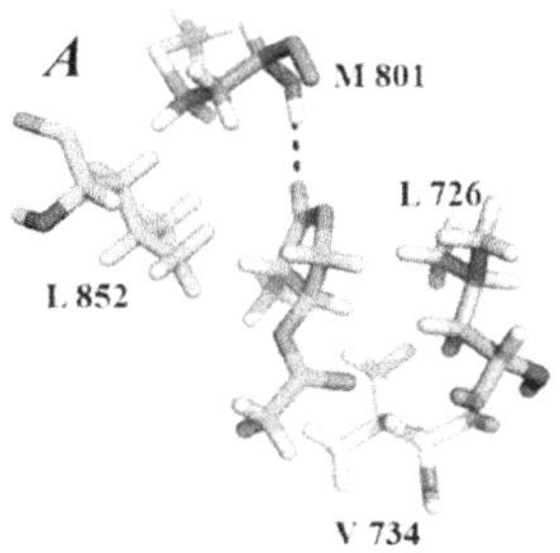

4-methyl-5-oxo-tetrahydrofuran-3yl acetate with EGFR. Reproduced from [62] with BMC permission.

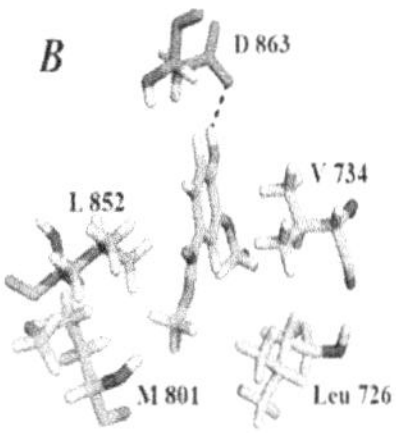

Methyl-4-hydroxy-3-methoxybenzoate with EGFR. Reproduced from [62] with BMC permission.

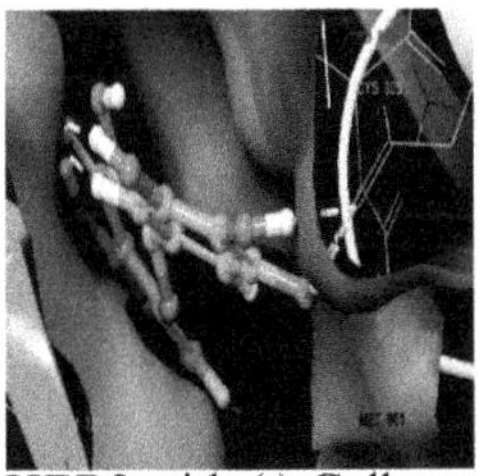

HER2 with (-)-Gallocatechin Ebenyi, HER2. Reproduced from [74] with permission from Taylor & Francis.

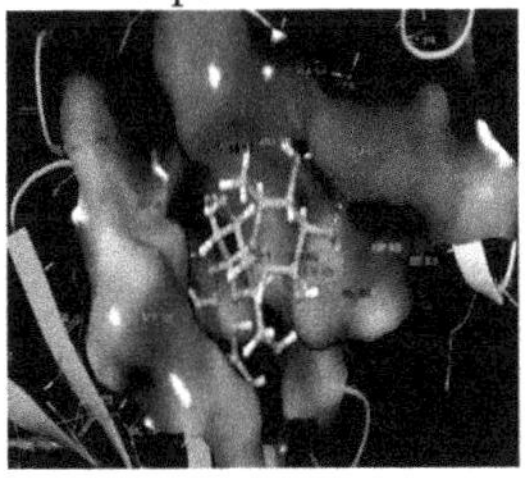

HER2 with tricetinidin Ebenyi, HER2. Reproduced from [74] with permission from Taylor & Francis.

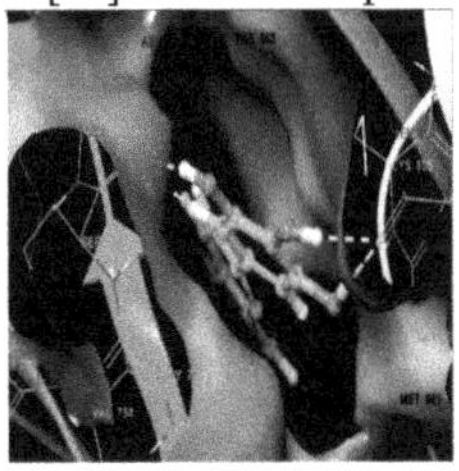

HER2 with Camellianin B Ebenyi, HER2. Reproduced from [74] with permission from Taylor & Francis.

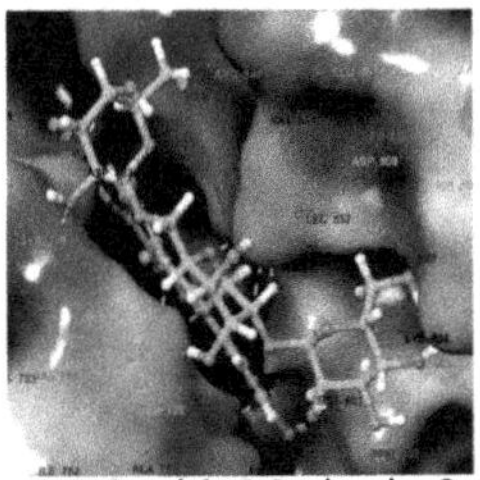

HER2 with Myricetin 3-Glucoside Ebenyi, HER2. Reproduced from [74] with permission from Taylor & Francis.

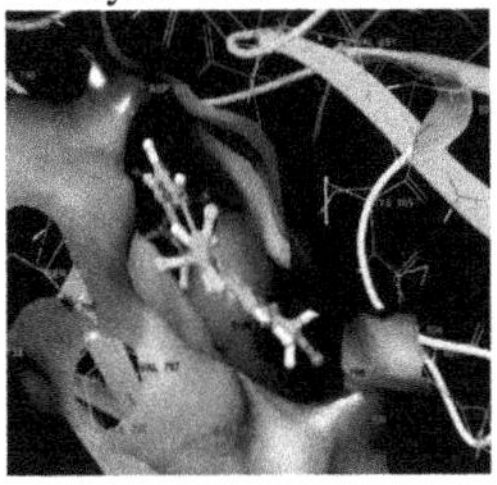

HER2 with Myricetin Ebenyi, HER2. Rerpoduced from [74] with permission from Taylor & Francis.

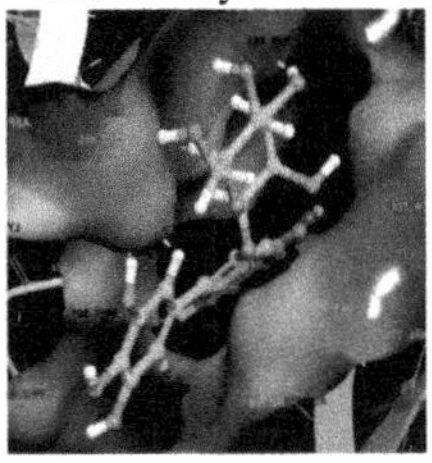

HER2 with Camelliaside A Ebenyi, HER2. Reproduced from [74] with permission from Taylor & Francis.

Table 11.4. (*Continued*)

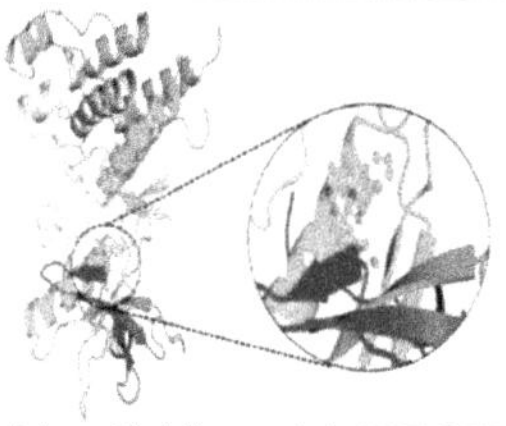	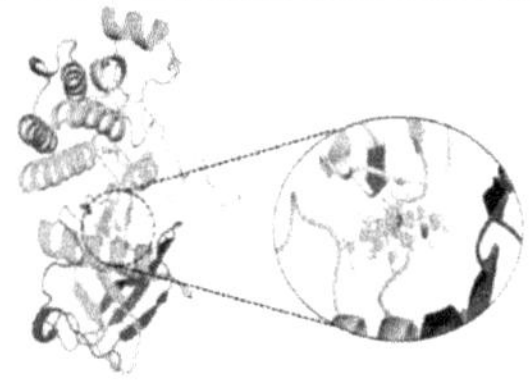	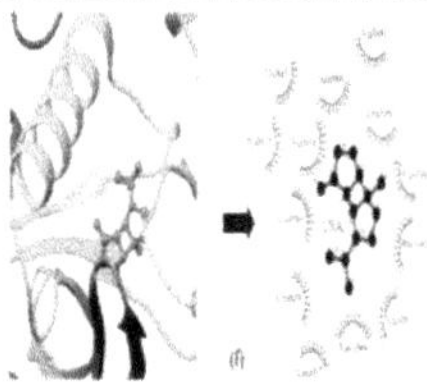
Ajmalicidine with VEGFR2. Reproduced from [52] with permission from Hindawi.	1, 2-dihydrovomilenine with VEGFR2. Reproduced from [52] with permission from Hindawi.	Beta-bourbonene with VEGFR2. Reproduced from [53] with permission from PLOS.

11.7.2 GLUT 4

GLUT 4, a glucose transporter, is the novel therapeutic target for the new development of drug formulation. It is reported that GLUT 4 and GLUT 1 are transcriptionally suppressed by a tumor suppressor gene, p53 which has an important role in cell cycle control and apoptosis. Scientists suggested that the inhibition of GLUT 4 by HIV protease can increase the growth arrest and hence, cause apoptosis. It is believed that alteration in the regulation of GLUT 4 can interrupt the DNA binding domain of p53 gene. Targeting p53 via indirectly blocking the GLUT 4 by phytochemicals can be successful for new anti-cancer drugs. Apigenin, lupeol, stigmasterol glucoside, caffiec acid, scopoletin, esculin and solasodine mimicking the reported anti-cancer drug, Doxorubicin with GLUT 4 protein [32].

11.7.3 NF-κβ

Nuclear factor-kappa B (NF-κβ) is a transcriptional factor, considered as an immunity regulator. It has been seen that NF-κβ regulates the expression of different genes which are involved in DNA synthesis, replication, immunological and inflammatory response and cell death. Recent studies showed that NF-κβ up-regulation causes the pathogenesis of breast cancer, lymphoma and colorectal cancer via activation of PI3K/Akt pathway and EGFR signaling. Cancer target VEGR and interleukin-8 (IL-8) are directly activated for angiogenesis and cancer formation. It can be a key target for the treatment of cancer. Phytochemcials blocking this protein might down-regulate further cancerous proteins like VEGFR, cyclin D, PI3K and CDK. Figure 11.2 shows interaction of Ixocarpalactone A with NF-κβ with a stable binding energy −9.3k kcal mol^{-1} and forming hydrophobic bond with key amino acids located in the binding site such as ARG105, CYS99, ALA42, PRO148, GLU149, VAL152, ILE165 [74].

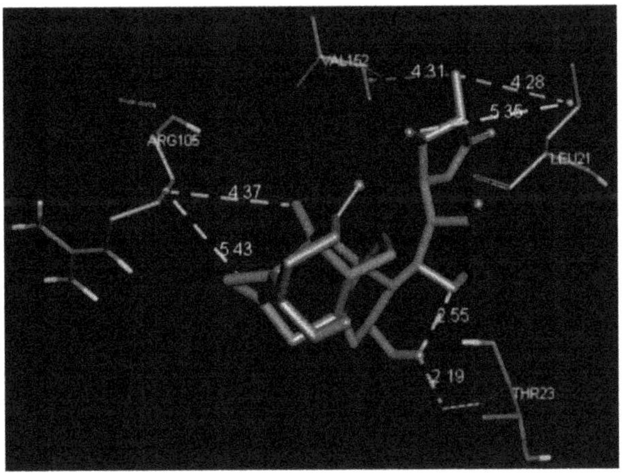

Figure 11.2. 3D docking interaction of Ixocarpalactone A in the active site of the NF-κβ protein. Reproduced from [74] with permission from Taylor & Francis.

11.7.4 BRCA2, estrogen and progesterone receptor

Everybody retrieves one copy of BRCA genes i.e., BRCA1 and BRCA2 from either of their parents. BRCA is tumor suppressor gene, and mutated BRCA gene leads to the pathogenesis of breast cancer. Breast cancer is one of the most frequent cancers found in women; the breast cancer statistics shows that one new case emerges every 18 seconds and approximately 18% women die of breast cancer. This is happening because of increasing population and speedy development of cancer in middle-aged (40–60 years of age) women. Death is varied in different cancer subtypes like HER2 positive having the highest death rate, followed by TNBC, Luminal A and Luminal B subtypes. BRCA2 gene mutation increases the susceptibility of early onset of breast cancer. BRCA2 encodes BRCA2 protein, which repairs the DNA damage via homologous recombination. The defective BRCA2 gene leads damaged DNA to be more prone to DNA interstrand cross-linking agents which further decreases the chance of DNA double-stranded break repair. Hence, more mutated DNA is generated which causes cancer. BRCA2 is the target for various drugs which have side effects and a resurgence of the tumor and resistance. Likewise, estrogen and progesterone receptors are also used as targets for breast cancer [41] (table 11.5).

11.7.5 Cyclin-dependent kinase (CDK)

Cyclin-dependent kinases (CDKs) are a group of the protein kinase family which belongs to the serine/threonine (S/T) kinase enzymes. CDK2 protein plays an important role in the growth cycle progression, they bind with cyclins when activated. Such proteins play a significant role in up-regulation or down-regulation of mitotic division, transcription and the post-transcriptional process. For example, CDK2 binds with Cyclin E in the S phase of the cell division cycle. This complex activates the phoshphorylation of Rb protein, transcription factors E2F protein. According to this, CDK2 became a potential drug target in the therapy of cancer.

Table 11.5. 3D docking representation of various phytochemicals with Estrogen and progesterone receptor.

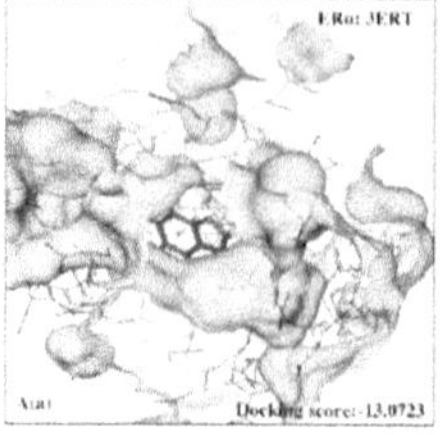 Bergapten and Estrogen receptor. Reproduced from [41] CC BY 4.0.	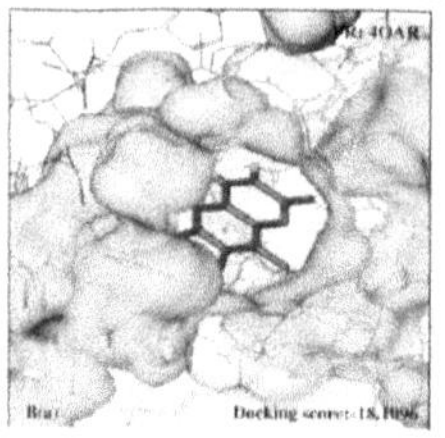 Xanthotoxol and progesterone receptor. Reproduced from [41] CC BY 4.0.	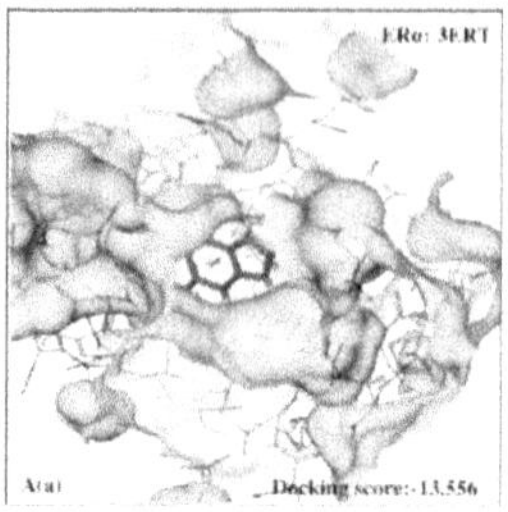 Xanthotoxol and Estrogen receptor. Reproduced from [41] CC BY 4.0.
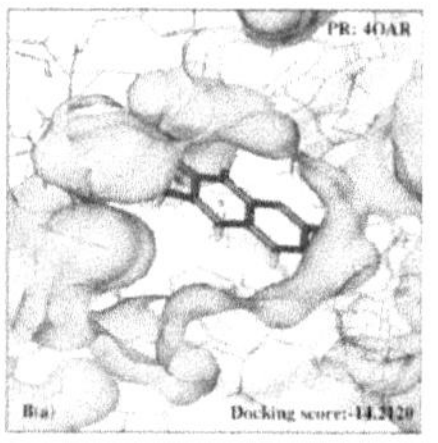 Psoralen and progesterone receptor. Reproduced from [41] CC BY 4.0.		

CDK2 also behaves like a channel for the signaling of growth factors in the PI3K/mTOR pathway. Downstream regulation of CDK2 leads to the p53 protein accumulation and activation of proto-oncogenic gene Src and their related Src pathway. Anti-cancer drugs like rapamycin that targets the mTOR pathway, xanthotoxol, psoralen, and epigallocatechin gallate were docked against mTOR protein and CDK2, respectively [41, 77, 79] (table 11.6).

11.7.6 P53–MDM2 pathway

In most types of cancer, Inactivation of P53 protein leads to up-regulation of murine double minute 2 (MDM2). MDM2 binds p53 for stabilization of P53 and also for cellular localization. This complex inhibits further p53 mediated transcriptional interaction and induces p53 proteasomal degradation. Thus, by blocking MDM2 protein binding with p53 gene results in the reactivation of p53 gene and its transcriptional pathways. Four phytochemicals, i.e., epigallocatechin gallate, alvaradoin and nordihydroguaiaretic acid were found to be potent inhibitors of p53–MDM2 complex. MDM2 involvement is seen in 7% malignancies like breast cancer, cervical cancer, ovarian cancer, colon cancer, prostate cancer and renal cancer. P53 gene is a tumor suppressor gene but the dysregulation of this gene exerts the stress signals which can either activate the apoptotic pathways or initiation of cancer formation. Figure 11.3 illustrates the 3D docking interaction of berberastine

Table 11.6. 2D and 3D docking interaction of phytochemicals with CDK2 and mTOR.

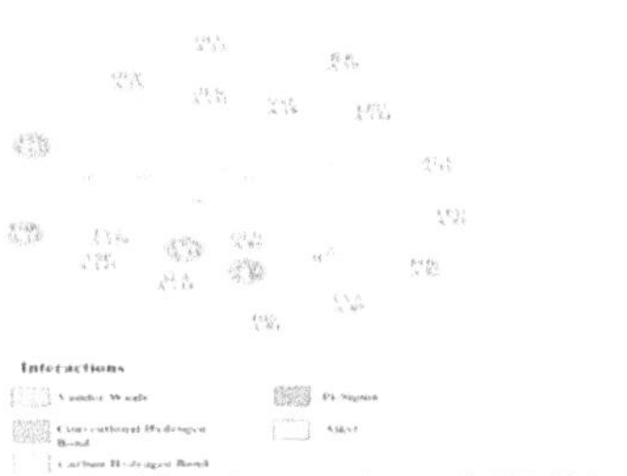 2D docking interaction of CDK2–schinilenol. Reproduced from [77] with permission from Taylor & Francis.	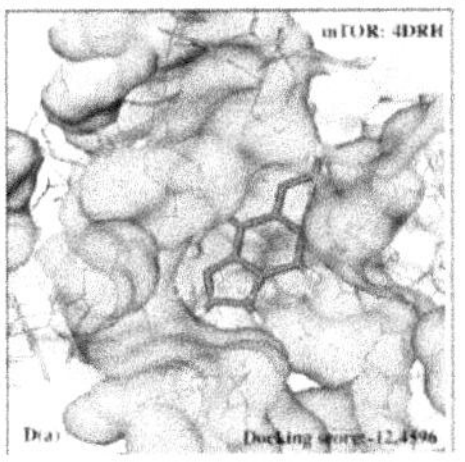 3D docking interaction of xanthotoxol and mTOR. Reproduced from [41] CC BY 4.0.	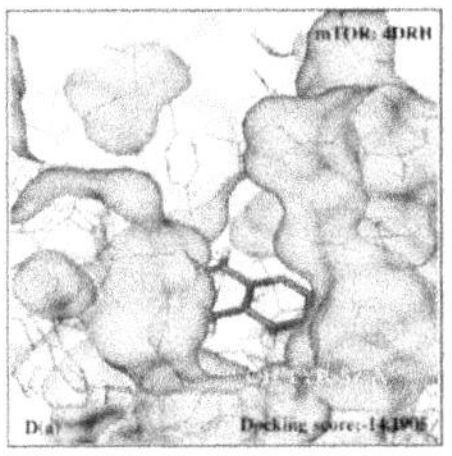 3D docking interaction of psoralen and mTOR. Reproduced from [41] CC BY 4.0.
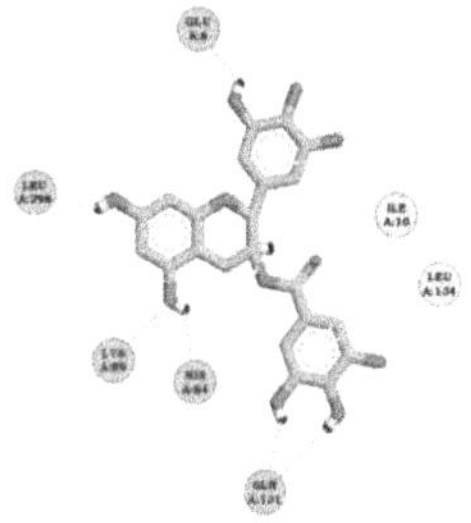 Epigallocatechin gallate and its receptor cyclin-dependent kinase-2. Reproduced from [79] with permission from Taylor & Francis.		

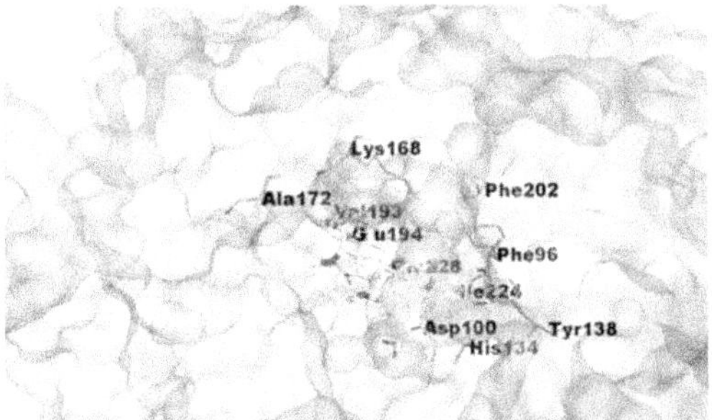

Figure 11.3. 3D docking interaction of Berberastine within the cavity of p53R2 3HF1. Reproduced from [74] with permission from Taylor & Francis.

within the cavity of p53R2 3HF1 blocking the p53 protein. Thereby, p53 or MDM2 protein makes a good target in treatment of cancer therapy.

11.7.7 COX inhibition

The first stage in the production of prostaglandins is catalysed by the enzymes cyclooxygenase-1 and -2 (COX-1/2). Their part in the development of cancer has recently become clearer. They play a significant part in the creation of carcinogens and have an impact on apoptosis, angiogenesis, and invasion. Typically, cancer cells express COX-2 at a high level. NSAIDS (non-steroidal anti-inflammatory medicines) and COX inhibitors have been demonstrated in large epidemiological studies of aspirin users and non-users to be beneficial in preventing the onset and progression of malignancies. Furthermore, selective COX-2 inhibitors have demonstrated effectiveness in reducing the number and size of colorectal polyps in patients with familial adenomatosis polyposis syndrome, according to clinical trials. Several preclinical investigations using combinations of either chemotherapy or radiation show promising results. In this chapter, a few phytochemicals (A—Girinimbine, B—Murrayanine, C—Murrastinine B and D—Mukolidine) were docked against COX-2 enzyme [38].

11.7.8 Tyrosine kinases and human topoisomerase

See table 11.7 for 2D and 3D docking interaction of phytochemicals with tyrosine kinases and human topoisomerase.

11.8 Conclusion

In the field of computer-based drug design, molecular docking tool shows great promise to screen the potential drug molecules by locking and scoring them in the active site of a protein. The present chapter includes the pharmacological properties, drug-likeness properties of phytochemicals and molecular docking of phytochemical constituents with cancer specific enzymes. Enzymes like EGFR, HER2, VEGFR2, BRCA, estrogen receptor and progesterone receptor are specific targets for breast cancer. Moreover, P53 protein, MDM2 protein, Cyclooxygenase 2 (COX) protein, tyrosine kinase, CDK, mTOR, GLUT 4, NFκβ are specific to various kinds of cancer like colorectal cancer, lung cancer, colon cancer, prostate cancer, stomach cancer, skin cancer, prostate cancer etc. Approximately 6000–8000 sites in human genes are thought to have promise as pharmaceutical potential targets. Only 400 of these encoded proteins have been demonstrated to be useful in the drug development process up to this point [75].

In addition to docking studies, computed drug likeness of phytochemicals also revealed that maximum compounds were in range of favorable candidates for good bioavailability as per the Lipinski Rule of Five. Therefore, the compilation of the docking analysis data of various phytochemicals allowed us to understand the mechanism behind cancer causing enzymes and their potential inhibitors (phytochemicals). The phytochemical constituents of medicinal plants behave as antagonists to cancer, which may further be investigated in *in vitro* and *in vivo* models.

Table 11.7. 2D and 3D docking interaction of phytochemicals with tyrosine kinases and human topoisomerase.

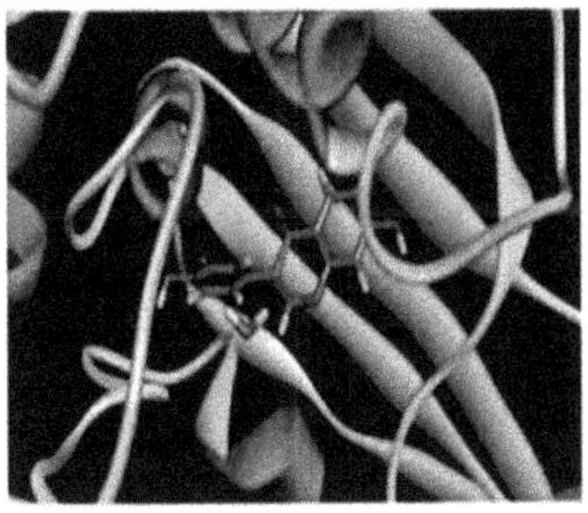	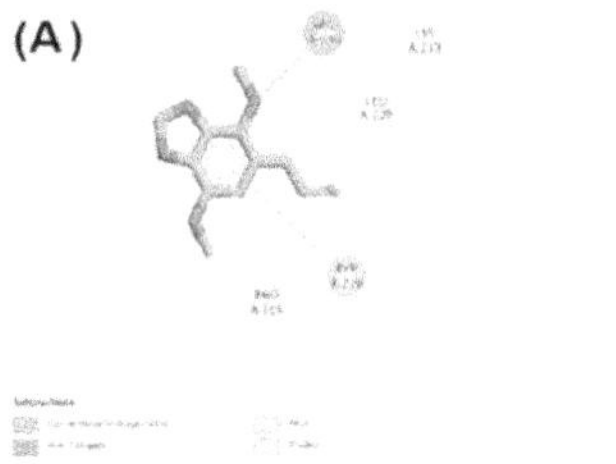	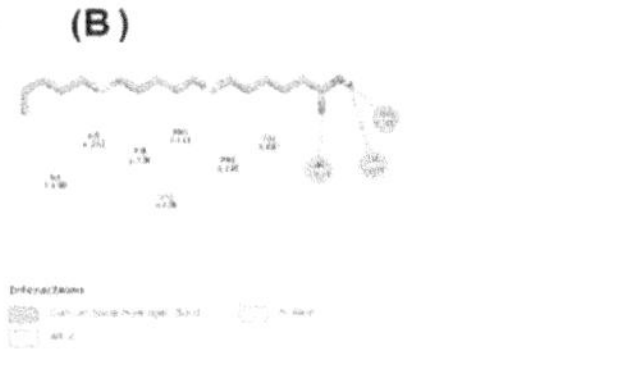
Daidzein and its receptor human topoisomerase II. Reproduced from [69] with permission from MDPI.	Apiol and tyrosine kinases. Reproduced from [66] with permission from Turkish Chemical Society.	Octadecadenoic acid and tyrosine kinases. Reproduced from [66] with permission from Turkish Chemical Society.
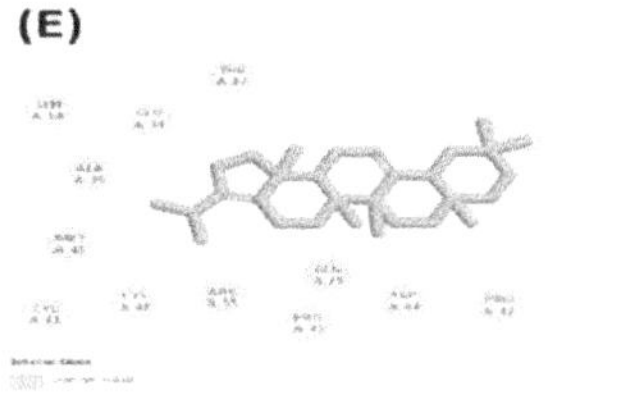	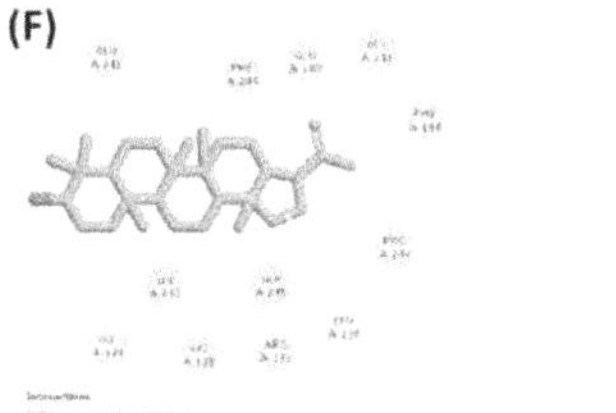	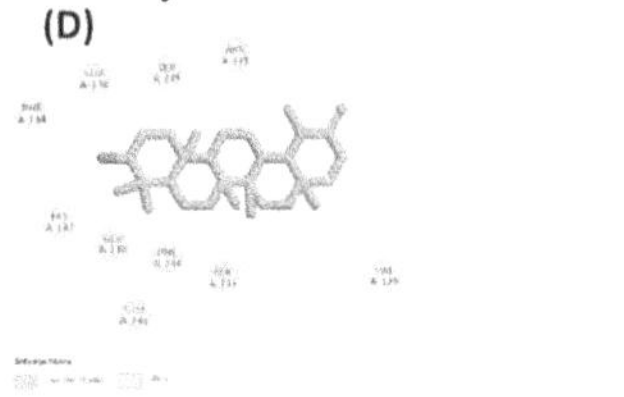
a-neooleana-3 and tyrosine kinases. Reproduced from [66] with permission from Turkish Chemical Society.	Hopa-22(29)-ene-3alpha-ol and tyrosine kinases. Reproduced from [66] with permission from Turkish Chemical Society.	Taraxasterol and tyrosine kinases. Reproduced from [66] with permission from Turkish Chemical Society.

References

[1] International Agency for Research on Cancer World Health Organization, PRESS RELEASE. Latest global cancer data: cancer burden rises to 18.1 million new cases and 9.6 million cancer deaths in 2018

[2] World Health Organization 2022 *Cancer* (Geneva: WHO)

[3] National Cancer Institute 2017 Statistics at a glance: the burden of cancer in the United States *Cancer Stat.*

[4] Sahayarayan J, Rajan K S and Vidhyavathi R *et al* 2020 In-silico protein-ligand docking studies against the estrogen protein of breast cancer using pharmacophore based virtual screening approaches *Saudi J. Biol. Sci.* **28** 400–7

[5] Ashraf M A 2020 Phytochemicals as potential anticancer drugs: time to ponder nature's bounty *BioMed. Res. Int.* **2020** 8602879

[6] Newman D J and Cragg G M 2016 Natural products as sources of new drugs from 1981 to 2014 *J. Nat. Prod.* **79** 629–61

[7] Huang M, Lu J J and Ding J 2021 Natural products in cancer therapy: past, present and future *Nat. Prod. Bioprospect* **11** 5–13
[8] Zhang H W, Lin Z X, Cheung F, Cho W C-S and Tang J-L 2018 Moxibustion for alleviating side effects of chemotherapy or radiotherapy in people with cancer *Cochrane Datab. Syst. Rev.* **11** 1465–858
[9] Duke J A 2002 *Handbook of Medicinal Herbs* (Boca Raton, FL: CRC Press)
[10] Hanahan D and Weinberg R A 2000 The hallmarks of cancer *Cell* **100** 57–70
[11] Lemjabbar-Alaoui H, Hassan O U, Yang Y W and Buchanan P 2015 Lung cancer: biology and treatment options *Biochim. Biophys. Acta.* **1856** 189–210
[12] Garg R, Benedetti L G, Abera M B, Wang H, Abba M and Kazanietz M G 2014 Protein kinase C and cancer: what we know and what we do not *Oncogene* **33** 5225–37
[13] Sohail S K, Sarfraz R, Imran M, Kamran M and Qamar S 2020 Estrogen and progesterone receptor expression in breast carcinoma and its association with clinicopathological variables among the Pakistani population *Cureus* **12** e9751
[14] Nabi M G, Ahangar A and Kaneez S 2016 Estrogen receptors, progesterone receptors and their correlation with respect to HER-2/neu status, histological grade, size of lesion, lymph node metastasis, lymphovascular involvement and age in breast cancer patients in a hospital in north India *Asian J. Med. Sci.* **7** 34
[15] Frame M C 2002 Src in cancer: deregulation and consequences for cell behaviour *Biochim. Biophys. Acta.* **1602** 114–30
[16] Baldanzi G and Graziani A 2014 Physiological signaling and structure of the HGF receptor MET *Biomedicines* **3** 1–31
[17] Summy J M and Gallick G E 2003 Src family kinases in tumor progression and metastasis *Cancer Metast. Rev.* **22** 337–58
[18] Harrison C, Kiladjian J J, Al-Ali H K, Gisslinger H and Waltzman R *et al* 2012 JAK inhibition with ruxolitinib versus best available therapy for myelofibrosis *N. Engl. J. Med.* **366** 787–98
[19] Timofeev O 2021 Mutant p53 in cancer progression and personalized therapeutic treatments *Front. Oncol.* **11** 740578
[20] Marei H E, Althani A and Afifi N *et al* 2021 p53 signaling in cancer progression and therapy *Cancer Cell Int* **21** 703
[21] Levine A J 2019 The many faces of p53: something for everyone *J. Mol. Cell. Biol.* **11** 524–30
[22] Sharma S, Kelly T K and Jones P A 2010 Epigenetics in cancer *Carcinogenesis* **31** 27–36
[23] Sigismund S, Avanzato D and Lanzetti L 2018 Emerging functions of the EGFR in cancer *Mol. Oncol.* **12** 3–20
[24] Lemmon M A and Schlessinger J 2010 Cell signaling by receptor tyrosine kinases *Cell* **141** 1117–34
[25] Roskoski R 2014 The ErbB/HER family of proteintyrosine kinases and cancer *Pharmacol. Res.* **79** 34–74
[26] Uribe M L, Marrocco I and Yarden Y 2021 EGFR in cancer: signaling mechanisms, drugs, and acquired resistance *Cancers (Basel)* **13** 2748
[27] Boulay P L, Mitchell L, Turpin J and Huot-Marchand J *et al* 2016 Rab11-FIP1C is a critical negative regulator in ErbB2-mediated mammary tumor progression *Cancer Res.* **76** 2662–74
[28] Bakhle Y S 2001 COX-2 and cancer: a new approach to an old problem *Br. J. Pharmacol.* **134** 1137–50

[29] Du J, Feng J, Luo D and Peng L 2022 Prognostic and clinical significance of COX-2 overexpression in laryngeal cancer: a meta-analysis *Front Oncol* **22** 854946
[30] Brooks A J and Putoczki T 2020 JAK-STAT signalling pathway in cancer *Cancers (Basel)* **12** 1971
[31] Gore M and Desai N S 2014 Computer-aided drug designing *Methods Mol. Biol.* **1168** 313–21
[32] Oyinloye B E, Adekiya T A, Aruleba R T, Ojo O A and Ajiboye B O 2019 Structure-based docking studies of GLUT4 towards exploring selected phytochemicals from solanum xanthocarpum as a therapeutic target for the treatment of cancer *Curr. Drug Discov. Technol.* **16** 406–16
[33] Qawoogha S S and Shahiwala A 2020 Identification of potential anticancer phytochemicals against colorectal cancer by structure-based docking studies *J. Recept. Signal Transduct. Res.* **40** 67–76
[34] De. Ruyck J, Brysbaert G, Blossey R and Lensink M F 2016 Molecular docking as a popular tool in drug design, an *in silico* travel *Adv. Appl. Bioinform. Chem.* **28** 1–11
[35] Moudi M, Go. R, Yien C Y and Nazre M 2013 Vinca alkaloids *Int. J. Prev. Med.* **4** 1231–5
[36] Sofowora A, Ogunbodede E and Onayade A 2013 The role and place of medicinal plants in the strategies for disease prevention *Afr. J. Tradit. Complement Altern. Med.* **10** 210–29
[37] Anand U U, Jacobo-Herrera N, Altemimi A and Lakhssassi N 2019 A comprehensive review on medicinal plants as antimicrobial therapeutics: potential avenues of biocompatible drug discovery *Metabolites* **9** 258
[38] Pandya P, Kumar P, Bhadresha K, Patel C, Patel S, Rawal R and Mankad A 2020 Identification of promising compounds from curry tree with cyclooxygenase inhibitory potential using a combination of machine learning, molecular docking, dynamics simulations and binding free energy calculations *Mol. Simul.* **46** 812–22
[39] Hou D X, Fujii M, Terahara N and Yoshimoto M 2004 Molecular mechanisms behind the chemopreventive effects of anthocyanidins *J. Biomed. Biotechnol.* **2004** 815182
[40] Wang L S and Stoner G D 2008 Anthocyanins and their role in cancer prevention *Cancer Lett.* **269** 281–90
[41] Acharya R, Chacko S, Bose P, Lapenna A and Pattanayak S P 2019 Structure based multitargeted molecular docking analysis of selected furanocoumarins against breast cancer *Sci Rep.* **9** 15743
[42] Lamichhane S, Rai R P and Khatri A *et al* 2021 Screening of phytochemicals as potential anti-breast cancer agents targeting HER2: an in-silico approach *J. Biomol. Struct. Dyn.* **26** 1–15
[43] Okagu I U, Ndefo J C, Aham E C and Udenigwe C C 2021 *Zanthoxylum* species: a comprehensive review of traditional uses, phytochemistry, pharmacological and nutraceutical applications *Molecules* **26** 4023
[44] Sharifi-Rad M, Pezzani R, Redaelli M, Zorzan M, Imran M, Ahmed Khalil A, Salehi B, Sharopov F, Cho W C and Sharifi-Rad J 2020 Preclinical pharmacological activities of epigallocatechin-3-gallate in signaling pathways: an update on cancer *Molecules* **25** 467
[45] Manda G, Rojo A I, Martínez-Klimova E, Pedraza-Chaverri J and Cuadrado A 2020 Nordihydroguaiaretic acid: from herbal medicine to clinical development for cancer and chronic diseases *Front. Pharmacol.* **11** 151
[46] Poschner S, Maier-Salamon A, Zehl M and Wackerlig J *et al* 2017 The impacts of genistein and daidzein on estrogen conjugations in human breast cancer cells: a targeted metabolomics approach *Front. Pharmacol* **8** 699

[47] Moghadasian M H 2000 Pharmacological properties of plant sterols *in vivo* and *in vitro* observations *Life Sci.* **67** 605–15

[48] Prasathkumar M, Anisha S, Dhrisya C, Becky R and Subramaniam S 2021 Therapeutic and pharmacological efficacy of selective Indian medicinal plants—a review *Phytomed. Plus* **1** 100029

[49] Roy N K, Parama D, Banik K and Bordoloi D *et al* 2019 An update on pharmacological potential of boswellic acids against chronic diseases *Int. J. Mol. Sci.* **20** 4101

[50] Ebenyi N, Lilian N and Chidinma A *et al* 2022 Identification of some bioactive compounds from camelia sinensis as possible inhibitors of HER2: a structure-based drug design for breast cancer treatment https://dx.doi.org/10.2139/ssrn.4078794

[51] Gouthami K, Veeraraghavan V and Nagaraja P 2022 In-silico characterization of phytochemicals identified from *Vitex negundo* (L) extract as potential therapy for WNT-signaling proteins *Egypt J. Med. Hum. Genet* **23** 3

[52] Abuzenadah A M, Al-Sayes F, Mahafujul Alam S S, Hoque M, Karim S, Hussain I M R and Tabrez S 2022 Elucidating antiangiogenic potential of *rauwolfia serpentina*: VEGFR-2 targeting-based molecular docking study *Evid. Based Complem. Alternat. Med.* **2022** 6224666

[53] Gurung A B, Ali M A, Lee J, Farah M A and Al-Anazi K M 2021 Molecular docking and dynamics simulation study of bioactive compounds from *Ficus carica* L. with important anticancer drug targets *PLoS One* **16** e0254035

[54] Islam M T *et al* 2019 Ponicidin as a promising anticancer agent: Its biological and biopharmaceutical profile along with a molecular docking study *Biotechnol. Appl. Biochem.* **66** 434–44

[55] Islam M T, Khalipha A B R, Bagchi R, Mondal M, Smrity S Z, Uddin S J, Shilpi J A and Rouf R 2019 Anticancer activity of thymol: a literature-based review and docking study with emphasis on its anticancer mechanisms *IUBMB Life* **71** 9–19

[56] Ahammad F, Alam R, Mahmud R, Akhter S, Talukder E K and Tonmoy A M *et al* 2021 Pharmacoinformatics and molecular dynamics simulation-based phytochemical screening of neem plant (*Azadirachta indica*) against human cancer by targeting MCM7 protein *Brief Bioinform* **22** bbab098

[57] Javed T, Raja S A, Rehman K U, Khalid S, Khalid N and Riaz S 2021 In silico bimolecular characterization of anticancer phytochemicals from *Fagonia indica Pak. J. Pharm. Sci.* **34** 883–9

[58] Liu X, Zhou Q G, Zhu X C, Xie L and Cai B C 2019 Screening for potential active components of fangji huangqi tang on the treatment of nephrotic syndrome by using integrated metabolomics based on 'correlations between chemical and metabolic profiles' *Front. Pharmacol.* **10** 1261

[59] Mohammed H A, Khan R A, Abdel-Hafez A A and Abdel-Aziz M *et al* 2021 Phytochemical profiling, *in vitro* and in silico anti-microbial and anti-cancer activity evaluations and staph gyraseB and *h*-TOP-IIβ receptor-docking studies of major constituents of *Zygophyllum coccineum* L. aqueous-ethanolic extract and its subsequent fractions: an approach to validate traditional phytomedicinal knowledge *Molecules* **26** 577

[60] Muhammad M, Kausar F, Hassan M, Javaid S and Malik A 2021 Anticancer activities of phenolic compounds from *Moringa oleifera* leaves: *in vitro* and in silico mechanistic study *Beni-Suef Univer. J. Basic Appl. Sci.* **10** 12

[61] Ullah A, Nazmul Islam P, Araf Y, Hossain S, Sarkar B and Saha A 2019 Molecular docking and pharmacological property analysis of phytochemicals from clitoria ternatea as potent

inhibitors of cell cycle checkpoint proteins in the cyclin/CDK pathway in cancer cells *Comput. Mol. Biosci.* **9** 81–94

[62] Mahnashi M H, Alqahtani Y S and Alyami B A *et al* 2021 Cytotoxicity, anti-angiogenic, anti-tumor and molecular docking studies on phytochemicals isolated from *Polygonum hydropiper* L *BMC Complement. Med. Ther.* **21** 239

[63] Pulipati S, Babu P and Dommati H 2021 Phytochemical, in-silico analysis and anticancer activity of a bioactive principle isolated from *Amaranthus tricolor* (L) *Res. J. Biotechnol.* **16** 122–33

[64] Sadeer N B, Sinan K I, Cziáky Z, Jekő J, Zengin G, Jeewon R, Abdallah H H, Rengasamy K R R and M F M 2020 Assessment of the pharmacological properties and phytochemical profile of *Bruguiera gymnorhiza* (L.) lam using *in vitro* studies, in silico docking, and multivariate analysis *Biomolecules* **10** 731

[65] Guha G, Rajkumar V, Ashok Kumar R and Mathew L 2011 Therapeutic potential of polar and non-polar extracts of cyanthillium cinereum *in vitro Evid. Based Complement. Alternat. Med.* **2011** 784826

[66] Ahmed M *et al* 2022 Comprehensive phytochemical profiling, biological activities, and molecular docking studies of *Pleurospermum candollei*: an insight into potential for natural products development *Molecules* **27** 4113

[67] Shakya A 2019 Natural phytochemicals: potential anti-HCV targets in silico approach *J. Appl. Pharm. Sci.* **9** 94–100

[68] Huang B 2009 MetaPocket: a meta approach to improve protein ligand binding site prediction *Omics* **13** 325–30

[69] Ismail S, Uzairu A, Sagagi B and Sabiu Muhammad S 2018 : Insilico molecular docking and pharmacokinetic studies of selected phytochemicals with estrogen and progesterone receptors as anticancer agent for breast cancer *J. Turkish Chem. Soc., A: Chem.* **5** 1337–50

[70] Roy A and Garg S 2021 Evaluation of different phytochemicals against BRCA2 Receptor *Biointerface Res. Appl. Chem.* **12** 1670–81

[71] Oyedele A K, Adelusi T I and Ogunlana A T *et al* 2022 Promising disruptors of p53-MDM2 dimerization from some medicinal plant phytochemicals: a molecular modeling study *J. Biomol. Struct. Dyn.* **13** 1–10

[72] Obaid A Y, Voleti S, Bora R S, Hajrah N H, Omer A M S, Sabir J S M and Saini K S 2017 Cheminformatics studies to analyze the therapeutic potential of phytochemicals from *Rhazya stricta Chem. Cent. J.* **11** 11

[73] Singh A N, Baruah M M and Sharma N 2017 Structure based docking studies towards exploring potential anti-androgen activity of selected phytochemicals against prostate cancer *Sci. Rep.* **7** 1955

[74] Purawarga Matada G S, Dhiwar P S, Abbas N, Singh E, Ghara A, Das A and Bhargava S V 2022 Molecular docking and molecular dynamic studies: screening of phytochemicals against EGFR, HER2, estrogen and NF-KB receptors for their potential use in breast cancer *J. Biomol. Struct. Dyn.* **40** 6183–92

[75] Jha V, Devkar S, Gharat K, Kasbe S, Matharoo D K, Pendse S, Bhosale A and Bhargava A 2022 Screening of phytochemicals as potential inhibitors of breast cancer using structure based multitargeted molecular docking *Anal. Phytomed. Plus* **2** 100227

[76] Iheagwam F N, Ogunlana O O, Ogunlana O E, Isewon I and Oyelade J 2019 Potential anti-cancer flavonoids isolated from *Caesalpinia bonduc* young twigs and leaves: molecular docking and *in silico* studies *Bioinform Biol. Insights* **13** 1177932218821371

[77] Sharma M, Sharma N, Muddassir M, Rahman Q I, Dwivedi U N and Akhtar S 2021 Structure-based pharmacophore modeling, virtual screening and simulation studies for the identification of potent anticancerous phytochemical lead targeting cyclin-dependent kinase 2 *J. Biomol. Struct. Dyn.* **40** 9815–32
[78] Riaz M, Ashfaq U A, Qasim M, Yasmeen E, Ul Qamar M T and Anwar: F 2017 screening of medicinal plant phytochemicals as natural antagonists of p53-MDM2 interaction to reactivate p53 functioning *Anticancer Drugs* **28** 1032–8
[79] Sarkar B, Ullah M A, Islam S S, Rahman M H and Araf Y 2021 Analysis of plant-derived phytochemicals as anti-cancer agents targeting cyclin dependent kinase-2, human topoisomerase IIa and vascular endothelial growth factor receptor-2 *J. Recept. Signal Transduct. Res.* **41** 217–33
[80] Anusha D, Sharanya S, Ramya R and David D 2019 Anticancer screening of the phytochemicals present in the medicinal plant vitex negundo against mutant anaplastic lymphoma kinase (ALK) protein: an in-silico approach *Biomed. Pharmacol. J.* **12** 993–1000

Chapter 12

Modern approaches to study the effects of phytochemicals on cellular epigenome

Rahul Kumar, Pankaj Keshari, Yashaswee Mishra and Ajay Kumar Sharma

Many phytochemicals exert anti-cancerous or cancer preventive effects on a mammalian cell by altering its epigenetic profile or the epigenome. These epigenetic signatures primarily include DNA methylation, histone modifications, non-coding RNAs and three-dimensional spatial structure of chromatin. All these epigenetic signatures also crosstalk with one another. Changes incurred by a particular phytochemical upon the cellular epigenome can be studied using various methods. These methods can be local, targeting a few known selected loci, or global, targeting the whole genome. These methods may further be divided into direct or indirect. Direct methods involve detection of individual epigenetic signatures. These methods require access to the site of modification. Chromatin immunoprecipitation (ChIP) is one of the most commonly used methods to study histone modifications. Bisulphite conversion technology is considered the gold standard in studying DNA methylation. Microarray technology and RNA sequencing technology are important in studying non-coding RNA profile of the cell. The three-dimensional spatial structure of chromatin can be studied using chromosome conformation capture (3C) technology. Indirect methods include detection of different proteins or their respective mRNAs, which are responsible for carrying out specific epigenetic changes inside a cell. These methods, whether direct or indirect, have been modified variously by different workers over time. These methods are also used in combination in an integrative manner to study multiple types of epigenetic modifications together. Most of these methods are now available with high-throughput technology to generate whole-genome-based data. The present chapter provides an illustrative account of some of the most important and popular methods used to study different epigenetic signatures associated with a particular cell or tissue.

doi:10.1088/978-0-7503-5252-9ch12

12.1 Introduction

The term epigenetics was coined by Conrad Waddington in 1942 for describing such changes which are inherited by an organism in its phenotype without changes in its genotype (Waddington 1959, Waddington 2012). The word is a portmanteau of two words, viz. 'epi' meaning 'above' and 'genetics' meaning 'pertaining to heredity'. The modern definition of epigenetics describes it as the study of heritable chemical changes which can modulate gene expression without any changes to the nucleotide sequence itself (Hughes 2014). Gene expression in mammals involves epigenetic regulations at multiple levels. The four most important ones are histone modifications, DNA methylation patterns, chromatin structural conformation changes and non-coding RNAs (Zhang and Pradhan 2014). The epigenome refers to the sum total of all such potential heritable changes across the genome (Bernstein *et al* 2007). Epigenetic regulations are important in controlling cell physiology and types (Margueron *et al* 2005). Epigenetic marks provide a signature of cancer development and progression. All cancers have altered epigenetic landscapes (Nebbioso *et al* 2018). We know that prevention is better than cure. Cancer prevention is a set of strategies which involves active measures to reduce cancer risk (Banerjee *et al* 2010, Sarkar *et al* 2009). Chemoprevention is the reversal or inhibition of carcinogenesis using chemical compounds which may be natural or synthetic in origin (Singh *et al* 2014). Dietary phytochemicals have been in use for thousands of years to cure and prevent different diseases including cancers in different cultures and civilizations, particularly in Asian countries (Shankar *et al* 2013). Phytochemicals can have inhibitory effects on the signaling pathways and epigenetic events involved in carcinogenesis (Singh *et al* 2014). Many dietary phytochemicals present in seasonal fruit, vegetables, medicinal herbs and spices have anti-cancerous activities. Many such phytochemicals have been purified and studied by various workers from all around the globe. Research and development on phytochemicals in disease prevention (or nutraceuticals) has become quite popular in recent years (Nwosu and Ubaoji 2020). Nutraceutical industries are becoming a high-demand business venture and phytochemical research is becoming popular under new disciplines like foodomics and nutri-epigenetics (Shankar *et al* 2013, Ortea 2022). The global market concerning this area has been estimated to be over 100 billion USD in a recent report (Nwosu and Ubaoji 2020). A recent estimate suggests that more than 40 % of global cancer related deaths may be related to malnutrition and deficiency of dietary factors (Aggarwal *et al* 2006). The last 20 years have witnessed a great deal of research providing evidence to show that phytochemicals are potent epigenetic regulators and can target or revert abnormal epigenetic modifications in different cancers (Gerhauser 2013). The anti-cancerous activities of these phytochemicals are attributed to their abilities to inhibit DNA methyltransferases (DNMTs), modify histones or affect the expression of non-coding RNAs (Shankar *et al* 2016). To study these effects, scientists use cultured cells or tissue samples of an animal after treatment with a specific dose of a particular phytochehmical or combination of phytochemicals. These cells or tissue samples are further subjected to epigenome profiling to study the effect of these treatments. Epigenome profiling may be local or global. Individual or local modifications can be studied by using antibodies against specific modifications. Many PCR-based methods have also been developed like bisulfite modification for studying DNA methylation pattern (Li 2021). Conventionally, FISH (fluorescence *In Situ* hybridization) has been used to probe non-coding RNA molecules in living cells (Hinten *et al* 2016, Vautrot *et al* 2021). Three-dimensional chromosomal conformation patterns are detected using chromosome confirmation capture technology (3C) (Li 2021). Modern technology allows us to profile all the epigenetic changes occurring inside a cell at a particular time point after phytochemical treatment. The present chapter deals with some of the most popular methods used for cellular epigenome profiling.

12.2 Methods in epigenome profiling

Epigenome profiling is conducted primarily to detect histone acetylation and methylation patterns, DNA methylation patterns, non-coding RNAs and three-dimensional spatial chromosomal conformations (Zentner and Henikoff 2014, Mehrmohamadi *et al* 2021). Various popular and important methods used for epigenome profiling are explained in subsequent paragraphs. These methods have been customized variously by different scientists. The basic operating principles of some of the most important methods used in epigenetic studies are discussed in the following.

12.2.1 Direct methods

Direct methods require direct access to the site of modification or the epigenetic changes. These methods are based on detecting the exact epigenetic signatures of the chromatin (DNA, histone and its three-dimensional conformation).

12.2.1.1 Methods to study histone modifications

Before knowing about the methods used in detection of histone modifications, let us understand first what these modifications are. Post-translational modifications of histone proteins are important epigenetic mechanisms controlling gene expression (Khan *et al* 2015). These modifications may reflect the active or repressed state of the chromatin. Acetylation, deacetylation and methylation of specific lysine residue of the histone tails are of prime importance in detecting epigenetic signatures. These modifications are primarily linked to chromatin remodeling. Acetylation is associated with transcriptional activation and deacetylation with transcriptional inactivation (Kouzarides 2007) (figure 12.1(A)). Acetylations are associated with lysine 9, 14, 18, 23 and 56 of histone H3. Acetylation of lysine 9 on the histone H3 (H3K9ac) is associated with gene activation. Methylations have been reported to occur at arginine 2, lysine 9, 14, 18, 23 and 56 of histone H3. Histone methylation has different effects based on the site of methylation. For example, trimethylation of the fourth lysine (K4) residue of histone H3 (H3K4me3) and monomethylation of lysine 20 on the histone H3 (H3K20me) leads to transcriptional activation, whereas methylation of the ninth lysine residue (K9) of histone H3 (H3K9me3) results in transcriptional silencing (figure 12.1(B)) (Hon *et al* 2009, Mills 2010, Hawkins *et al* 2011, Leszinski *et al* 2012, Bag and Bag 2018). An important group of enzymes

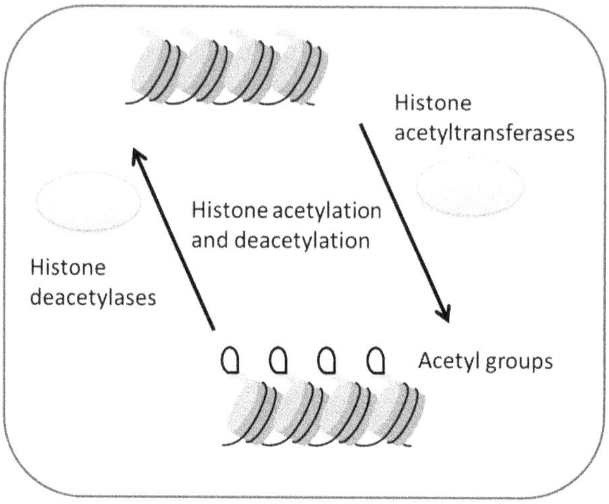

(A)

Modifications	Acetylation	Deacetylation	Methylation
	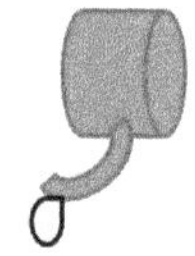	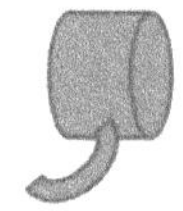	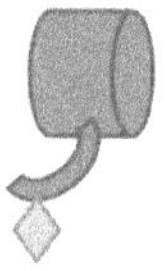
Effect of H3K9 modification	Transcriptional activation	Transcriptional inactivation	Transcriptional silencing

(B)

Figure 12.1. Epigenetic histone modifications. (A) Acetylation and deacetylation of histones. All histone associated epigenetic modifications take place on histone tails on specific sites. Site specific modifications have specific effects. (B) Example of transcriptional regulation by histone modifications. H3K9 refers to third lysine residue of histone H3 protein in the nucleosome. H3K9 methylation is linked to transcriptional silencing and H3K9 acetylation is associated with transcriptional activation. Deacetylation of H3K9 marks transcriptional inactivation.

responsible for these modifications are histone deacetylases (HDACs), histone acetyltransferases (HATs) and histone methyltransferases (HMTs) (Li 2021). These enzymes are the main targets of the dietary phytochemicals which affect the process of chromatin remodeling (Shankar *et al* 2013). Examples of such phytochemicals are curcumin, resveratrol, diindolylmethane, etc (Liu *et al* 2005, Chen *et al* 2007, Bora-Tatar *et al* 2009, Li *et al* 2010, Roy *et al* 2011). Histone modification patterns are altered in most cancers and many dietary phytochemicals can prevent as well as reverse such alterations (Shankar *et al* 2016).

Chromatin immunoprecipitation (ChIP) is the most popular method to study chromatin modifications and DNA–protein interactions (Collas 2010). ChIP is considered a fundamental technique in studying chromatin structure and histone modifications (Li 2021). ChIP assay is based on recognition of particular histone modification markers, epigenetic modulators, transcription factors or any other protein associated with DNA using specific antibodies. It allows assignment of locus-specific functions of histone modifications by providing information about the DNA sequence bound to the histones with specific modifications (Gade and Kalvakolanu 2012). For specific target DNA sequences bound to histones with a specific modification, ChIP is followed by PCR. The amplicon can further be sequenced using the primers used for PCR for additional sequence information. But if the targets are undefined, ChIP is followed by large-scale high-throughput sequencing (ChIP-seq) or microarray profiling (ChIP-chip) (Pillai and Chelappan 2009, Collas 2010). These later methods are used for global epigenome profiling of DNA sequences associated with a particular histone modification. Microarray technology and ChIP-seq have been described in detail in subsequent sections. ChIP-seq is widely used in profiling the genome-wide histone modification landscape (Albert *et al* 2007, Barski *et al* 2007, Johnson *et al* 2007, Mikkelsen *et al* 2007, Li 2021).

In a standard ChIP experiment, interactions between histones and DNA sequences are fixed by treating cells with formaldehyde. Formaldehyde mediates crosslinking of proteins with DNA. In this way, it freezes the interactions as it is. After crosslinking, nuclei are extracted from these cells. These nuclei are lysed to release the chromatin. Chromatin is then fragmented using sonication. The chromatin fragments are incubated with antibodies against a particular histone modification. The non-target fragments are washed away. Antibodies allow the target chromatin fragment to be pulled down separately. This process of immuno-precipitaion is followed by reverse-crosslinking of chromatin and purification of DNA segments out of chromatin fragments using standard phenol-chloroform based purification of DNA. These DNA are sheared due to sonication. Therefore, repairing of sheared ends is done. This DNA is further used for PCR, sequencing or microarray to identify the regions bound to histones with particular modifications. The basic steps of a standard ChIP experiment are shown in figure 12.2. For large-scale sequencing, adapters are ligated to ends of DNA followed by PCR-based amplification using primers designed to bind with the adapter sequences. The PCR product is then subjected to sequencing for whole-genome-based histone modification profiling follows by data analysis (Ricci *et al* 2020).

12.2.1.2 Methods to study DNA methylation

DNA methylation is among the most extensively studied epigenetic modifications. DNA methylation in human beings predominantly involves methylation of the fifth carbon of cytosine. This methyl group comes from S-adenosyl-L-methionine (SAM) (Thakur *et al* 2014). This transfer of methyl group leads to formation of 5-methyl-cytosine (5mC). The process of methylation of cytosine is catalyzed by a group of enzymes known as DNA methyltransferases (figure 12.3) (Smith and Meissner 2013, Yong *et al* 2016). CpG dinucleotide are most common targets of these enzymes in adults. During embryonic development, non-CpG dinucleotides are also methylated

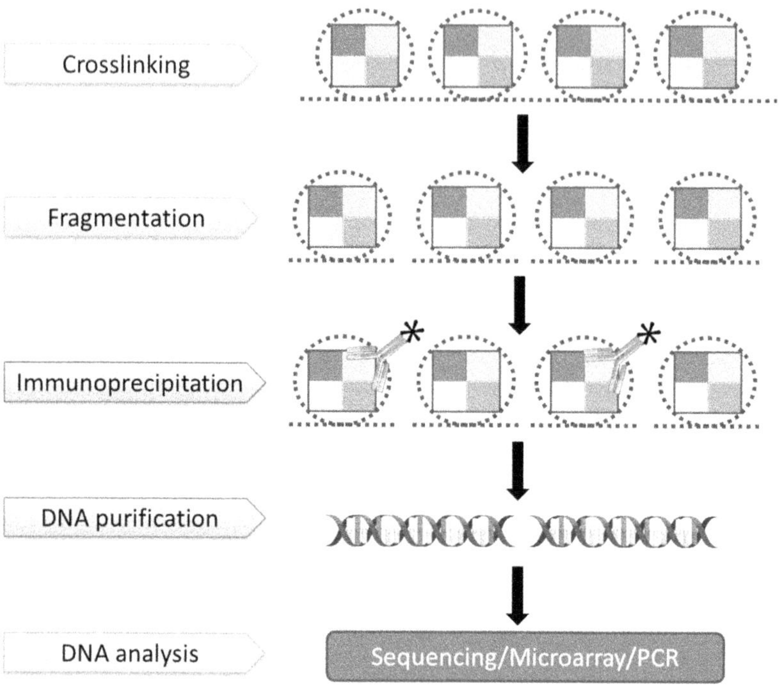

Figure 12.2. Chromatin immunoprecipitation procedure. DNA–histone interactions are frozen using cross-linking agents like formaldehyde. Chromatin fragmentation is done using sonication. Antibodies raised against the modified histones are used for immunoprecipitation. DNA is purified from the pulled-down antibody-chromatin complexes followed by its analysis using PCR, sequencing or microarray.

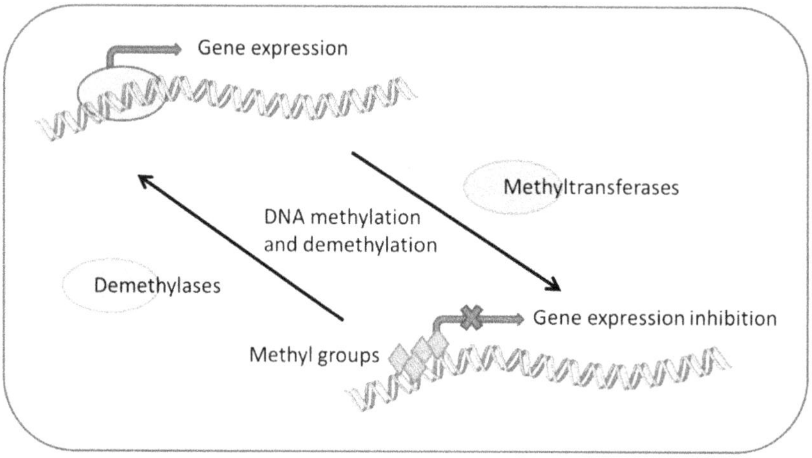

Figure 12.3. Process of DNA methylation. DNA methylation are mostly inhibitory towards gene expression. Methyltransferases and demethylases carry out DNA methylation and demethylation processes, respectively.

like CpA and CpT (Ramsahoye *et al* 2000). 5mC forms about 1% of all DNA bases of the human genome. It represents 70%–80% of all CpG dinucleotides (Ehrlich *et al* 1982). CpG dinucleotides are not evenly distributed throughout the genome. Rather, these are found to be clustered together in some regions which are known as CpG islands (Kim *et al* 2009). DNA methylation plays a crucial role during the mammalian embryonic development process. It is necessary for normal development and structural-functional integrity of the chromatin (Derreumaux *et al* 2001). It is involved in the process of X-chromosome inactivation and genomic imprinting (Leonhardt *et al* 1999, Robertson and Jones 2000). DNA methylation also plays an important role in development of cancer and tumorigenesis (Jones and Liard 1999, Momparler and Bovenzi 2000). DNA methylation in the promoter region of a gene suppresses gene activity by inhibition of binding of transcription factors to their binding sites (Tate and Bird 1993). Excess methylation of CpG islands present in the promoter regions of many genes can have deleterious effects. For example, hypermethylation of promoters of tumor suppressor genes can lead to cancer. In contrast, DNA hypomethylation has been found to be associated with genomic instability (Gama-Sosa *et al* 1983, Goelz *et al* 1985, Thakur *et al* 2014). Many anti-cancerous phytochemicals target DNMTs to affect the process of DNA methylation. A few examples of such phytochemicals are apigenin, curcumin, epigallocatechin-3-gallate, genistein, quercetin, resveratrol, etc (Shankar *et al* 2016).

A variety of DNA methylation profiling methods are available. There are methods for the study of the locus-specific DNA methylation patterns as well as the whole-genome DNA methylation (methylome) signatures. All of these methods are grouped under four broad categories (table 12.1). These are restriction enzyme-based methods, affinity enrichment based methods, bisulfite conversion-based methods and others (Yong *et al* 2016). Among these methods bisulfite conversion is considered the gold standard for studying DNA methylation pattern (Li 2021). In this method, genomic DNA is treated with sodium bisulfite. Bisulfite treatment leads to deamination of unmethylated cytosines to uracil. This treatment does not affect the methylated cytosine residues in the genome, which allows 5mCs to be distinguished all across the genomic DNA (Frommer *et al* 1992, Jones 2012). After PCR, uracil converts to thymine and all the cytosines in the template indicate the locations of the methylated ones (Yong *et al* 2016) (figure 12.4). This basic and fundamental technique has been customized differently for locus-specific DNA methylation studies and whole genome methylome profiling (Yong *et al* 2016, Li 2021). For locus-specific studies, direct bisulfite PCR product sequencing is done. For whole genome methylome profiling, bisulfite conversion is coupled with methylome specific arrays or high-throughput sequencing (Leti *et al* 2018, Li 2021).

12.2.1.3 Methods to study non-coding RNAs

Recent studies have demonstrated that expression of different non-coding RNAs (ncRNAs) play a pivotal role in cancer pathophysiology and many phytochemicals (e.g., curcumin) can modulate these RNAs to inhibit cancers (Shankar *et al* 2016, Adriaens and Marine 2017, Caracciolo *et al* 2019, Ganapathy and Ezekiel 2019, Saghafi *et al* 2019, Tokgun *et al* 2019). ncRNAs can be classified into infrastructural

Table 12.1. Examples of different methods used for studying DNA methylation pattern.

S. No.	DNA methylation technology	Examples of the available methods
1	Restriction enzyme-based methods	Locus-specific restriction digestion Comprehensive high-throughput arrays for relative methylation (CHARM)
2	Affinity enrichment based methods	Methylated DNA immunoprecipitation (MeDIP)
3	Bisulfite conversion-based methods	Locus-specific bisulfite conversion Methylation array Whole-genome bisulfite sequencing (WGBS) Reduced-representation bisulfite sequencing (RRBS) Oxidative bisulfite sequencing (OxBS-seq) TET-assisted bisulfite sequencing (TAB-seq) Single-cell methylome
4	Other methods	Methylation-specific PCR Genome-wide 5-hydroxylmethylation profiling Single-molecule real-time sequencing Nanopore sequencing

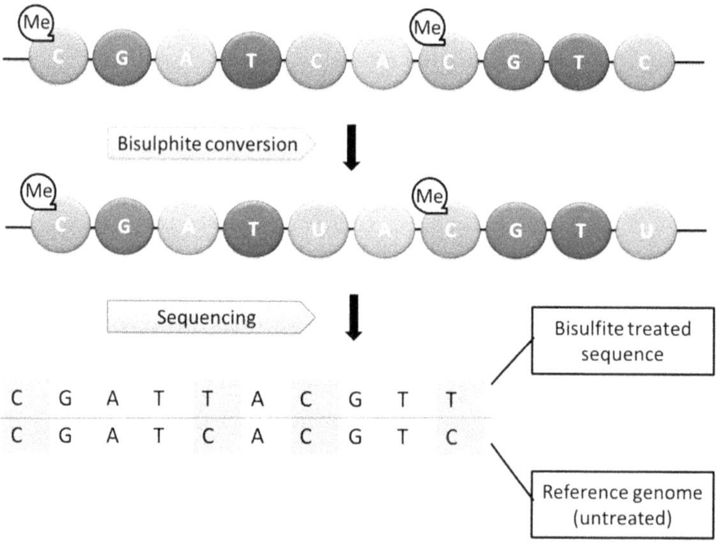

Figure 12.4. Bisulfite conversion technology. DNA is treated with sodium bisulfite. Bisulfite deaminates unmethylated cytosines to uracils without affecting the methylated cytosine residues. PCR converts to uracil to thymine and all cytosines present in the PCR products are at the place of the ones which were methylated.

ncRNAs and regulatory ncRNAs. Infrastructural ncRNAs include constitutively expressed RNAs like ribosomal RNA (rRNA), transfer RNA (tRNA), small nuclear RNA (snRNA) and small nucleolar RNA (snoRNA) (Kaikkonen *et al* 2011). Many workers do not include infrastructural ncRNAs under ncRNAs and snoRNA has been classified under long non-coding RNAs which will be discussed subsequently. Henceforth, regulatory ncRNAs will be referred as ncRNAs only in subsequent paragraphs in this chapter.

Regulatory ncRNAs or simply the ncRNAs may be divided into long ncRNA (lncRNA) and small (or short) ncRNA based on their size (Han Li and Chen 2015). lncRNAs are longer than 200 nucleotides (Statello *et al* 2021). Small ncRNAs are shorter than 200 nucleotides (Han Li and Chen 2015). lncRNAs include long-intervening RNA (lincRNA), small nucleolar RNA (snoRNA) and circular RNA (circRNA) (Elia and Quintavalle 2017). Small ncRNAs include micro RNA (miRNA), piwi-interacting RNA (piRNA) and short-interfering RNA (siRNA) (Elia and Quintavalle 2017). Some of the important examples of ncRNAs with established role in cellular epigenetic regulation processes are given in table 12.2. Among all ncRNAs, roles of micro RNA and long non-coding RNA have been explored in-depth. These ncRNAs play an important role in gene regulation at various levels. Different ncRNAs have been found to be associated with regulation of transcriptional silencing, mRNA stability, protein expression, DNA methylation, histone modifications, chromatin structure, etc and therefore have important implications in tumor biology (figure 12.5) (Storz *et al* 2004, Wierzbicki 2012, Böhmdorfer *et al* 2014, Böhmdorfer and Wierzbicki 2015, Daniel *et al* 2015, Fan *et al* 2015, Amodio *et al* 2018, Tang *et al* 2019). Thus it is important to profile the

Table 12.2. Examples of some non-coding RNAs involved in epigenetic regulation.

S. No.	Non-coding RNA	Role	References
1	miR-29b	Interacts with DNMTs, influencing DNA methylation	Zhang *et al* (2018)
3	miR-377	Targets 3'-UTR of DNMT1 mRNA, miR-377-DNMT1-p53 axis plays a pivot role in skin senescence	Xie *et al* (2017)
4	miR-29	Interplay with DNMT3A affects genome methylation	Palmbos *et al* (2015)
5	miR-34a	Interplay with HDAC1 leading to enhanced H3K9 acetylation	Zhao *et al* (2017)
6	miR-138	Targets KDM5B causing histone demethylation in cancer	Denis *et al* (2016)
7	lncPRESS1	Acts as decoy and sequester the histone deacetylase sirtuin 6 (SIRT6)	Jain *et al* (2016)
8	lncRNA TARID	Forms R loop, recruits GADD45A to facilitate TCF21 expression which is inactivated in many cancers due to promoter methylation	Arab *et al* (2019)

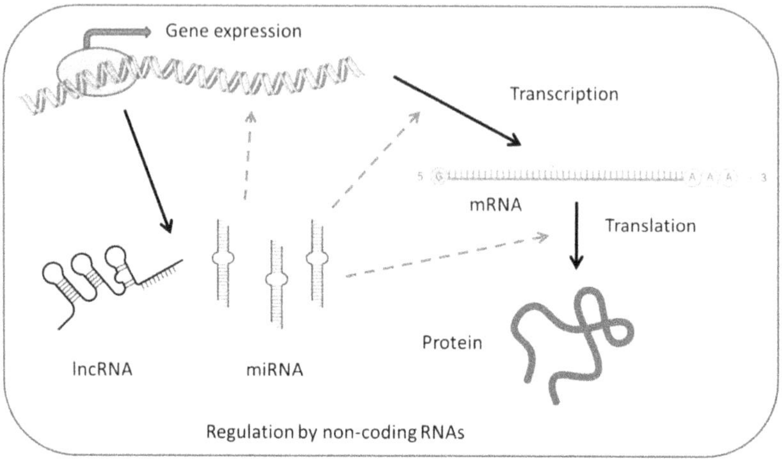

Figure 12.5. Non-coding RNAs in gene regulation. Non-coding RNAs can affect gene expression both at the level of transcription and translation. The regulatory role of these RNAs is also linked to DNA and histone modifications. Long non-coding RNA (lncRNA) and micro RNA (miRNA) form a major group of regulatory non-coding RNAs in epigenetics.

large-scale expression of ncRNAs to understand and identify useful ncRNAs which could be novel biomarkers of cancer development and progression, and could be potential targets of different phytochemicals.

Usually, ncRNAs are expressed in lower abundance as compared to mRNA and high-throughput technologies such as microarray have emerged as a major method to quantify expression of ncRNAs (Pritchard *et al* 2012). A typical microarray procedure starts with total RNA isolation from cells or tissue. Total RNA is reverse transcribed into cDNA, which are then labeled with a fluorescent dye such as Cy5 and Cy3. The labeled reverse transcribed product is then hybridized to the probes of known RNAs tethered on a chip (or glass slide) for 16–24 h. The chip is scanned and fluorescence signal is recorded. The experimental and the control cDNAs are labeled with different dyes. The experimental sample may be the cells or the tissue treated with a particular phytochemical, while the control sample is the untreated one. Florescent signals from different dyes are of different colors. For example, if the experimental sample is labeled with Cy5 it would fluoresce red while the control sample labeled with Cy3 would fluoresce green. More intensty of red color indicates the presence of more RNA from the experimental sample relative to the control (up-regulation), whereas more intensity of green color indicates the presence of more RNA from the control sample relative to the experimental (down-regulation). If RNA from both samples is in similar quantity, yellow color is obtained. Signal strength is directly proportional to the quantity of RNA in the original sample. The relative intensity of fluorescence (experimental versus control) is recorded for individual spots to determine expression level of each non-coding RNA (Khan *et al* 1999, Kurian *et al* 1999, Schulze and Downward 2001, Glanzer *et al* 2004) (figure 12.6). Microarray-based expression profiling is performed differently for small ncRNA and lncRNA because small ncRNA such as miRNA lacks polyA tail,

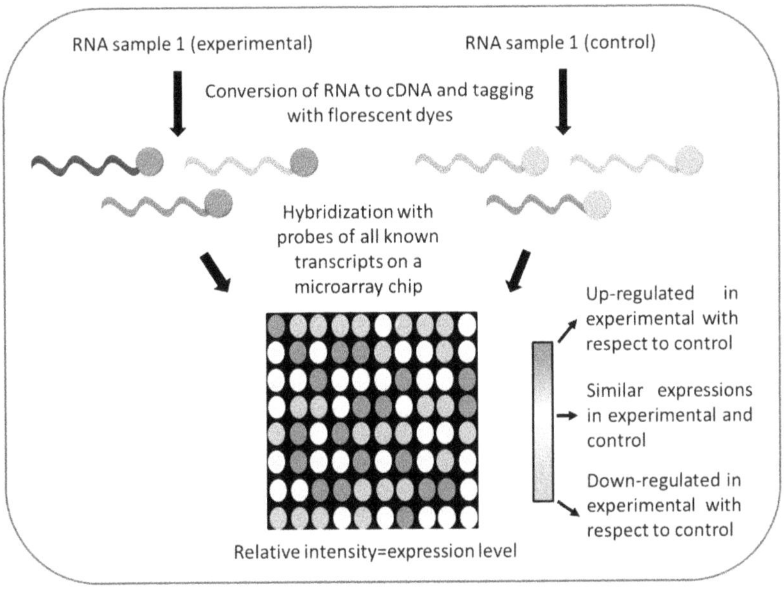

Figure 12.6. A simplified schematic of microarray technology. Whole genome profiling of non-coding RNAs can be performed using microarray technology. For microarray-based studies, RNA is extracted from the experimental and the control sample. Experimental sample may be the cells or the tissue treated with a particular phytochemical. Control sample is the untreated one. RNAs are converted to cDNAs and the resulting cDNAs are labeled with fluorescent dyes. The experimental and the control cDNAs are labeled differently. The labeled cDNA molecules are hybridized with the probe tethered on a chip at different spots. The relative intensity of fluorescence (experimental versus control) is recorded for individual spots to determine expression level of each non-coding RNA.

whereas the majority of lncRNA show similarities with mRNA in having a poly-A tail. Terminal poly-A tails play an important role during cDNA-probe hybridization within most microarray experiments. Thus, lncRNA profiling can be performed along with mRNAs, whereas small ncRNA requires a different approach. One such approach is to tag the 3′ end of small ncRNAs like miRNA with biotin and the probes are labeled with streptavidin. The miRNA binds to its probe through streptavidin-biotin interaction (Liang *et al* 2005). Although microarray technology is highly useful for large-scale quantification, it is limited to the known sequences as it requires oligonucleotide probe preparation.

As compared to microarray technology, RNA sequencing (RNA-seq) provides a comprehensive picture of the entire transcriptome at any given time point. It is a probe/labeling-free method having the advantage of identification of novel/unknown RNA as well as isoforms of RNAs and RNAs that differ even in a single nucleotide. A typical RNA sequencing begins with the isolation of total RNA from control and experimental samples followed by an assessment of the quality of RNA samples for sequencing using instruments like a bioanalyzer, which produces an RNA Integrity Number (RIN). It produces a RIN score between 1–10 with 10 being the highest quality for sequencing. RIN scores below 6 are considered to be of the low quality of

RNA preparation and may affect the downstream processes of sequencing output. Tissues such as paraffin-embedded samples and autopsy samples yield lower RIN score RNA and further analysis of RNA sequencing results should be considered carefully in such cases (Tomita *et al* 2004, Thompson *et al* 2007, Rudloff *et al* 2010). Following RNA isolation, cDNA library is prepared by reverese transcription and adapter ligation. Various strategies have been developed to either enrich RNAs of a particular type by selective depletion of certain RNAs such as the removal of rRNA. Similarly to selecting small RNA, a separate strategy is preferred (Morin *et al* 2010). Usually, small RNAs are enriched by size fractionation using silica-based columns or by running agarose gel electrophoresis and cutting the gel in the 15–30 nucleotide region for purification followed by precipitation to increase the concentration of small ncRNAs. Library preparation is followed by sequencing and data analysis of the transcriptome. Large-scale sequencing data analysis is driven by RNA-Seq data analysis pipelines. Data is generated as FASTQ-format reads and these reads are aligned to reference annotated genome followed by quantification of the expression of different RNAs. The number of sequencing reads represents the level of expression of a particular non-coding RNA. Special care has to be taken during alignment due to many reads spanning the splice junction. Usually, it is done by supplementing the reference genome with exon-exon splice junction annotated known sequences. Following alignment and mapping of reads, transcripts are assembled for quantification of ncRNAs (Mortazavi *et al* 2008). The number of sequencing reads represents the level of expression of a particular non-coding RNA (figure 12.7). Massive amounts of data are generated in this process which is difficult to analyze and requires special expertise. Bioinformaticians and computational biologists play an important role in analyzing such high-throughput data.

12.2.1.4 Methods to study three-dimensional spatial structure of chromatin

Spatial organization of the genome plays an important role in gene expression. There are chromatin regulatory loops which bring enhancer and associated transcription factors in close proximity to the specific promoter to affect gene expression (Pongubala and Murre 2021). The cancer genome is structurally distinct from normal genomes. Altered chromosome folding has been reported in cancer (Wang *et al* 2022). Both DNA methylation and histone modifications are associated with changes in the chromatin structure and packaging (Ikegami *et al* 2009). Therefore, by affecting DNA methylation and histone modifications, phytochemicals may alter the spatial structure of chromatin. Three-dimensional organization of chromatin can be studied using x-ray crystallography conventionally (Subirana and Martínez 1976). Advanced cryo-electron microscopy may provide greater insights into chromatin structure (Bhoopathi *et al* 2020). These tools involve many complex steps during sample processing spanning over days but provide information about the biomolecular structural details at high resolution. To study *in vivo* genomic organization, chromosome conformation capture (3C) technology is one of the most useful techniques (Hagège *et al* 2007). Direct physical interactions between DNA segment of a gene (mostly the promoter region) and distantly placed regulatory

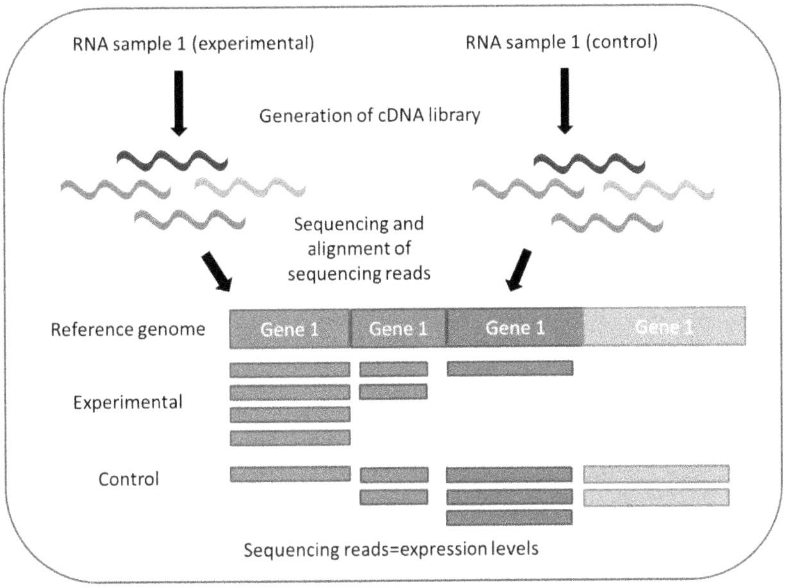

Figure 12.7. A simplified schematic of RNA sequencing technology. Whole genome profiling of non-coding RNAs can be performed using RNA sequencing. For RNA sequencing, RNA is extracted from the experimental and the control sample. Experimental sample may be the cells or the tissue treated with a particular phytochemical. Control sample is the untreated one. RNAs are converted to cDNAs. Each cDNA is then sequenced and aligned with the reference genome. The number of sequencing reads represents the level of expression of a particular non-coding RNA.

elements may mediate long-range control of gene expression. Chromosome conformation capture can detect such 'looping' interactions (Dekker 2006).

The basic idea behind 3C or 3C based methods is to quantify the frequencies of physical interactions between different far placed DNA segments in a cell population (Dekker *et al* 2002). The first step of 3C procedure involves crosslinking the interacting proteins bound to DNA. It is achieved by fixing the cells using formaldehyde solution. After crosslinking, the chromatin is extracted from the cells. The chromatin is then subjected to restriction digestion. Mostly, the enzyme producing sticky ends are used for facilitating easy ligation. Ligation of the sticky ends produced after restriction digestion is done. The different DNA fragments connected to one another via crosslinked interacting proteins ligate and form chimeric DNA. Ligation is followed by reversal of crosslinking to release interacting proteins and retain the chimeric DNA only. The chimeric DNA fragments are then detected by PCR or sequencing. This approach is targeted and requires PCR primers to be designed for which the template information should be available (Losuwers *et al* 2009, Han *et al* 2018) (figure 12.8).

For genome scale assays, there are high-throughput methods derived from the basic 3C which have been developed by combining it with other techniques. Chromosome conformation capture on-chip (4C), chromosome conformation capture carbon copy (5C), chromatin interaction analysis by paired-end tag

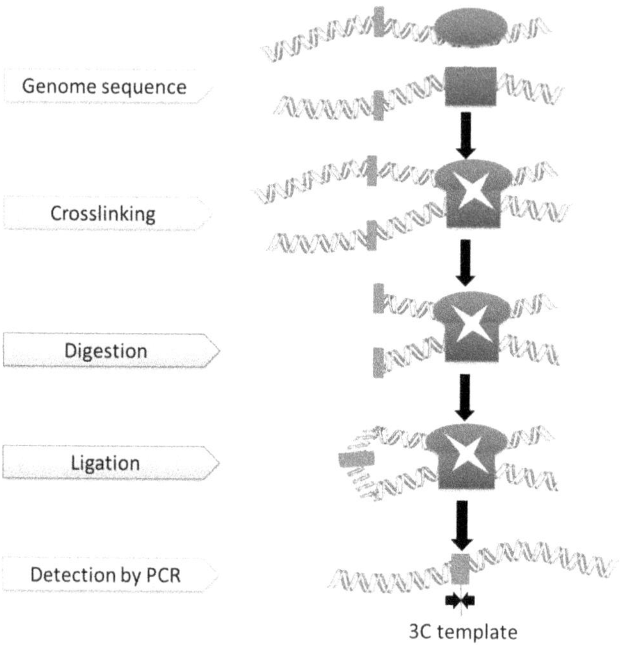

Figure 12.8. Chromosome conformation capture (3C) technology. The first step of 3C technology involves fixation of cells using formaldehyde. Formaldehyde fixation leads to crosslinking of interacting proteins along with the bound DNA. Fixation is followed by restriction digestion using a common restriction enzyme followed by ligation of the digested ends. The final step is detection of the bound DNA sequence using polymerase chain reaction (PCR). Sequencing can also be done for detection.

sequencing (ChIA-PET) and Hi-C technology are a few such advanced methods derived from basic 3C which generate high-throughput chromatin interaction data. Among these methods, Hi-C technology was the first and is still one of the most popular high-throughput methods to be developed which does not require specific primers. In Hi-C, the method is similar up to restriction digestion in the case of 3C. This means, Hi-C also requires cell fixation to facilitate crosslinking, chromatin extraction and restriction digestion. But after restriction digestion, the generated sticky ends are filled with biotin-labeled nucleotides. End filling is followed by blunt-end ligation. The chromatin is then sheared and purified using a chromatography column filled with streptavidin beads. Streptavidin has affinity for biotin. Therefore, it binds to the biotin-labeled DNA fragments helping in their separation. The purified DNA fragments are subjected to high-throughput sequencing. It generates genome-wide interaction maps (Lieberman-Aiden *et al* 2009, van Berkum *et al* 2010) (figure 12.9).

12.2.2 Indirect methods

Indirect methods do not require direct access to the site of modification or the epigenetic changes. Indirect methods involve studying the proteins and other biomolecules which carry out or lead to epigenetic changes. This method is based on expression profile of the transcripts or detection of the proteins themselves which

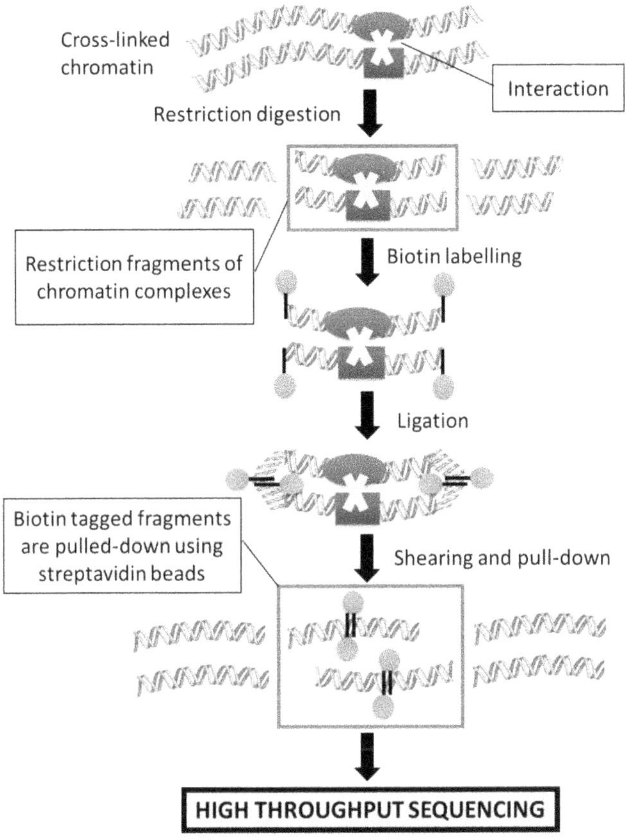

Figure 12.9. Hi-C technology. In Hi-C technology, crosslinking and restriction digestion steps are similar to the basic 3C. The major difference is tagging DNA fragments with biotin and pulling down the tagged fragments using streptavidin beads followed by high-throughput sequencing.

are involved in a particular epigenetic modification process inside a cell. These proteins are HATs, HDACs, histone methyltransferases DNMTs, many transcription factors and other proteins involved in the process of chromatin remodeling. Many of these proteins as well as interactions between different proteins are cell-type specific (Emig and Albrecht 2011, Ibarguren and Villamarin 2017). Downstream targets of these proteins are equally important. Histones are not the sole substrate of many histone methyltransferases. Many other non-histone proteins are also targets of these enzymes. Methylation of these proteins plays an important role in regulation of protein stability and degradation (Zhang and Pradhan 2014). Therefore, not only these enzymes but gene expression pattern of their downstream target proteins or the level of these target proteins at a time also provide important clues about the upstream events like level of translation of these enzymes as these enzymes are also associated with histone modifications.

Antibody-based detection techniques like western blotting and ELISA may provide quantitative data about a particular protein. Differential level of proteins in a cell relative to time and space provides much useful information about the role of that protein. Likewise, expression profile of different mRNA transcripts coding for these proteins is also useful. qRT-PCR is an important method for quantitative assessment of the expression profile of different mRNAs. These tools are employed for the study of specific mRNAs and proteins. For global transcriptome profiling microarray-based tools and high-throughput RNA sequencing are popular methods (Heller 2002, Tachibana 2015). Protein chip technology, two-dimensional gel electrophoresis and advanced mass spectroscopy-based methods like isotope coded affinity tag (ICAT)-based mass spectroscopy are used for global proteome profiling (Weston and Hood 2004). Whole genome transcriptome and proteome data provide indirect evidence of the ongoing processes of epigenetic modifications across the genome inside a cell at a particular time.

A standard transcriptome profiling workflow involves RNA extraction from the cells or tissue treated with a particular phytochemical. cDNA is synthesized from the RNA. Then it can directly be subjected to sequencing or it may be labeled by fluorescent dyes for microarray profiling. The resulting data is whole genome data which needs to be analyzed for gene ontology and pathway analysis to understand its functional relevance. Expression of selected genes from this data can further be validated using qRT-PCR (Xu 2017) (figure 12.10).

Like transcriptome profiling, the initial step for standard proteome profiling is protein extraction followed by sample fractionation or enrichment of post-translationally modified proteins if we are interested in specific protein or a particular post-translation modification in the protein. The extracted and purified protein sample can be analyzed using various methods. A purified sample containing only one protein can be identified directly using mass spectroscopy. For whole cell protein mixture, typically, two alternative approaches are followed. The first is a top-down

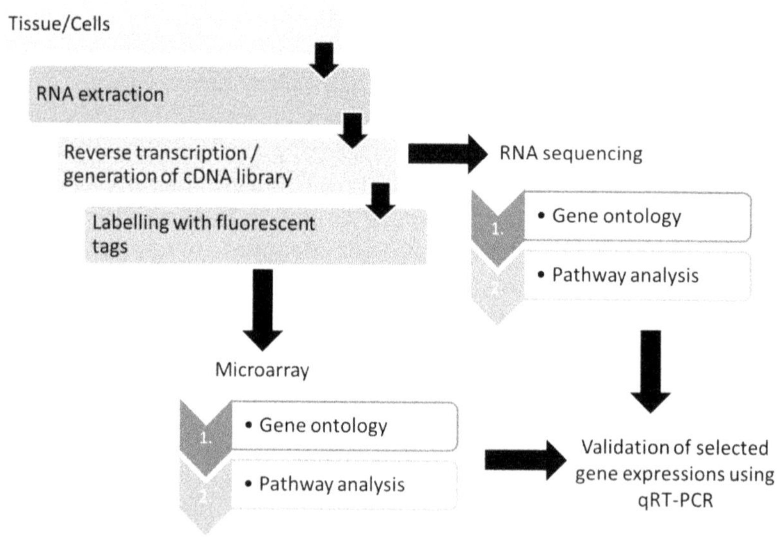

Figure 12.10. Simplified outline of a standard transcriptome profiling workflow.

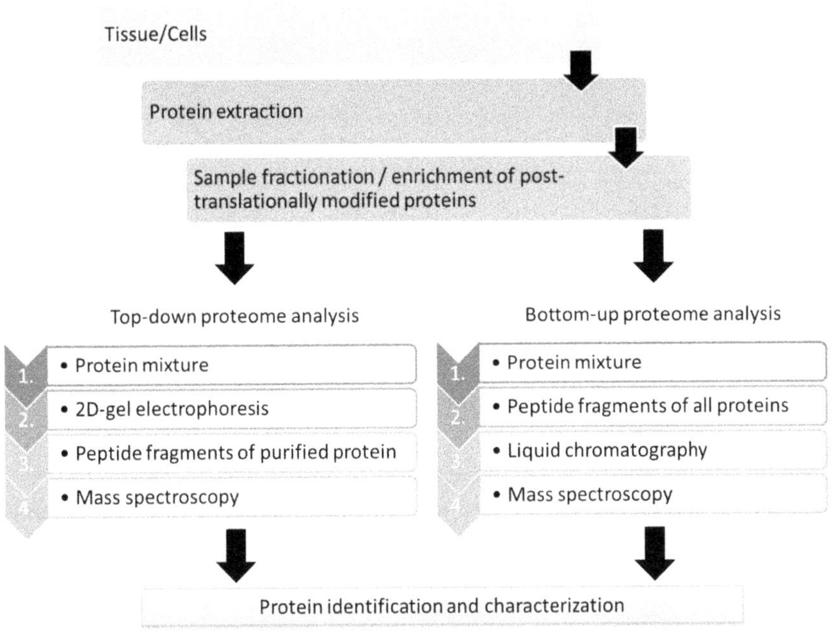

Figure 12.11. Simplified outline of a standard proteome profiling workflow.

approach where whole extracted protein is subjected to two-dimensional (2D) gel electrophoresis to separate individual proteins followed by in-gel digestion of proteins localized at the specific spots over 2D gel. In-gel digestion generates peptide fragments which are further identified using mass spectroscopy. The other approach is the bottom-up approach where whole protein mixture is fragmented and separated using liquid chromatography. Each separated peptide is then identified using mass spectroscopy (Megger *et al* 2014) (figure 12.11). Fragmentation is usually achieved through digestion of proteins using the enzyme trypsin. There are various modifications of both top-down and bottom-up approaches in proteomics. In the case of genes of unknown functions, functional characterization is required. Functional characterization may involve overexpression of a particular protein or silencing of a particular gene of interest and studying the effects of these alterations on cellular epigenome.

12.2.3 Integrative approach

Dynamic equilibrium exists between different epigenetic events (Li 2021). Cross talks happen between DNA methylation and histone modification. The processes work in conjunction to affect the transcription process. Genomic conformation change is also influenced by these two processes and vice versa (Kondo 2009, Li 2021). On one hand, CpG methylation may provide a signal for histone modifications, on the other hand DNMTs can be recruited by histone methylation (Fujita *et al* 2003, Lehnertz *et al* 2003). Many miRNAs target DNMTs (Sato *et al* 2011, Zhang *et al* 2013, Veek and Esteller 2010).

There are some methods which can be used to study the dynamic interactions between DNA methylation and histone modifications. These methods can identify allele-specific DNA methylation with specific histone modification. There is a method called ChIP-bisulfite methylation sequencing (ChIP-BMS) which can be used to determine the methylation status of a particular DNA sequence pulled down using antibodies against a particular histone modification (Li and Tollefsbol 2011). This method is used for the study of locus-specific epigenetic modifications. For global profiling, there is another method called BisChIP-seq which is based on chromatin immunoprecipitation after bisulfite treatment followed by high-throughput sequencing (Statham *et al* 2012). These combinatorial approaches are coupled with fluorescence-based single molecular imaging for co-localization of different epigenetic marks on the level of a single nucleosome in SCAN (single chromatin molecule analysis in nanochannels) (Murphy *et al* 2013).

12.3 Conclusion

Different phytochemicals may affect the epigenetic profile of a cell differently. These may alter one or more than one kind of epigenetic signatures. These signatures are mainly in the form of DNA methylation pattern, histone modifications, non-coding RNAs and three-dimensional spatial chromatin structure. The present chapter provides an overview of important techniques used to study the effects of phytochemicals on the cellular epigenome. Each of these techniques have their own advantages and disadvantages. Some of these techniques are suitable for the study of local epigenetic changes only, whereas some are used for global epigenomic profiling. Various modifications and customizations over many basic techniques are being done to devise new tools derived from the existing ones for global epigenetic studies which were otherwise being used for local studies only. Modern technology focuses on development of such tools which can be used to record and analyze all kinds of epigenetic changes simultaneously in an integrative manner. The field of research and development pertaining to the effects of phytochemicals on the epigenetic signature of a cell in light of cancer prevention and treatment is a field with great possibilities and these studies cannot be conducted without the aid of modern techniques, as discussed in the present chapter. The area of epigenetics research has already advanced significantly in recent years and is still growing at a fast pace. This growth is attributed to the modern technologies which have been developed to study the cellular epigenome or which are still being developed to make the study of the cellular epigenome more precise and accurate. Most modern methods now utilize high-throughput technology to yield whole-genome-based data. This data requires advanced computational and bioinformatics-based tools for proper analysis and interpretation. Parallel innovation in bioinformatics and computational biology coupled with the development of new techniques used in epigenomic profiling have led to the creation of methods which are more powerful and robust. Many more such technologies are expected to arrive in the near future.

References

Adriaens C and Marine J C 2017 NEAT1-containing paraspeckles: central hubs in stress response and tumor formation *Cell Cycle* **16** 137–8

Albert I, Mavrich T N, Tomsho L P, Qi J, Zanton S J, Schuster S C and Pugh B F 2007 Translational and rotational settings of H2A. Z nucleosomes across the *Saccharomyces cerevisiae* genome *Nature* **446** 572–6

Amodio N, Stamato M A, Juli G, Morelli E, Fulciniti M, Manzoni M and Tassone P 2018 Drugging the lncRNA MALAT1 via LNA gapmeR ASO inhibits gene expression of proteasome subunits and triggers anti-multiple myeloma activity *Leukemia* **32** 1948–57

Arab K, Karaulanov E, Musheev M, Trnka P, Schäfer A, Grummt I and Niehrs C 2019 GADD45A binds R-loops and recruits TET1 to CpG island promoters *Nat. Genet.* **51** 217–23

Bag A and Bag N 2018 Tea polyphenols and prevention of epigenetic aberrations in cancer *J. Nat. Sci., Biol., Med.* **9** 2

Banerjee S, Padhye S, Azmi A, Wang Z, Philip P A, Kucuk O and Mohammad R M 2010 Review on molecular and therapeutic potential of thymoquinone in cancer *Nutr. Cancer* **62** 938–46

Barski A, Cuddapah S, Cui K, Roh T Y, Schones D E, Wang Z and Zhao K 2007 High-resolution profiling of histone methylations in the human genome *Cell* **129** 823–37

Bernstein B E, Meissner A and Lander E S 2007 The mammalian epigenome *Cell* **128** 669–81

Böhmdorfer G, Rowley M J, Kuciński J, Zhu Y, Amies I and Wierzbicki A T 2014 RNA-directed DNA methylation requires stepwise binding of silencing factors to long non-coding RNA *Plant J.* **79** 181–91

Böhmdorfer G and Wierzbicki A T 2015 Control of chromatin structure by long noncoding RNA *Trends Cell Biol.* **25** 623–32

Boopathi R, Dimitrov S, Hamiche A, Petosa C and Bednar J 2020 Cryo-electron microscopy of the chromatin fiber *Curr. Opin. Struct. Biol.* **64** 97–103

Bora-Tatar G, Dayangaç-Erden D, Demir A S, Dalkara S, Yelekçi K and Erdem-Yurter H 2009 Molecular modifications on carboxylic acid derivatives as potent histone deacetylase inhibitors: activity and docking studies *Bioorg. Med. l. Chem.* **17** 5219–28

Caracciolo D, Di Martino M T, Amodio N, Morelli E, Montesano M, Botta C and Tassone P 2019 miR-22 suppresses DNA ligase III addiction in multiple myeloma *Leukemia* **33** 487–98

Chen Y, Shu W, Chen W, Wu Q, Liu H and Cui G 2007 Curcumin, both histone deacetylase and p300/CBP-specific inhibitor, represses the activity of nuclear factor kappa B and Notch 1 in Raji cells *Basic Clin. Pharmacol. Toxicol.* **101** 427–33

Collas P 2010 The current state of chromatin immunoprecipitation *Mol. Biotechnol.* **45** 87–100

Daniel C, Lagergren J and Öhman M 2015 RNA editing of non-coding RNA and its role in gene regulation *Biochimie* **117** 22–7

Dekker J 2006 The three 'C's of chromosome conformation capture: controls, controls, controls *Nat. Methods* **3** 17–21

Dekker J, Rippe K, Dekker M and Kleckner N 2002 Capturing chromosome conformation *Science* **295** 1306–11

Denis H, Van Grembergen O, Delatte B, Dedeurwaerder S, Putmans P, Calonne E and Deplus R 2016 MicroRNAs regulate KDM5 histone demethylases in breast cancer cells *Mol. Biosyst.* **12** 404–13

Derreumaux S, Chaoui M, Tevanian G and Fermandjian S 2001 Impact of CpG methylation on structure, dynamics and solvation of cAMP DNA responsive element *Nucleic Acids Res.* **29** 2314–26

Ehrlich M, Gama-Sosa M A, Huang L H, Midgett R M, Kuo K C, McCune R A and Gehrke C 1982 Amount and distribution of 5-methylcytosine in human DNA from different types of tissues or cells *Nucleic Acids Res.* **10** 2709–21

Elia L and Quintavalle M 2017 Epigenetics and vascular diseases: influence of non-coding RNAs and their clinical implications *Front. Cardiovasc. Med.* **4** 26

Emig D and Albrecht M 2011 Tissue-specific proteins and functional implications *J. Proteome Res.* **10** 1893–903

Fan J, Xing Y, Wen X, Jia R, Ni H, He J and Fan X 2015 Long non-coding RNA ROR decoys gene-specific histone methylation to promote tumorigenesis *Genome Biol.* **16** 1–17

Frommer M, McDonald L E, Millar D S, Collis C M, Watt F, Grigg G W and Paul C L 1992 A genomic sequencing protocol that yields a positive display of 5-methylcytosine residues in individual DNA strands *Proc. Natl Acad. Sci.* **89** 1827–31

Fujita M, Enomoto T and Murata Y 2003 Genetic alterations in ovarian carcinoma: with specific reference to histological subtypes *Mol. Cell. Endocrinol.* **202** 97–9

Gade P and Kalvakolanu D V 2012 Chromatin immunoprecipitation assay as a tool for analyzing transcription factor activity *Transcriptional Regulation: Methods and Protocols* (Cham: Springer) pp 85–104

Gama-Sosa M A, Slagel V A, Trewyn R W, Oxenhandler R, Kuo K C, Gehrke C W and Ehrlich M 1983 The 5-methylcytosine content of DNA from human tumors *Nucl. Acids Res.* **11** 6883–94

Ganapathy A and Ezekiel U 2019 Phytochemical modulation of MiRNAs in colorectal cancer *Medicine* **6** 48

Gerhauser C 2013 Cancer chemoprevention and nutriepigenetics: state of the art and future challenges *Natural Products in Cancer Prevention and Therapy* (Berlin: Springer) pp 73–132

Glanzer J G, Haydon P G and Eberwine J H 2004 Expression profile analysis of neurodegenerative disease: advances in specificity and resolution *Neurochem. Res.* **29** 1161–8

Goelz S E, Vogelstein B, Hamilton S R and Feinberg A P 1985 Hypomethylation of DNA from benign and malignant human colon neoplasms *Science* **228** 187–90

Hagege H, Klous P, Braem C, Splinter E, Dekker J, Cathala G and Forné T 2007 Quantitative analysis of chromosome conformation capture assays (3C-qPCR) *Nat. Protoc.* **2** 1722–33

Han J, Zhang Z and Wang K 2018 3C and 3C-based techniques: the powerful tools for spatial genome organization deciphering *Mol. Cytogen.* **11** 1–10

Han Li C and Chen Y 2015 Small and long non-coding RNAs: novel targets in perspective cancer therapy *Curr. Genom.* **16** 319–26

Hawkins R D, Hon G C, Yang C, Antosiewicz-Bourget J E, Lee L K, Ngo Q M and Ren B 2011 Dynamic chromatin states in human ES cells reveal potential regulatory sequences and genes involved in pluripotency *Cell Res.* **21** 1393–409

Heller M J 2002 DNA microarray technology: devices, systems, and applications *Annu. Rev. Biomed. Eng.* **4** 129–53

Hinten M, Maclary E, Gayen S, Harris C and Kalantry S 2016 Visualizing long noncoding RNAs on chromatin *Long Non-Coding RNAs: Methods and Protocols* (New York: Springer) pp 147–64

Hon G C, Hawkins R D and Ren B 2009 Predictive chromatin signatures in the mammalian genome *Hum.Mol. Genet.* **18** R195–201

Hughes V 2014 Epigenetics: the sins of the father *Nature* **507** 22–4

Ibarguren I and Villamarín A 2017 Different cells make different proteins: a laboratory exercise illustrating tissue-specific protein expression in animals *J. Biol. Educ.* **51** 284–94

Ikegami K, Ohgane J, Tanaka S, Yagi S and Shiota K 2009 Interplay between DNA methylation, histone modification and chromatin remodeling in stem cells and during development *Int. J. Dev. Biol.* **53** 203–14

Jain A K, Xi Y, McCarthy R, Allton K, Akdemir K C, Patel L R and Barton M C 2016 LncPRESS1 is a p53-regulated LncRNA that safeguards pluripotency by disrupting SIRT6-mediated de-acetylation of histone H3K56 *Mol. Cell* **64** 967–81

Johnson D S, Mortazavi A, Myers R M and Wold B 2007 Genome-wide mapping of *in vivo* protein–DNA interactions *Science* **316** 1497–502

Jones P A 2012 Functions of DNA methylation: islands, start sites, gene bodies and beyond *Nat. Rev. Genet.* **13** 484–92

Jones P A and Laird P W 1999 Cancer-epigenetics comes of age *Nat. Genet.* **21** 163–7

Kaikkonen M U, Lam M T and Glass C K 2011 Non-coding RNAs as regulators of gene expression and epigenetics *Cardiovasc. Res.* **90** 430–40

Khan J, Saal L H, Bittner M L, Chen Y, Trent J M and Meltzer P S 1999 Expression profiling in cancer using cDNA microarrays *Electrophoresis* **20** 223–9

Khan S A, Reddy D and Gupta S 2015 Global histone post-translational modifications and cancer: Biomarkers for diagnosis, prognosis and treatment? *World J. Biol. Chem.* **6** 333

Kim J H, Shin S H, Kwon H J, Cho N Y and Kang G H 2009 Prognostic implications of CpG island hypermethylator phenotype in colorectal cancers *Virchows Archiv.* **455** 485–94

Kondo Y 2009 Epigenetic cross-talk between DNA methylation and histone modifications in human cancers *Yonsei Med. J.* **50** 455–63

Kouzarides T 2007 Chromatin modifications and their function *Cell* **128** 693–705

Kurian K M, Watson C J and Wyllie A H 1999 DNA chip technolgy *J. Pathol.* **187** 267–71

Lehnertz B, Ueda Y, Derijck A A, Braunschweig U, Perez-Burgos L, Kubicek S and Peters A H 2003 Suv39h-mediated histone H3 lysine 9 methylation directs DNA methylation to major satellite repeats at pericentric heterochromatin *Curr. Biol.* **13** 1192–200

Leonhardt H, Rahn H P and Cardoso M C 1999 Functional links between nuclear structure, gene expression, DNA replication, and methylation *Crit. Rev. Eukaryot. Gene Expr.* **9** 3–4

Leszinski G, Gezer U, Siegele B, Stoetzer O and Holdenrieder S 2012 Relevance of histone marks H3K9me3 and H4K20me3 in cancer *Anticancer Res.* **32** 2199–205

Leti F, Llaci L, Malenica I and DiStefano J K 2018 Methods for CpG methylation array profiling via bisulfite conversion *Disease Gene Identification: Methods and Protocols* (New York: Springer) pp 233–54

Li Y 2021 Modern epigenetics methods in biological research *Methods* **187** 104–13

Li Y, Li X and Guo B 2010 Chemopreventive agent 3, 3′-diindolylmethane selectively induces proteasomal degradation of class I histone deacetylases *Cancer Res.* **70** 646–54

Li Y and Tollefsbol T O 2011 DNA methylation detection: bisulfite genomic sequencing analysis *Epigenetics Protocols* (New York: Springer) pp 11–21

Liang R Q, Li W, Li Y, Tan C Y, Li J X, Jin Y X and Ruan K C 2005 An oligonucleotide microarray for microRNA expression analysis based on labeling RNA with quantum dot and nanogold probe *Nucleic Acids Res.* **33** e17–7

Lieberman-Aiden E, Van Berkum N L, Williams L, Imakaev M, Ragoczy T, Telling A and Dekker J 2009 Comprehensive mapping of long-range interactions reveals folding principles of the human genome *Science* **326** 289–93

Liu H L, Chen Y, Cui G H and Zhou J F 2005 Curcumin, a potent anti-tumor reagent, is a novel histone deacetylase inhibitor regulating B-NHL cell line Raji proliferation *Acta Pharmacol. Sin.* **26** 603–9

Louwers M, Splinter E, Van Driel R, De Laat W and Stam M 2009 Studying physical chromatin interactions in plants using chromosome conformation capture (3C) *Nat. Protoc.* **4** 1216–29

Margueron R, Trojer P and Reinberg D 2005 The key to development: interpreting the histone code? *Curr. Opin. Genet. Develop.* **15** 163–76

Megger D A, Naboulsi W, Meyer H E and Sitek B 2014 Proteome analyses of hepatocellular carcinoma *J. Clin. Transl. Hepatol.* **2** 23

Mehrmohamadi M, Sepehri M H, Nazer N and Norouzi M R 2021 A comparative overview of epigenomic profiling methods *Front. Cell Dev.l Biol.* **9** 714687

Mikkelsen T S, Ku M, Jaffe D B, Issac B, Lieberman E, Giannoukos G and Bernstein B E 2007 Genome-wide maps of chromatin state in pluripotent and lineage-committed cells *Nature* **448** 553–60

Mills A A 2010 Throwing the cancer switch: reciprocal roles of polycomb and trithorax proteins *Nat. Rev. Cancer* **10** 669–82

Momparler R L and Bovenzi V 2000 DNA methylation and cancer *J. Cell. Physiol.* **183** 145–54

Morin R D, Zhao Y, Prabhu A L, Dhalla N, McDonald H, Pandoh P and Marra M 2010 Preparation and analysis of microRNA libraries using the Illumina massively parallel sequencing technology *RNAi and microRNA-Mediated Gene Regulation in Stem Cells: Methods, Protocols, and Applications* (New York: Humana Press) pp 173–99

Mortazavi A, Williams B A, McCue K, Schaeffer L and Wold B 2008 Mapping and quantifying mammalian transcriptomes by RNA-Seq *Nat. Methods* **5** 621–8

Murphy P J, Cipriany B R, Wallin C B, Ju C Y, Szeto K, Hagarman J A and Soloway P D 2013 Single-molecule analysis of combinatorial epigenomic states in normal and tumor cells *Proc. Natl Acad. Sci.* **110** 7772–7

Nebbioso A, Tambaro F P, Dell'Aversana C and Altucci L 2018 Cancer epigenetics: moving forward *PLoS Genet.* **14** e1007362

Nwosu O K and Ubaoji K I 2020 Nutraceuticals: history, classification and market demand *Functional Foods and Nutraceuticals: Bioactive Components, Formulations and Innovations* (New York: Springer) pp 13–22

Ortea I 2022 Foodomics in health: Advanced techniques for studying the bioactive role of foods *TrAC, Trends Anal. Chem.* **150** 116589

Palmbos P L, Wang L, Yang H, Wang Y, Leflein J, Ahmet M L and Simeone D M 2015 ATDC/TRIM29 drives invasive bladder cancer formation through miRNA-mediated and epigenetic mechanisms *Cancer Res.* **75** 5155–66

Pillai S and Chellappan S P 2009 ChIP on chip assays: genome-wide analysis of transcription factor binding and histone modifications *Chromatin Protocols* (New York: Springer) 2nd pp 341–66

Pongubala J M and Murre C 2021 Spatial organization of chromatin: Transcriptional control of adaptive immune cell development *Front. Immunol.* **12** 633825

Pritchard C C, Cheng H H and Tewari M 2012 MicroRNA profiling: approaches and considerations *Nat. Rev. Genet.* **13** 358–69

Ramsahoye B H, Biniszkiewicz D, Lyko F, Clark V, Bird A P and Jaenisch R 2000 Non-CpG methylation is prevalent in embryonic stem cells and may be mediated by DNA methyltransferase 3a *Proc. Natl Acad. Sci.* **97** 5237–42

Ricci W A, Levin L and Zhang X 2020 Genome-wide profiling of histone modifications with ChIP-Seq *Cereal Genomics: Methods and Protocols* (New York: Springer) pp 101–17

Robertson K D, Jones A and P 2000 DNA methylation: past, present and future directions *Carcinogenesis* **21** 461–7

Roy S K, Chen Q, Fu J, Shankar S and Srivastava R K 2011 Resveratrol inhibits growth of orthotopic pancreatic tumors through activation of FOXO transcription factors *PLoS One* **6** e25166

Rudloff U, Bhanot U, Gerald W, Klimstra D S, Jarnagin W R, Brennan M F and Allen P J 2010 Biobanking of human pancreas cancer tissue: impact of ex-vivo procurement times on RNA quality *Ann. Surg. Oncol.* **17** 2229–36

Saghafi T, Taheri R A, Parkkila S and Zolfaghari Emameh R 2019 Phytochemicals as modulators of long non-coding RNAs and inhibitors of cancer-related carbonic anhydrases *Int. J. Mol. Sci.* **20** 2939

Sarkar F H, Li Y, Wang Z and Kong D 2009 Cellular signaling perturbation by natural products *Cell. Signal.* **21** 1541–7

Sato F, Tsuchiya S, Meltzer S J and Shimizu K 2011 MicroRNAs and epigenetics *FEBS J.* **278** 1598–609

Schulze A and Downward J 2001 Navigating gene expression using microarrays? A technology review *Nat. Cell Biol.* **3**

Shankar E, Kanwal R, Candamo M and Gupta S 2016 Dietary phytochemicals as epigenetic modifiers in cancer: promise and challenges *Seminars in Cancer Biology* 40 (New York: Academic) pp 82–99

Shankar S, Kumar D and Srivastava R K 2013 Epigenetic modifications by dietary phytochemicals: implications for personalized nutrition *Pharmacol. Ther.* **138** 1–17

Singh B N, Singh H B, Singh A, Naqvi A H and Singh B R 2014 Dietary phytochemicals alter epigenetic events and signaling pathways for inhibition of metastasis cascade: phytoblockers of metastasis cascade *Cancer Metastasis Rev.* **33** 41–85

Smith Z D and Meissner A 2013 DNA methylation: roles in mammalian development *Nat. Rev. Genet.* **14** 204–20

Statello L, Guo C J, Chen L L and Huarte M 2021 Gene regulation by long non-coding RNAs and its biological functions *Nat. Rev. Mol. Cell Biol.* **22** 96–118

Statham A L, Robinson M D, Song J Z, Coolen M W, Stirzaker C and Clark S J 2012 Bisulfite sequencing of chromatin immunoprecipitated DNA (BisChIP-seq) directly informs methylation status of histone-modified DNA *Genome Res.* **22** 1120–7

Storz G, Opdyke J A and Zhang A 2004 Controlling mRNA stability and translation with small, noncoding RNAs *Curr. Opin. Microbiol.* **7** 140–4

Subirana J A and Martinez A B 1976 Model studies of chromatin structure based on X-ray diffraction data *Nucleic Acids Res.* **3** 3025–42

Tachibana C 2015 Transcriptomics today: microarrays, RNA-seq, and more *Science* **349** 544–6

Tang Q, Zheng F, Liu Z, Wu J, Chai X, He C and Hann S S 2019 Novel reciprocal interaction of lncRNA HOTAIR and miR-214-3p contribute to the solamargine-inhibited PDPK1 gene expression in human lung cancer *J. Cell. Mol. Med.* **23** 7749–61

Tate P H and Bird A P 1993 Effects of DNA methylation on DNA-binding proteins and gene expression *Curr Opin Genet. Dev.* **3** 226–31

Thakur V S, Deb G, Babcook M A and Gupta S 2014 Plant phytochemicals as epigenetic modulators: role in cancer chemoprevention *AAPS J.* **16** 151–63

Thompson K L, Pine P S, Rosenzweig B A, Turpaz Y and Retief J 2007 Characterization of the effect of sample quality on high density oligonucleotide microarray data using progressively degraded rat liver RNA *BMC Biotechnol.* **7** 1–12

Tokgun P E, Tokgun O, Kurt S, Tomatir A G and Akca H 2019 MYC-driven regulation of long non-coding RNA profiles in breast cancer cells *Gene* **714** 143955

Tomita H, Vawter M P, Walsh D M, Evans S J, Choudary P V, Li J and Bunney W E 2004 Effect of agonal and postmortem factors on gene expression profile: quality control in microarray analyses of postmortem human brain *Biol. Psychiatry* **55** 346–52

van Berkum N L, Lieberman-Aiden E, Williams L, Imakaev M, Gnirke A, Mirny L A and Lander E S 2010 Hi-C: a method to study the three-dimensional architecture of genomes *J. Vis. Exp.* **6** e1869

Vautrot V, Heckler G, Aigueperse C and Behm-Ansmant I 2021 Fluorescence *in situ* hybridization of small non-coding RNAs *Small Non-Coding RNAs: Methods and Protocols* (New York: Springer) pp 73–85

Veeck J and Esteller M 2010 Breast cancer epigenetics: from DNA methylation to microRNAs *J. Mammary Gland Biol. Neoplasia* **15** 5–17

Waddington C H 1959 Canalization of development and genetic assimilation of acquired characters *Nature* **183** 1654–5

Waddington C H 2012 The epigenotype *Int. J. Epidemiol.* **41** 10–3

Wang M, Sunkel B D, Ray W C and Stanton B Z 2022 Chromatin structure in cancer *BMC Mol. Cell Biol.* **23** 1–10

Weston A D and Hood L 2004 Systems biology, proteomics, and the future of health care: toward predictive, preventative, and personalized medicine *J. Proteome Res.* **3** 179–96

Wierzbicki A T 2012 The role of long non-coding RNA in transcriptional gene silencing *Curr. Opin. Plant Biol.* **15** 517–22

Xie H F, Liu Y Z, Du R, Wang B, Chen M T, Zhang Y Y and Li J 2017 miR-377 induces senescence in human skin fibroblasts by targeting DNA methyltransferase 1 *Cell Death Dis.* **8** e2663–3

Xu S 2017 Transcriptome profiling in systems vascular medicine *Front. Pharmacol.* **8** 563

Yong W S, Hsu F M and Chen P Y 2016 Profiling genome-wide DNA methylation *Epigenet. Chromatin* **9** 1–16

Zentner G E and Henikoff S 2014 High-resolution digital profiling of the epigenome *Nat. Rev. Genet.* **15** 814–27

Zhang G and Pradhan S 2014 Mammalian epigenetic mechanisms *IUBMB Life* **66** 240–56

Zhang W C, Liu J, Xu X and Wang G 2013 The role of microRNAs in lung cancer progression *Med. Oncol.* **30** 1–9

Zhang Z, Cao Y, Zhai Y, Ma X, An X, Zhang S and Li Z 2018 Micro RNA-29b regulates DNA methylation by targeting Dnmt3a/3b and Tet1/2/3 in porcine early embryo development *Dev. Growth. Differ.* **60** 197–204

Zhao Q, Li S, Li N, Yang X, Ma S, Yang A and Jiang Y 2017 miR-34a targets HDAC1-regulated H3K9 acetylation on lipid accumulation induced by homocysteine in foam cells *J. Cell. Biochem.* **118** 4617–27

Chapter 13

Advancement in phytochemical delivery systems for improved anti-cancer activity

Pramod Kumar Singh and B Rai

Despite their significant anti-cancer pharmacological properties, natural compounds are limited by their low bioavailability and selectivity. The current therapeutic regimens depend on selective drug targeting to increase their effectiveness against cancer cells and minimize their toxicity against normal cells. A nanotechnology-driven approach to the development of drugs and drug delivery systems is being used to better treat and manage cancer. Additionally, nanoparticles extend drug half-lives in the blood, reduce non-target organ adverse effects, and concentrate drug effectiveness on cancer cells as well as improving drug solubility and stability. The use of organic and inorganic materials, synthetics as well as natural, has been explored in order to identify plant ingredients with various physical, biological, and functional properties. In this area, developing cost-effective methods for scaling up production and delivering plant-derived bioactive compounds remains a challenge. To facilitate the commercialization of formulated plant delivery systems containing bioactive constituents, large-scale production methods need to be developed in the future.

13.1 Introduction

Worldwide, cancer is a major health concern that affects both industrialized and developing countries alike. Approximately 18.1 million new cases of cancer are estimated to occur in the world in 2018, and 23.6 million are predicted to occur by 2030 (Bray *et al* 2018). The disease is well-known and well-treated, but there is only a bit of success when it comes to curing it. Radiation therapy for the extensive accumulated cancer biomass is the current standard of care for patients with cancer, with systemic chemotherapy usually being administered once the cancer has been surgically removed. Chemotherapy has a number of drawbacks, such as recurrence, drug resistance, and potentially harmful side effects on tissues that aren't being

doi:10.1088/978-0-7503-5252-9ch13

treated. This may reduce patient quality of life and the use of anti-cancer medications. In an effort to address the problems with current cancer treatment, novel, promising anti-cancer drugs are being searched for.

Plant-based phytochemicals and their derivatives have promise for increasing cancer patients' response rates and reducing side effects. Nature contains a number of phytochemicals that have significant anti-cancer properties and are biologically active substances. Natural extracts (from dry or wet plant matter) will be evaluated for potential anti-cancer biological activity as a first step in developing a side-effect-free, effective phytochemical anti-cancer therapy, followed by purification and *in vitro* and *in vivo* effectiveness using bioassay-guided fractionation. A number of epidemiological studies suggest that plant-based foods are associated with lower cancer risk (Gullett *et al* 2010). According to a recent study published in the journal Cancer Research (2010), plant-derived bioactive compounds are relatively inexpensive, well tolerated, and effective for the treatment of multiple diseases, including cancer (Kaur *et al* 2018). There are several phytochemical groups that are promising for cancer prevention and treatment, including alkaloids, terpenoids, polyphenols, and organosulfur compounds (Kaur *et al* 2018). A naturally occurring quinoline alkaloid, Camptothecin obtained from plant leaves *Camptotheca acuminata* inhibits DNA topoisomerase I show spectrum activity on neoplastic cells (Rothwell *et al* 2017). In a study published in 2019 by Zhang *et al* (2019), it was suggested that terpenoids (celastrol) are capable of inhibiting tumor growth through a number of biological functions including the regulation of transcription factors, proteases, angiogenesis, cell cycle, and apoptosis. A soy phytoestrogen called genistein has been extensively studied as a cancer therapy in prostate and lung cancer trials (Shanmugam *et al* 2016), often in combination with standard chemotherapy. As a result of the toxin's action on estrogen receptors, tumor suppressors, and transcription factors, the isoflavone inhibited cancer cells (Pool *et al* 2018) (figure 13.1).

13.2 Mechanism of action of phytochemicals

13.2.1 Effects of detoxifying carcinogens

There are several polyphenols, such as curcumin, epigallocatechin-3-gallate (EGCG), and resveratrol, that are powerful antioxidants and anti-inflammatory agents that help prevent the development of cancer and metastatic disease (Sinha *et al* 2017). According to Taniguchi and Karin (2018), reactive oxygen species (ROS) and chronic inflammation contribute to multistage, multiorgan cancer development, as well as transcriptional reprogramming caused by a genetic abnormality. As a result of the use of antioxidants and anti-inflammatory phytochemicals in healthy cells, carcinogenesis can be prevented by reducing ROS production, minimizing DNA damage, inhibiting nuclear factor-kB (NF-kB) pathways, and activating antioxidant responses through nuclear factor erythroid 2-related factor 2 (NRF2). It has been shown that cancer initiates an increase of inflammation, driven by aberrantly activated NF-kB in the tumor microenvironment, which influences genes that induce proliferative and anti-apoptotic growth

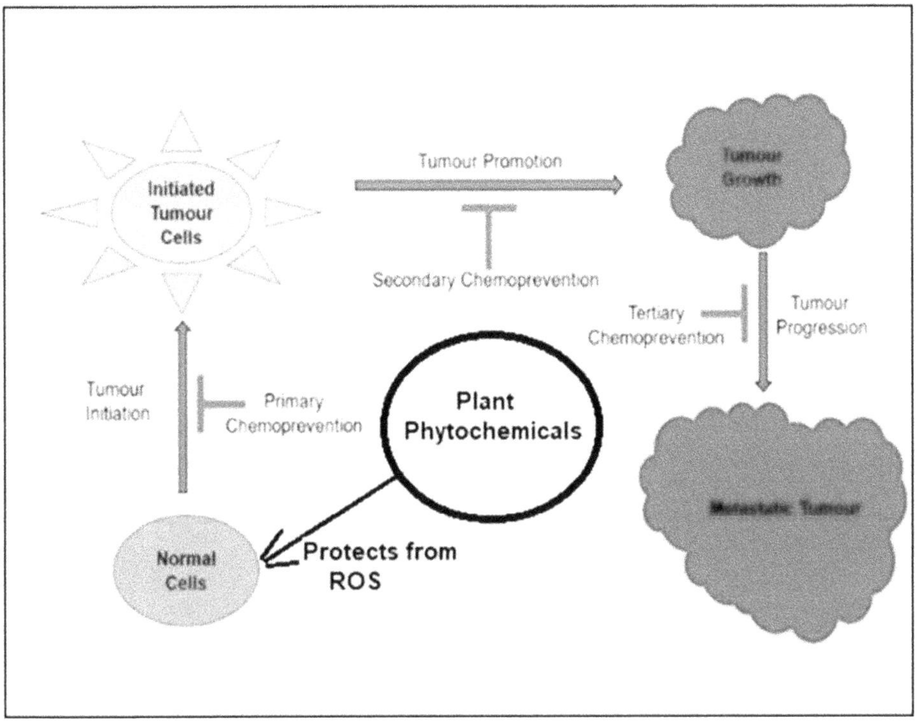

Figure 13.1. Phytochemicals and their anti-cancer effect. (Adapted and modified from George *et al* 2021)

(Rengasamy *et al* 2019). It was found that curcumin, resveratrol, lycopene, EGCG, and genistein suppressed NF-kB signaling in tumor microenvironments. These compounds are useful for controlling tumor growth and preventing cancer (Rengasamy *et al* 2019). There are also a variety of phytochemicals whose effects can enhance the metabolism of xenobiotics (e.g., cytochrome P450) and reduce the effectiveness of phase I enzymes that metabolize xenobiotics (e.g., cytochrome P450) as well as increase phase II enzymes that detoxify xenobiotics, thus minimizing the time period that carcinogens can be active (Asensi *et al* 2011). Several compounds containing polyphenols such as isothiocyanate, indole, and EGCG protocatechuic acid and tannic acid induce phase II and antioxidant gene expression via the Nrf2 pathway (Shanmugam *et al* 2016). It has been reported that Nrf2 is capable of triggering the expression of a number of detoxifying and antioxidant enzymes, such as hemeoxygenase (HO), glutathione S-transferase (GST), superoxide dismutase (SOD), and catalase (Shanmugam *et al* 2016). It is thought that ROS promote cancer cell proliferation and migration, which contributes to the growth and metastasis of tumors. The anti-cancer therapeutic and preventive potential of phytochemicals that inhibit ROS, particularly at mitochondrial levels, has been widely recognized (Sznarkowska *et al* 2017).

13.2.2 Regulation of different cell death pathways

Some phytochemicals, such as etoposide, camptothecin, and polyphenols, can act as prooxidants in the same way as traditional anti-cancer drugs, such as doxorubicin and mitomycin C (Suphim *et al* 2010, Kaur *et al* 2018) ROS levels can be elevated and cause cell death. The pro-oxidative behavior of polyphenols depends on several conditions, namely pH, levels of transition metal ions and O_2, but it seems that only extremely high concentrations of polyphenols induce cell necrosis to cancer cells (Rengasamy *et al* 2019). Apoptosis was triggered by EGCG in a variety of cancer models by increasing the Bax/Bcl-2 protein ratio(Khan *et al* 2014). It has been reported that Bcl-2 and Bcl-xL are anti-apoptotic proteins of the Bcl-2 family. They bind to pro-apoptotic Bax and Bad in mitochondria and inhibit mitochondrial release of cytochrome c (Maji *et al* 2018). It has been reported that gallic acid can activate both intrinsic and extrinsic pathways of apoptosis in cancer cell lines, as evidenced by increases in initiator caspase-8 and caspase-9 (Kaur *et al* 2018). Celastrol has also been shown to induce apoptosis both *in vitro* and *in vivo*, through multiple pathways, including up-regulation of Bax and p53 and inhibition of Bcl-2 and NF-k B signaling (Taniguchi and Karin 2018). A functional genomics approach provides important insight into chemo-preventative and anti-cancer effects of phytochemicals. It has been reported that resveratrol alters the expression of genes associated with apoptosis, cell cycle control, and the androgen pathway similarly to the p53 pathway, while further research on epigenetic modification and micro RNA profiling is required (Huminiecki and Horbańczuk 2018). Low concentrations of curcumin that cause apoptosis or inhibit NF-kB signaling in cholangiocarcinoma decrease Bcl-xL level and partially depolarize the mitochondria, but with no detectable ROS and intracellular GSH levels, (Suphim *et al* 2010). As a result of curcumin's action at the same concentrations, Bax and p53 pro-apoptotic proteins were also increased, whereas higher concentrations failed to alter these proteins but caused ROS generation, mitochondrial collapse, and massive cell death. A number of studies related EGCG's cytotoxicity to relatively high, pro-oxidant concentrations (Lambert and Elias 2010, Branco *et al* 2015), albeit its activity against melanoma cells is apparently stronger than curcumin's. A relatively high concentration of polyphenols is usually necessary for their effective antitumor activity, even though low concentrations can modulate cell signaling pathways implicated in carcinogenesis and migration. Since high doses of these compounds also raise safety concerns, for example, tea catechins may cause liver damage (Lambert and Elias 2010, Kaur *et al* 2018, Rengasamy *et al* 2019), targeted delivery to cancer cells and tumor sites seems to be a desirable option. The bioactive components of different plant chemicals, including celastrol, curcumin, resveratrol, thymoquinone, tocotrienol, and ursolic acid, have been linked to autophagy in a variety of cancer models (Deng *et al* 2019). Besides apoptosis and autophagy, non-canonical programmed cell death mechanisms are also capable of providing efficient therapeutic outcomes (Diederich and Cerella 2016).

13.2.3 Targeting angiogenesis by phytochemicals

Angiogenesis is the development and growth of new blood vessels that ensure wound healing, cell growth, and reproduction. A leading cause of death worldwide is angiogenesis, which plays a crucial role in cancer progression. Therefore, inhibiting angiogenesis may be an effective anti-cancer therapy. It is closely regulated and a variety of inhibitors and stimulators keep it in balance (Folkman 2007). The angiogenesis balance is disturbed by up-regulation of stimulators in tumors, which results in tumor growth and metastasis (Folkman 2006). Tumor blood vessels have a different structure with irregular branches and they are more heterogeneous than normal blood vessels (Shang *et al* 2012). Angiogenesis is up-regulated by pathways such as VEGF, EGF, FGF and HGF (Wahl *et al* 2011). Phytochemicals might be effective anti-cancer drugs if combined with therapies targeting multiple components of angiogenesis (Wahl *et al* 2011). Secondary plant metabolites are valuable sources of small molecules and numerous drugs have been identified from plants. A number of studies have shown that curcumin, EGCG, and resveratrol have been found to reduce VEGF and HIF1 production as well as angiogenesis (Reuben *et al* 2012).

13.2.4 Synergistic effects of phytochemicals in combinations with classical antineoplastic agents

Synergy is the process by which substances combine to produce a greater effect than their individual properties. This strategy is based on the natural' 'straight' approach, which has evolved for the purpose of achieving greater efficiency at a lower cost over time. Flavonoids such as quercetin or apigenin combined with low concentrations of doxorubicin or etoposide led to reduced ATP levels, increased apoptosis (caspase-3, caspase-8, and caspase-9 activation), and cell cycle arrests in malignant cells (Mahbub *et al* 2015). Together, these combinations reduced glutathione levels and increased DNA damage synergistically, while the drugs alone had only moderate effects on these parameters. A number of antioxidant polyphenols have been studied in combination with chemotherapy, including emodin, cis-stilbene, and rhein, however, their anti-cancer effects were a bit less pronounced than those found in flavonoids (Mahbub *et al* 2015). These polyphenols appeared to cause synergistic effects on the cancer cells due to activation of caspase-9, thus intrinsic apoptosis, though the cell lines were p53 null, suggesting that they affect mitochondrial targets in the cells, as also hypothesized for menadione and quercetin (Baran *et al* 2014). In addition to reducing the adverse toxic effects of chemo- and radiotherapies, antioxidants and natural compounds may also play a role in improving drug results at target tissues through delivery systems (Asensi *et al* 2011). Recently, studies on the cardiotoxicity of chemotherapeutic agents have shown that controlled release of thymoquinone and ginsenoside Rg3 could mitigate early markers of doxorubicin cardiotoxicity, including heart lipid peroxidation and creatine kinase leakages (El-Ashmawy *et al* 2017). In combination with classical antineoplastic agents, phytochemicals can reduce the resistance of cancer cells to chemo- and radio-resistant molecules, including multidrug resistance proteins, P-glycoprotein, breast cancer resistance protein, and many other pathways involved in chemo- and radio-resistance of cancer cells (Mercader and Pomilio 2012). Phytochemicals can inhibit diverse oncogenes and promote tumor suppressor genes, which may explain their chemo-preventive and therapeutic properties. The role of p53 regulation has received significant attention, and several compounds have been found to be effective in promoting the expression of p53 and facilitating apoptosis in cancer cells (Suphim *et al* 2010).

13.3 Delivery systems for enhanced bioavailability of phytochemicals

A number of diseases, including cancer, have historically been treated with the help of plants, with 60% of modern anti-cancer drugs derived from plants. According to Song *et al* (2014), half of all anti-cancer drugs approved in foreign markets are natural products or derivatives of natural substances. Several significant limitations exist in most clinically used anti-cancer drugs. Several challenges encountered when using plant bioactive ingredients as anti-cancer drugs in pharmaceuticals are summarized in this section.

13.3.1 Solubility

The lack of soluble plant bioactive ingredients in water and oil makes it difficult to incorporate them directly into foods, beverages, cosmetics, and pharmaceuticals. It is more difficult to add ingredients that do not dissolve readily in water (e.g., carotenoids) to aqueous-based products while oil-based products could easily incorporate ingredients that do not dissolve readily in water (McClements 2014).

13.3.2 Bioavailability

In order to create novel delivery systems for plants' bioactive ingredients, it is essential that their bioavailability be enhanced. Bioactive compounds are affected by several factors, including their molecular and physicochemical properties, their interactions with other ingredients, and their solubility and stability during digestive processes. This means that many plant ingredients are poorly absorbed and metabolized and accumulate poorly in the target tissues (Bilia *et al* 2018). As mentioned above, it is possible to overcome these limitations by modifying the design of carriers, enhancing the bioavailability of plant ingredients, and resulting in formulations that are more stable, solubilized, pharmacologically active, and toxic (Dang *et al* 2015). An effective delivery system involves controlling particle size, the surface properties of the particles, and the rate and dosage of encapsulated ingredients toward site-specific activity (Gunasekaran *et al* 2014). The most common formulations used to increase the bioavailability of plant molecules have been lipid-based systems, especially liposomes, which are based on the physicochemical nature and chemistry of the molecules to be encapsulated.

13.3.3 Stability

Plant-derived ingredients, isolated compounds, extracts, or essential oils, may be limited by their stability in the food, medicinal, and cosmetic industries. Compounds of this type are vulnerable to degradation when processed, stored, or absorbed in the gut by the digestive system when oxidized, hydrolyzed, crystallized, or deteriorated by enzymes. There are a variety of factors that influence their stability, including oxygen, temperature, pH, additives, metal ions, etc (Thakur *et al* 2011). Different bioactive compounds are protected and stabilized through encapsulation. It is possible to hide the increased instability of plant ingredients using nanoemulsions, liposomes, pyrosomes, ethosomes, and nanoparticles, including zedoary turmeric oil (Saraf 2010), verbascoside (Isacchi *et al* 2017), and tea polyphenols (Dang *et al* 2015).

13.3.4 Release

To achieve accurate effectiveness, delivery systems should allow active ingredients to be released at specific sites for action, whether by controlling the rate or by responding to an environmental trigger (e.g., pH, temperature). The trigger can be either during the storage of food (such as releasing an antimicrobial) or throughout the body (such as during the release of substances into the mouth, stomach, small intestine, or colon). A successful delivery system must consider the release followed by the carrier biodegradation. Several mechanisms have been proposed for releasing plant metabolites from carriers. They involve: (a) the desorption of the metabolite(s); (b) the diffusion of the metabolite(s) through the matrix (and in some cases, diffusion through the carrier wall in nanocapsules); (c) matrix decomposition; and (d) all of these. Using a sustained-release formulation, which releases metabolites continuously from the carrier, allows for predictable and reproducible drug-metabolism interactions (Natarajan *et al* 2014). A synchronized release may also apply to complex systems rather than isolated metabolites, such as plant extracts or essential oils. Therefore, multiple metabolites must be released within a specified time period while maintaining a ratio between the metabolites. As a consequence, such systems need to utilize this approach because asynchronous and non-controllable releases of plant metabolites usually result in decreased bioactivity (Lu *et al* 2007) (figure 13.2).

13.4 Delivery systems of phytochemicals

13.4.1 Lipid-based delivery systems

Most nanocarriers are lipid-based, and this category has been the subject of considerable research. There have been a number of formulations developed by using liposomes and similar carrier structures, including ethosomes, transfersomes, solid liposomes, nanostructured lipid carriers, and lipid-based drugs (Shukla *et al* 2018). The toxicity profiles of these carriers tend to be lower than those of polymeric carriers, and their costs tend to be lower (Chen *et al* 2010). The encapsulation efficiency is also improved, the release is controlled, they are biodegradable, easy to

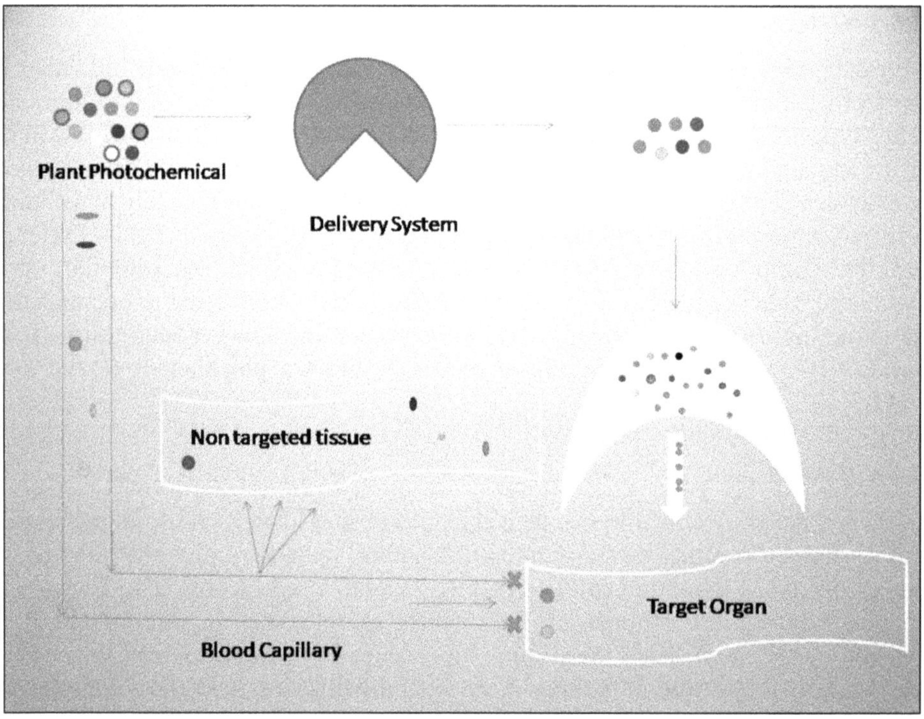

Figure 13.2. Mechanism of the delivery system.

manufacture, highly bioavailable, easy to manufacture and are possible to administer it in a variety of ways (oral, intravenous, topical, pulmonary, etc), as well as with targeted delivery through peripheral group modification. A variety of lipids can be used to prepare lipidic nanosystems. These particles must be biodegradable, biocompatible, stable, and possess low polydispersity index, high loading capacity, and have no toxic properties (Pathak *et al* 2011). Triglycerides, partial glycerides, fatty acids, and sterols are the most commonly used lipids for such purposes. In addition, selecting lipids should consider the physicochemical characteristics of the ingredient(s) to be encapsulated, along with the formulation's desired characteristics. In addition to particle size, release profile, delivery route, encapsulation method, and product cost, a number of factors must be considered (Anu Bhushani and Anandharamakrishnan 2014).

13.4.2 Vesicular systems

In vesicular carriers, phytochemicals self-assemble into concentric bilayers, resulting in the formation of amphiphilic building blocks. In order to transport and target encapsulated materials, such systems can prove to be extremely beneficial. Liposomes are the most extensively studied and developed category, while newer systems are continually being developed that can carry and deliver plant ingredients (Jain *et al* 2014). It is possible that these ingredients can be stabilized, protected, and

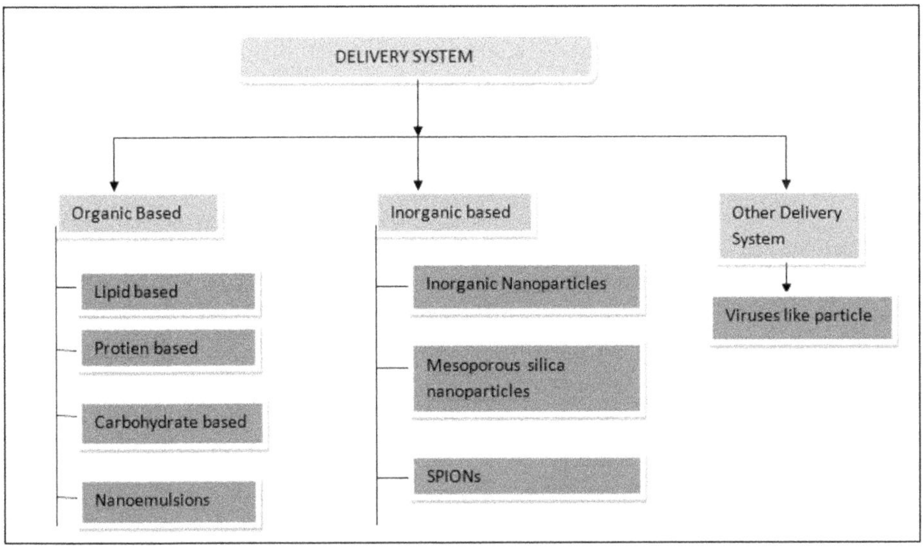

Figure 13.3. Types of delivery system.

prolonged in the systemic circulation when they are encapsulated in vesicular structures, which reduces the risk of toxicity (Biju *et al* 2006) (figure 13.3).

13.4.3 Liposomes

This technique was first developed in the year 1960. The term 'lipos' means fat and 'soma' means body (Shukla *et al* 2018). In addition to being highly efficient, liposomes are relatively easy to construct and are highly effective in encapsulating and delivering hydrophilic and lipophilic molecules. Liposomal formulations are mainly composed of phospholipids or sphingolipids. Liposomes can be prepared in several ways (Has and Sunthar 2020). A temperature above the lipid phase transition is required for all of them. It is reported that traditional methods like hydration, sonication, and micro emulsification are still being used, while newer, more efficient methods are being developed (e.g., spray drying, freeze drying, membrane-conductor method, etc) (Has and Sunthar 2020). Liposomes are classified according to their diameters and layers as multilamellar vesicles (MLVs) or unilamellar vesicles. According to Akbarzadeh *et al* (2013), the latter type is further subdivided into small unilamellar vesicles and large unilamellar vesicles. It is generally expensive to produce liposomal carriers due to their high production cost. Such systems must also be thermodynamically stable.

13.4.4 Transfersomes, ethosomes, phytosomes, and niosomes

Transferosomes have a liposomal structure, but the primary difference lies in the use of surfactants. In addition to providing flexibility, surfactants act as softeners and destabilizers of membranes (Kumar 2018). A transfer loaded with apigenin was found to have enhanced stability, permeability, and extended-release properties

(Jangdey *et al* 2017). In addition, a formulation encapsulated within transfersomes and containing epigallocatechin-3-gallate (from Camellia sinensis) was found to be skin-solubilizing, stable, and permeable, as well as anti-aging (Jangdey *et al* 2017). Among the components of ethosomes are phospholipids, water, and high concentrations of alcohol (ethyl alcohol or isopropanol), which are responsible for the elastic properties of the membranes and their ability to retain lipophilic molecules (Niu *et al* 2019). A preparation of caffeic acid-containing ethosomes was developed by Hallan *et al* in 2020, in order to achieve transdermal delivery. A longer period of antioxidant activity was maintained after encapsulating caffeine acid during this study compared to other systems described in the literature.

An interaction between metabolites within plant extracts and phosphatidylcholine produces phytosomes. In addition to their high solubility and bioavailability, the formulations are also highly stable (Lu *et al* 2019). It is thought that phytosomes are the result of complexing compounds (such as silymarin and curcumin) with extracts (like milk thistle, grape seed, tea leaf, and *Ginkgo biloba*).

The niosome is made up of lipids and surfactants that are non-ionic (Bhardwaj *et al* 2020). In addition to increasing solubility, niosome formulations could lead to better bioavailability, controlled release, and stability for plant ingredients (Gharbavi *et al* 2018). The low solubility and permeability of *Myrtus communis* extract in particular limit its application. While free extracts were found to have less antimicrobial activity, they exhibited higher antimicrobial activity when they were incorporated into multilamellar niosomes. Agarwal *et al* (2018) found that niosomes containing lipophilic flavin morusin were more soluble, encapsulated more efficiently, and released with a controlled rate of release, as well as having an anti-cancer effect.

13.4.5 Non-vesicular systems

Nanocarriers based on solid lipids are used in non-vesicular delivery systems. It is a colloidal particle whose size ranges from 50 to 1000 nm (Agarwal *et al* 2018) and can be prepared with low-energy methods like solvents and microemulsions/double emulsions, or high-energy methods like high-pressure homogenizations, high-speed homogenizations, emulsifications–evaporations, and ultrasound (Pucek *et al* 2020). It has been studied that non-vesicular lipid nanocarriers can be used to help transfer genes, perform bioimaging, and treat bacterial infections (Agarwal *et al* 2018). In addition to being oral, intravenous, and topically effective, the drugs are highly biocompatible (Agarwal *et al* 2018).

13.4.6 Solid lipid nanoparticles

As a colloidal carrier, solid lipid nanoparticles (SLNs) are created by mixing non-ionic emulsifiers with melted liquid to stabilize dispersion at room temperature as well as within the human body. Over the past few years, SLNs have drawn attention because of their large surface area, high encapsulation efficiency, controlled release, and targeted delivery (Scioli Montoto *et al* 2020). There are a number of benefits associated with SLN formulations. The use of these additives could improve the stability of plant ingredients, reduce the possibility of adverse effects, be non-toxic, highly biodegradable, and may be formulated in a variety of sizes and surfaces for increased cellular uptake (Rahman *et al* 2020). The formulations can also be produced at a large scale and enhance stability while facilitating industrial logistics (Mishra *et al* 2018). The SLNs can be classified into three types: Type I is a homogeneous matrix, which distributes the bioactive compounds evenly throughout the lipid core. There are two types of drug-enriched models, Type II and Type III. Type II is where the bioactive compound(s) are present both in the solid shell and the lipid core, while Type III is based on lipid core solubility near saturation. Consequently, a lipid cover forms over the core due to its precipitation. SLNs can be transformed dramatically by changes to the manufacturing process, allowing them to be used for any purpose (Borges *et al* 2020).

13.4.7 Nanostructured lipid carriers

Colloidal delivery systems, like solid lipid delivery systems, are primarily composed of lipids that are solid at room temperature and liquid at room temperature. Consequently, an unorganized matrix becomes formed with a few layers or sheets covering it (Chauhan *et al* 2020). Using a low-order matrix results in high encapsulation efficiency and prevents early compound release. In a recent study, a nanostructured lipid carrier (NLC) was prepared to encapsulate silymarin, a lipophilic compound with a low bioavailability (Bhise *et al* 2017). A study of quercetin loaded into NLCs and SLNs for brain delivery found that NLC formulations showed better loading efficiency and bioavailability (Kumar *et al* 2016).

13.4.8 Protein-based delivery systems

As well as being nutritionally valuable, proteins are macromolecules that can encapsulate hydrophilic or hydrophobic bioactive ingredients, including phenols, carotenoids, polyunsaturated fatty acids, and vitamins. Depending on the properties of biocompatibility, biodegradability, self-association, emulsion, foaming, and gelation, they are biocompatible, biodegradable, self-association, and emulsification. Many protein-based delivery systems have been reported in the literature, such as hydrogels, micro- and nanoparticles, and films. There are a number of different types of proteins typically used in food-grade delivery systems, including casein, whey protein, gelatand soy, cereals (such as zein), and legumes (such as pea) (Rather *et al* 2019).

13.4.9 Systems for delivering carbohydrates

Natural macromolecules like carbohydrates and lipids are used in delivery systems as building blocks. A few of their unique properties include being water-soluble, biocompatible, biodegradable, and able to entrap both hydrophilic and hydrophobic molecules due to functional groups and molecular structures. A further advantage of carbohydrates is their thermal stability, which makes them a better delivery method than lipids and proteins. (Fathi *et al* 2014). Carbohydrate-based delivery methods have many uses in the food, drug, and cosmetic sectors. Various carbohydrates have been used thus far to create delivery systems, either in their original state or changed after being subjected to physical, chemical, or enzymatic treatment (Khaleel Basha *et al* 2019). It is especially important to mention the biodegradable, biocompatible, and inexpensive properties of starch as a storage carbohydrate. It is composed of two macromolecules, linear amylose and branching amylopectin. As an encapsulating substance, starch has several uses. However, due to its hydrophilic nature, it cannot be used to encapsulate hydrophobic chemicals. Furthermore, it cannot be used for other purposes because of the sensitivity to the amylase activity in the mouth. To overcome these limitations and increase its commercial usefulness, it can be modified via enzymatic (such as αamylase), physical (such as extrusion), or chemical (such as acid hydrolysis) approaches (Fathi *et al* 2018). It has been demonstrated that a variety of starch-based delivery systems can be produced with various techniques, including self-assembly, nanoprecipitation, ultrasonication, electrospinning, extrusion, and micro fluidization (Rostamabadi *et al* 2019). Another therapeutic approach of starch is the formation of compounds maltodextrins due to partial hydrolysis. The hydrophilicity of this maltodextrin is greater than that of starch. Maltodextrins are biocompatible biopolymers that are widely used as the wall component of several bioactive chemical delivery systems.

References

Agarwal S, Mohamed M S, Raveendran S, Rochani A K, Maekawa T and Kumar D S 2018 Formulation, characterization and evaluation of morusin loaded niosomes for potentiation of anticancer therapy *RSC Adv.* **8** 32621–36

Akbarzadeh A, Rezaei-sadabady R, Davaran S, Joo S W and Zarghami N 2013 Liposome: classification, preparation, and applications *Nanoscale Res. Lett.* **8** 102

Anu Bhushani J and Anandharamakrishnan C 2014 Electro spinning and electro spraying techniques: potential food based applications *Trends Food Sci. Technol.* **38** 21–33

Asensi M, Ortega A, Mena S, Feddi F and Estrela J M 2011 Natural polyphenols in cancertherapy *Crit. Rev. Clin. Lab. Sci.* **48** 197–216

Baran I, Ionescu D, Filippi A, Mocanu M and Iftime A *et al* 2014 Novel insights into theantiproliferative effects and synergism of quercetin and menadione in human leukemia Jurkat T cells *Leuk. Res.* **38** 836–49

Bhardwaj P, Tripathi P, Gupta R and Pandey S 2020 Niosomes: a review on niosomal research in the last decade *J. Drug Deliv. Sci. Technol.* **56** 101581

Bhise K, Kashaw S K, Sau S and Iyer A K 2017 Nanostructured lipid carriers employing polyphenols as promising anticancer agents:quality by design (QbD) approach *Int. J. Pharm.* **526** 506–15

Biju S S, Talegaonka S, Mishra P R and Kharshoum R M 2006 Vesicular systems: an overview *Indian J. Pharm. Sci.* **68** 141–53

Bilia A R, Piazzini V, Asprea M, Risaliti L, Vanti G and Bergonzi M C 2018 Plants extractsloaded in nanocarriers: an emergent formulating approach *Nat. Prod. Commun.* **13** 1157–60

Borges A, de Freitas V, Mateus N, Fernandes I and Oliveira J 2020 Solid lipid nanoparticles as carriers of natural phenolic compounds *Antioxidants* **9** 998

Branco C, Lima É, Rodrigues T, Scheffel T and Scola G *et al* 2015 Mitochondria and redoxhomoeostasis as chemotherapeutic targets of *Araucaria angustifolia* (Bert.) O. Kuntze inhuman larynx HEp-2 cancer cells *Chem. Biol. Interact.* **231** 108–18

Bray F, Ferlay J, Soerjomataram I, Siegel R L, Torre L A and Jemal A 2018 Global cancer statistics 2018: GLOBOCAN estimates of incidence and mortality worldwide for 36 cancers in 185 countries *CA Cancer J. Clin.* **68** 394–424

Chauhan I, Yasir M, Verma M and Singh A P 2020 Nanostructured lipid carriers: a groundbreaking approach for transdermal drug delivery *Adv. Pharm. Bull.* **10** 150–65

Chen C C, Tsai T H, Huang Z R and Fang J Y 2010 Effects of lipophilic emulsifiers on the oral administration of lovastatin from nanostructured lipid carriers: physicochemical characterization and pharmacokinetics *Eur. J. Pharm. Biopharm.* **74** 474–82

Dang S, Gupta S, Bansal R, Ali J and Gabrani R 2015 Nano-encapsulation of a naturalpolyphenol, green tea catechins: way to preserve *Free Radicals in Human Health and Disease* ed V Rani and U Yadav (Chennai: Springer) pp 397–415

Deng S, Shanmugam M K, Kumar A P, Yap C T, Sethi G and Bishayee A 2019 Targetingautophagy using natural compounds for cancer prevention and therapy *Cancer* **125** 1228–46

Diederich M and Cerella C 2016 Non-canonical programmed cell death mechanisms triggeredby natural compounds *Semin. Cancer Biol.* **40–41** 4–34

El-Ashmawy N, Khedr E, Ebeid E Z, Salem M, Zidan A A and Mosalam E 2017 Enhanced anticancer effect and reduced toxicity of doxorubicin in combination withthymoquinone released from poly-N-acetyl glucosamine nanomatrix in mice bearing solid Ehrlish carcinoma *Eur. J. Pharm. Sci.* **109** 525–32

Fathi M, Donsi F and McClements D J 2018 Protein-based delivery systems for the nanoencapsulation of food ingredients *Compr. Rev. Food Sci. Food Saf.* **17** 920–36

Fathi M, Martín Á and McClements D J 2014 Nano encapsulation of food ingredients using carbohydrate based delivery systems *Trends Food Sci. Technol.* **39** 18–39

Folkman J 2006 Angiogenesis *Annu. Rev. Med.* **57** 1–18

Folkman J 2007 Angiogenesis: an organizing principle for drug discovery? *Nat. Rev. Drug Discov.* **6** 273–86

George B P, Chandran R and Abrahamse H 2021 Role of phytochemicals in cancer chemoprevention: insights *Antioxidants* **10** 1455

Gharbavi M, Amani J, Kheiri-Manjili H, Danafar H and Sharafi A 2018 Niosome: a promising nanocarrier for natural drug delivery through blood-brain barrier *Adv. Pharmacol. Sci.* 2018

Gullett N P, Ruhul Amin A R, Bayraktar S, Pezzuto J and Shin D *et al* 2010 Cancer preventionwith natural compounds *Semin. Oncol.* **37** 258–81

Gunasekaran T, Haile T, Nigusse T and Dhanaraju M D 2014 Nanotechnology: an effective tool for enhancing bioavailability and bioactivity of phytomedicine *Asian Pac. J. Trop. Bio Med.* **4** S1–7

Hallan S S, Sguizzato M, Mariani P, Cortesi R, Huang N, Simelière F, Marchetti N, Drechsler M, Ruzgas T and Esposito E 2020 Design and characterization of ethosomes for transdermal delivery of caffeic acid *Pharmaceutics* **12** 740

Has C and Sunthar P A 2020 Comprehensive review on recent preparation techniques of liposomes *J. Liposome Res.* **30** 336–65

Huminiecki L and Horbańczuk J 2018 The functional genomic studies of resveratrol in respectto its anti-cancer effects *Biotechnol. Adv.* **36** 1699–708

Isacchi B, Bergonzi M C, Iacopi R, Ghelardini C, Galeotti N and Bilia A R 2017 Liposomal formulation to increase stability andprolong ant neuropathic activity of verbascoside *Planta Med.* **83** 412–9

Jain S, Jain V and Mahajan S C 2014 Lipid based vesicular drug delivery systems *Adv. Pharm.* **2014** 574673

Jangdey M S, Gupta A and Saraf S 2017 Development and optimization of apigenin-loaded transfersomal system for skin cancer delivery: *in vitro* evaluation *Artif. Cells Nanomed. Biotechnol.* **45** 1452–62

Kaur V, Kumar M, Kumar A, Kaur K, Dhillon V and Kaur S 2018 Pharmacotherapeuticpotential of phytochemicals: implications in cancer chemoprevention and futureperspectives *Biomed. Pharmacother.* **97** 564–86

Khaleel Basha S, Syed Muzammil M, Dhandayuthabani R and Sugantha Kumari V 2019 Polysaccharides as excipient in drug delivery system *Mater. Today Proc.* **36** 280–9

Khan N, Bharali D, Adhami V, Siddiqui I and Cui H *et al* 2014 Oral administration ofnaturally occurring chitosan-based nanoformulated green tea polyphenol EGCG effectivelyinhibits prostate cancer cell growth in a xenograft model *Carcinogenesis* **35** 415–23

Kumar A 2018 Transferosome: a recent approach for transdermal drug delivery *J. Drug Deliv. Ther.* **8** 100–4

Kumar P, Sharma G, Kumar R, Singh B, Malik R, Katare O P and Raza K 2016 Promises of a biocompatible nanocarrier in improved brain delivery of quercetin: biochemical, pharmacokinetic and bio distribution evidences *Int. J. Pharm.* **515** 307–14

Lambert J D and Elias R J 2010 The antioxidant and pro-oxidant activities of green teapolyphenols: a role in cancer prevention *Arch. Biochem. Biophys.* **501** 65–72

Lu C, Lu Y, Chen J, Zhang W and Wu W 2007 Synchronized and sustained release of multiple components in silymarin from erodibleglycerylmonostearate matrix system *Eur. J. Pharm. Biopharm.* **66** 210–9

Lu M, Qiu Q, Luo X, Liu X, Sun J, Wang C, Lin X, Deng Y and Song Y 2019 Phyto-phospholipid complexes (phytosomes): a novel strategy to improve the bioavailability of active constituents *Asian J. Pharm. Sci.* **14** 265–74

Mahbub A, Le Maitre C, Haywood-Small S, Cross N and Jordan-Mahy N 2015 Polyphenolsact synergistically with doxorubicin and etoposide in leukaemia cell lines *Cell Death Discov.* **1** 15043

Maji S, Panda S, Samal S K, Shriwas O and Rath R *et al* 2018 Bcl-2 antiapoptotic familyproteins and chemoresistance in cancer *Advances in Cancer Research* (New York: Academic)vol 137 pp 37–75

McClements D J 2014 *Nanoparticle- and Microparticle-Based Delivery Systems: Encapsulation, Protection and Release of Active Compounds* (Boca Raton, FL: CRC Press)

Mercader A and Pomilio A 2012 (Iso)flav(an)ones, chalcones, catechins, and theaflavins asanticarcinogens: mechanisms, anti-multidrug resistance and QSAR studies *Curr. Med. Chem.* **19** 4324–47

Mishra V, Bansal K K, Verma A, Yadav N, Thakur S, Sudhakar K and Rosenholm J M 2018 Solid lipid nanoparticles: emerging colloidal nano drug delivery systems *Pharmaceutics* **10** 191

Natarajan J V, Nugraha C, Ng X W and Venkatraman S 2014 Sustained-release from nanocarriers: a review *J. Control. Release* **193** 122–38

Niu X Q, Zhang D P, Bian Q, Feng X F, Li H, Rao Y F, Shen Y M, Geng F N, Yuan A R and Ying X Y *et al* 2019 Mechanism investigation of ethosomes transdermal permeation *Int. J. Pharm.* X **1** 100027

Pathak K, Keshri L and Shah M 2011 Lipid nanocarriers: influence of lipids on product development and pharmacokinetics *Crit. Rev. Ther. Drug Carrier Syst.* **28** 357–93

Pool P, Campos-Vega R, Herrera-Hernández M, García-Solis P and García-Gasca T *et al* 2018 Development of genistein-PEGylated silica hybrid nanomaterials with enhanced antioxidant and antiproliferative properties on HT29 human colon cancer cells *Am. J. Transl. Res.* **10** 2306–23

Pucek A, Tokarek B, Waglewska E and Bazylinska U 2020 Recent advances in the structural design of photosensitive agent formulations using 'soft' colloidal nanocarriers *Pharmaceutics* **12** 587

Rahman H S, Othman H H, Hammadi N I, Yeap S K, Amin K M, Samad N A and Alitheen N B 2020 Novel drug delivery systems for loading of natural plant extracts and their biomedical applications *Int. J. Nanomed.* **15** 2439–83

Rather S A, Masoodi F A, Rather J A, Akhter R and Ganaie T A 2019 Protein-based delivery systems *Food Hydrocolloids as Encapsulating Agents in Delivery Systems* ed G Adil, F Masoodi, U Shah and A Shah (Boca Raton, FL: CRC Press) pp 159–76

Rengasamy K, Khan H, Gowrishankar S, Lagoa R and Mahomoodally F *et al* 2019 Therole of flavonoids in autoimmune diseases: therapeutic updates *Pharmacol. Ther.* **194** 107–31

Reuben S C, Gopalan A, Petit D M and Bishayee A 2012 Modulation of angiogenesis bydietary phytoconstituents in the prevention and intervention of breast cancer *Mol. Nutr. Food Res.* **56** 14–29

Rostamabadi H, Falsafi S R and Jafari S M 2019 Starch based nanocarriers as cutting-edge natural cargos for nutraceutical delivery *Trends Food Sci. Technol.* **88** 397–415

Rothwell J, Knaze V and Zamora-Ros R 2017 Polyphenols: dietary assessment and role in theprevention of cancers *Curr. Opin. Clin. Nutr. Metab. Care* **20** 512–21

Saraf S 2010 Applications of novel drug delivery system for herbal formulations *Fitoterapia* **81** 680–9

Scioli Montoto S, Muraca G and Ruiz M E 2020 Solid lipid nanoparticles for drug delivery: pharmacological and biopharmaceutical aspects *Front. Mol. Biosci.* **7** 587997

Shang B, Cao Z and Zhou Q 2012 Progress in tumor vascular normalization for anticancer therapy: challenges and perspectives *Front Med.* **6** 67–78

Shanmugam M, Lee J, Chai E, Kanchi M and Kar S *et al* 2016 Cancer prevention andtherapy through the modulation of transcription factors by bioactive natural compounds *Semin. Cancer Biol.* **40–41** 35–47

Shukla T, Upmanyu N, Prakash Pandey S and Gosh D 2018 *Lipid Nanocarriers* (Amsterdam: Elsevier)

Sinha D, Biswas J, Nabavi S and Bishayee A 2017 Tea phytochemicals for breast cancer prevention and intervention: from bench to bedside and beyond *Semin. Cancer Biol.* **46** 33–54

Song Y H, Sun H, Zhang A, Yan G, Han Y and Wang X 2014 Plant derivednatural products as leads to anti-cancer drugs *J. Med. Plant Herb. Ther. Res.* **2** 6–15

Suphim B, Prawan A, Kukongviriyapan U, Kongpetch S, Buranrat B and Kukongviriyapan V 2010 Redox modulation and human bile duct cancer inhibition by curcumin *Food Chem. Toxicol.* **48** 2265–72

Sznarkowska A, Kostecka A, Meller K and Bielawski K P 2017 Inhibition of cancerantioxidant defense bynatural compounds *Oncotarget.* **8** 15996–6016

Taniguchi K and Karin M 2018 NF-κB, inflammation, immunity and cancer: coming of age *Nat. Rev. Immunol.* **18** 309–24

Thakur L, Ghodasra U, Patel N and Dabhi M 2011 Novel approaches for stability improvement in natural medicines *Pharmacogn. Rev.* **5** 48–54

Wahl O, Oswald M, Tretzel L, Herres E and Arend J *et al* 2011 Inhibition of tumor angiogenesis by antibodies, synthetic small molecules and natural products *Curr. Med. Chem.* **18** 3136–55

Zhang Q, Tian X and Cao X 2019 Transferrin-functionalised microemulsion co-delivery of β-elemene and celastrol for enhanced anti-lung cancer treatment and reduced systemic toxicity *Drug Deliv. Transl.* **9** 667–78

IOP Publishing

Phytochemicals as an Epigenetic Modifier in Cancer Prevention

Nidhi Puranik, Deepa Yadav and Sangeeta Shukla

Chapter 14

Potential role of nanophytochemicals in breast cancer therapy

Amit Sonkar and Priyanka Sonkar

Breast cancer is the most common form of cancer type caused in women and leading to the majority of cancer deaths among women worldwide. The rapid increase in breast cancer occurrences in recent years affects different physical, mental, and social aspects of women's lives. Although the exact mechanism of breast cancer is still unidentified, its associated risks were recognized. These risk factors include aging, menarche history, genetic changes, breast cancer in family history, race, obesity, and alcohol consumption. The current treatment of breast cancer relies upon surgery, radiation therapy, and chemotherapy or more targeted strategies including anti-estrogens and aromatase inhibitors. Although there has been significant developments in diagnostic methods, and specific and targeted chemotherapies over the past decades, there are still many challenges related to overall breast cancer management. So, the development of effective therapeutics is a top priority to overcome drug resistance. There has been growing interest in plant-based chemicals that have the potential as anti-cancer agents. These chemicals can act directly on both estrogen-dependent and estrogen-independent cell proliferation, making them promising candidates for therapeutic use. Collected research data analysis demonstrated the encouraging anti-cancer effects of phytochemicals inhibiting proliferation and malignant transformation of the cells. These plant-derived chemicals are non-toxic and play multiple roles in human health. These phytochemicals may positively affect the cell signaling processes and cell cycle regulation.

This chapter provides an overview of breast cancer and its various risk factors and explores the potential of phytochemicals in both preventing and treating breast cancer. Additionally, the chapter emphasizes the importance of dietary interventions in lowering the risk of breast cancer and highlights the association between intake of a plant-based diet and a lower incidence of breast cancer. Furthermore, the chapter explores the use of nanotechnology-based delivery systems for phytochemicals in breast cancer treatment, which can help to overcome issues such as poor

doi:10.1088/978-0-7503-5252-9ch14

bioavailability and stability of phytochemicals. However, it also highlights the need for careful consideration of the potential effects and safety implications of nano-formulations. Overall, the review provides valuable insights into the potential of phytochemicals and nanotechnology in breast cancer treatment and highlights the importance of ongoing research in this field.

Abbreviations

The following abbreviations are used in this manuscript:

WHO	World Health Organization
BCSCs	Breast cancer stem cells
HER2	Human epidermal growth factor receptor 2
ER	Estrogen receptor
EGCG	Nano-epigallocatechin-3-gallate
QT	Quercetin
MCF-7 cells	Michigan Cancer Foundation-7 breast cancer cells
TNBC	Triple-negative breast cancer
NPs	Nanoparticles

14.1 Introduction

According to the report of the World Health Organization (WHO), 2021, breast cancer is the most frequently diagnosed cancer among women globally, and the second most common type of cancer overall. There were approximately 2.3 million new cases of breast cancer diagnosed worldwide in 2020, which accounted for 11.7% of all new cancer cases [1]. Additionally, breast cancer is the primary cause of cancer-related deaths among women, with approximately 685 000 deaths reported [2]. However, early detection and treatment can significantly improve breast cancer outcomes, and WHO recommends regular breast cancer screening for women in all age groups. Breast cancer typically develops without noticeable symptoms and is commonly detected through regular screening. The progression of breast cancer is classified into four stages, with stage zero denoting the initial stage (carcinoma *in situ*) and stages I to IV representing the advancement of the disease. Treatment for stage I breast cancer, which is confined to the breast, has a 100% survival rate [3]. However, breast cancer tends to spread to other areas of the body, including the lungs, liver, bones, and brain, through a process known as metastasis [4].

Breast cancer is divided into three subtypes based on the presence or absence of specific receptors [3, 5]:

(i) Hormone receptor-positive [estrogen receptor-positive (ER+] (HER-positive);
(ii) Human epidermal growth factor receptor (EGFR) 2 (HER2-positive);
(iii) Triple-negative tumors.

The first subtype of breast cancer is known as HER-positive, which is characterized by the presence of estrogen receptors and is part of the epidermal growth factor (EGF) receptor family. The second subtype is referred to as HER2-positive, which is distinguished by the presence of HER2, another member of the EGF receptor family. The third subtype is referred to as triple-negative, which lacks the three primary receptors—estrogen, HER2, and progesterone. The treatment of breast cancer depends on factors such as the stage and type of cancer [6, 7]. Considerable efforts have been made in the development of breast cancer treatment options. Currently, the main treatment for breast cancer relies upon surgery, radiotherapy, combinations of therapies, and hormonal therapy [8]. Surgery and radiotherapy are the most commonly used treatments for cancer, including breast cancer, as they aim to remove or control cancerous cell growth in a specific area. Different types of surgery are performed depending on the type and stage of the breast cancer tumor. Typically, radiation therapy is performed after surgery, as it is an integral part of breast-conserving therapy [9, 10].

In addition to surgery and radiation, systematic treatment of breast cancer may involve chemotherapy. Chemotherapy consists of the use of anti-cancer drugs to obstruct the growth of cancerous cells [3]. Anti-cancer drugs can be administered orally or through intravenous/intramuscular injection. Chemotherapeutic agents may be given as a single drug or in combination, depending on the needs of the patient [11]. One of the significant challenges in breast cancer treatment is the problem of drug resistance, especially in HER-positive breast cancer [5]. There are several reasons for the development of drug resistance, including mutations that lead to resistance against the drugs.

Although there have been significant advancements in chemotherapeutic agents for breast cancer treatment in the past decade, the issue of drug resistance remains a challenge. As a result, researchers are actively searching for more effective treatments for breast cancer. One promising avenue is the use of naturally occurring compounds, which have been utilized for thousands of years and have demonstrated effectiveness against various types of cancer. Additionally, these compounds possess disease-preventing properties. By exploring the therapeutic potential of natural compounds, researchers hope to develop new and innovative treatments for breast cancer that are both effective and safe [5]. Researchers have been investigating dietary phytochemicals to better understand their chemical and biological properties. The mechanisms of action of phytochemicals have been explored through *in vitro* (at cellular, molecular, and genomic level trials) and *in vivo* studies, revealing abundant evidence of their strong anti-cancer properties [3, 12–15]. Many phytochemicals including capsaicin, cucurbitacin B, isoflavones, catechins, lycopene, phenethyl isothiocyanate, and piperlongumine, have been found to inhibit the growth of transformed cells, suggesting their potential as chemopreventive agents [16]. Studies have extensively investigated the effectiveness of various dietary components, such as quercetin, epigallocatechin-3-gallate, genistein, kaempferol, capsaicin, and lycopene in combating various types of cancer. However, the low absorption rate, limited solubility, and quick metabolism of these phytochemicals have hindered their utilization in cancer treatment. To overcome these challenges, modern nanotechnology may be utilized [17]. Implementing the techniques for nanoformulation results in improvements in biodistribution, bioavailability, pharmacokinetics, and drug transport specificity to the cancer site [20].

14.2 Breast cancer

14.2.1 Epidemiology

Breast cancer is a prevalent disease affecting women worldwide. In the United States, around 12.4% of women will develop invasive breast cancer during their lifetime. On a global scale, approximately 1.7 million new cases of breast cancer are reported each year. Breast cancer incidence rates vary widely around the world. Incidence rates of breast cancer tend to be higher in regions with higher income levels compared to those with lower income levels [21]. The incidence of breast cancer rises with age, and the majority of cases are diagnosed in women over the age of 50. However, breast cancer can develop in women of any age. The 5-year survival rates for breast cancer are significantly greater in high-income countries, where they can exceed 90%, compared to low- and middle-income countries like India and South Africa, where survival rates are considerably lower, ranging from 40% to 66%.

14.2.2 Risk factors

Generally, the breast cancer risk factors that manifest the cancerous lesions [22] can be classified into two categories: non-modifiable and modifiable. Non-modifiable risk factors denote factors that cannot be changed, such as genetic factors and epigenetic alterations, which can lead to sporadic breast cancer development among women worldwide. Changes in DNA methylation have been linked to the dysregulation of many pathological processes, including the development of breast cancer tumors. Modifiable risk factors, on the other hand, are factors that can be altered, such as environmental factors, sedentary lifestyle, and improper dietary habits, all these factors accelerate carcinogenesis and their clinical onset [23, 24]. The development of cancerous tissue transformation is a complex process that involves various factors such as DNA damage caused by oxidative stress, chronic inflammation, and cellular crosstalk between adjoining tissues [22, 24]. Modifiable risk factors have a significant impact on cancer development and prevention. Maintaining a stable balance between reactive oxygen species (ROS) and adequate response by detoxification pathways is crucial for efficient cancer prevention. The majority of all cancer types are sporadic and based on modifiable risk factors, making them highly preventable [25]. Therefore, these modifiable risk factors play an essential role in anti-cancer protection [26].

14.3 Phytochemicals

The term 'Phytochemicals' refers to biologically active substances found in plant-based foods that do not provide essential nutrients but can have beneficial effects on human health. These compounds are also known as phytonutrients and plant-derived chemicals [27]. Plants produce these phytochemicals as a means of protecting themselves from various environmental stresses, including microbial infections, exposure to pollutants, changes in temperature, and drought [28]. These properties make phytochemicals promising candidates for developing interventions that can improve health and extend longevity in various heterotrophic organisms [28]. Fruit, vegetables, and grains contain around 8000 different phytochemicals, though a significant portion remain unidentified [30]. Phytochemicals can be classified in various ways including chemical structure, botanical origin, and biological properties. Based on their chemical structure, they are categorized into phenolics, alkaloids, carotenoids, organosulfur compounds, and nitrogen-containing compounds [27, 29], as shown in figure 14.1. Among these carotenoids, phenolics, and organosulfur are the most commonly studied dietary phytochemicals compounds.

Phytochemicals, which are biologically active compounds found in plants, have been shown to have anti-cancer properties. One way in which they may act is by up-regulating the expression of tumor suppressor genes, which help prevent the formation and spread of cancer cells. At the same time, phytochemicals may down-regulate the expression of oncogenes, which promote the growth and proliferation of cancer cells. This dual action can help to prevent the development and progression of cancer. However, it is important to note that the specific mechanisms by which phytochemicals exert their anti-cancer effects can vary depending on the compound and the type of cancer being studied. They have beneficial effects in suppressing and inhibiting the growth of various human cancers. These plant compounds have been found to modulate immune responses, support

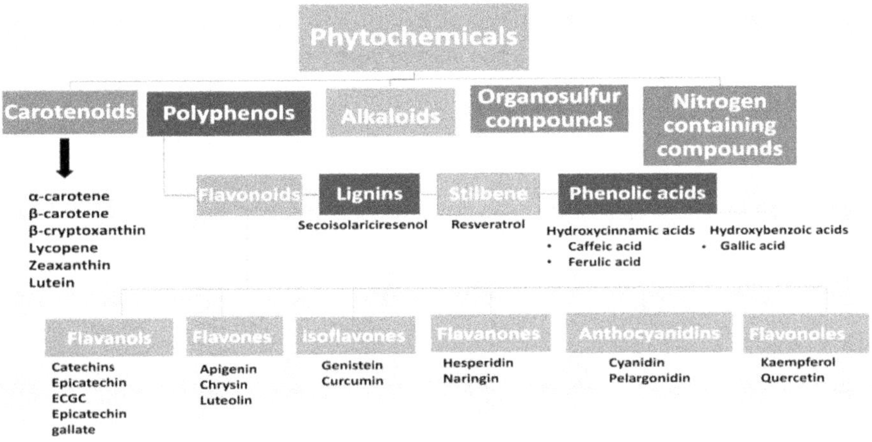

Figure 14.1. Classification of phytochemicals based on their chemical structure.

and replace cellular functions and reduce inflammation. These compounds have demonstrated protective effects against cancer and have been found to positively impact several cancer-related pathways. A diverse range of fruit and vegetables can provide nutrients and bioactive compounds, including phytochemicals (phenolics, flavonoids, and carotenoids), and their regular consumption may reduce the risk of different types of cancer [22, 31–33]. Scientific evidence strongly suggests that about one-third of all cancers can be prevented through proper dietary habits [27]. Carotenoids, flavonoids, and a subclass of polyphenols have been investigated for their potential use in the treatment of breast cancer [34]. Flavonoids such as flavanone, isoflavone, flavone, flavanol, and catechin have all demonstrated anti-cancerous properties, and have been used for the prevention and treatment of breast cancer [34]. The efficacy of these compounds varies depending on the cancer type, the concentration of doses, and the cell lines tested.

14.3.1 Carotenoids

Carotenoids or tetraterpenoids are organic pigments that are produced by plants and algae and typically exhibit yellow, red, or orange colors. These pigments assist in the absorption of light energy during the photosynthesis process. Since carotenoids are fat-soluble, they are absorbed in our bodies with fats [22]. Various fruit and vegetables, such as carrots, tomatoes, and pumpkins, obtain their characteristic color from carotenoids. Carotenoids are the most prevalent pigments and more than 750 structurally different carotenoids are found in nature. They consist of 40 carbon skeletons of isoprene structural units and they may be cyclized at one end or both ends, may possess different hydrogenation levels, or have functional groups (oxygen-containing) [35]. Based on the conversion of provitamin A they are classified into two groups.

14.3.1.1 Provitamin A carotenoids

Provitamin A carotenoids are a type of carotenoid that can be converted into vitamin A in the body. They are called 'provitamin A' because they can be converted into vitamin A, but they are not the active form of vitamin A itself. The most common provitamin A carotenoids are α-carotene, β-carotene, and β-cryptoxanthin. These carotenoids are found in a variety of plant-based foods, such as carrots, pumpkins, and leafy greens. When we consume these foods, the provitamin A carotenoids are absorbed by the body and converted into retinol, the active form of vitamin A, which plays a critical role in vision, immune function, and other important bodily processes. Consuming a diet rich in provitamin A carotenoids is important for maintaining good health and preventing deficiencies of vitamin A.

14.3.1.2 Non-provitamin A carotenoids

Non-provitamin A carotenoids are a group of carotenoids that cannot be converted into vitamin A in the body. Some common non-provitamin A carotenoids include lycopene, lutein, and zeaxanthin, which are found in foods such as tomatoes, watermelon, peppers, and spinach. Although these carotenoids do not contribute to vitamin A status, they still have important health benefits. For example, lutein and zeaxanthin are known to accumulate in the macula of the eye, where they act as antioxidants and may help protect against age-related macular degeneration. Lycopene is also a potent antioxidant and has been associated with a reduced risk of certain types of cancer, such as breast cancer.

Carotenoids have multiple functions, but their most important role is as provitamins and antioxidants [27]. Carotenoids neutralize free radicals and single oxygen atoms that can harm cells, making them effective as antioxidants [36]. Carotenoids have strong anti-cancer properties [35].

14.3.2 Phenolic acids

Phenolic compounds are referred to as secondary metabolites in plants. Phenolic acids are divided into two categories namely hydroxybenzoic acids and hydroxycinnamic acid, as displayed in figure 14.1. The first group is designated as hydroxybenzoic acid derivatives which include p-hydroxybenzoic, protocatechuic, vanillic, syringic, and gallic acids [22, 27]. They are often present in a bound form, which means they are chemically linked to other molecules and are part of complex structures such as lignins and hydrolyzable tannins. Phenolics, including phenolic acids, have been studied for their potential role in the treatment of breast cancer. Some studies suggest that phenolic compounds have been shown to possess anti-cancer properties. They may achieve this by inhibiting the proliferation of cancer cells and promoting apoptosis in cancer cells. For example, *in vitro* studies have shown that certain phenolic compounds, such as gallic acid and caffeic acid, can prevent the growth of breast cancer cells [12, 13]. Some research studies have suggested that consuming a diet rich in phenolic compounds, which can be found in whole grains, fruit and vegetables, may help to lower the risk of breast cancer. This is thought to be due to the anti-inflammatory and antioxidant properties of phenolic compounds, which may help to reduce oxidative stress and inflammation, two factors that are associated with an increased risk of cancer [25]. However, more research is needed to fully identify the role of phenolics in breast cancer prevention and treatment, as well as the optimal dosages and sources of these compounds for therapeutic purposes.

14.3.3 Flavonoids

Flavonoids are a diverse group of polyphenolic compounds found in plants, known for their antioxidant properties. Flavonoids are found in a wide variety of plant-based foods such as tea, wine, berries, citrus fruits, and dark chocolate. Around 4000 different flavonoids have been identified, and they can be classified into six major subclasses: anthocyanidins, flavanols, flavonols, flavanones, flavones, and isoflavones [27] as displayed in figure 14.1. Studies have suggested that flavonoids may have the potential to act as anti-cancer agents by modulating various cell signaling pathways. Flavonoids have been found to promote apoptosis, a process of programmed cell death [15], prevent angiogenesis (the formation of new blood vessels that can feed tumors), and suppress inflammation (which can contribute to cancer development) [34]. Some specific flavonoids, such as quercetin and kaempferol, have been studied for their potential anti-cancer effects [14, 37]. These flavonoids have been shown to inhibit the growth of different cancers, including breast, colon, prostate, and lung cancer cells [38]. Overall, flavonoids are a promising area of research for their potential role in cancer prevention and treatment, but more studies are needed to fully understand their mechanisms.

14.3.4 Alkaloids

Alkaloids are a class of organic compounds that are primarily found in plants, although they can also be found in some animals and fungi [39]. They are typically bitter-tasting and have a wide range of physiological effects on humans and other animals [40]. Some of the most well-known alkaloids include caffeine, nicotine, morphine, and quinine. Capsaicin is a potent alkaloid and the active compound found in chili peppers, which belong to the capsicum plant genus and are used for cancer prevention [41]. Some alkaloids have shown potential activity in breast cancer treatment, such as taxol (paclitaxel), which is derived from the Pacific yew tree and has also been utilized in the treatment of breast cancer [42]. Taxol works by stabilizing microtubules, preventing them from breaking down during cell division, and ultimately leading to cell death. While alkaloids have shown promise in the treatment of breast cancer, they can also have toxic side effects and are often used in combination with other chemotherapy drugs. Ongoing research is exploring the potential of alkaloids and other natural compounds for the complete understanding of the mechanism of action and their role and potential side effects in the treatment of breast cancer.

14.3.5 Organosulfur compounds

Organic compounds that possess sulfur atoms within their molecular structure are referred to as organosulfur compounds. Research has been conducted on the potential of organosulfur compounds for both the prevention and treatment of breast cancer. Some studies have suggested that certain organosulfur compounds, such as allyl sulfides found in garlic and onions, may have anti-cancer properties. The compound allicin has been found to cause a reduction in breast cancer cell viability (MCF-7 and HCC-70) and has shown anti-proliferative effects. These effects are believed to occur through the activation of caspases-3, 8, and 9, as well as the loss of mitochondrial membrane potential ($D\Psi m$), which leads to cancer cell apoptosis [43, 44].

14.4 Phytochemicals and their role in breast cancer prevention

Numerous reports and substantial evidence suggest that dietary phytochemicals have health benefits and disease-preventive properties. Research has shown that phytochemicals exhibit anti-cancer and anti-mutagenic properties, thereby playing a crucial role in reducing different types of cancers, as displayed in figure 14.2 [27, 45]. Furthermore, these chemicals act synergistically with a range of vitamins, nutrients, and minerals present in plant-derived foods. As a result, a diverse plant-rich diet is

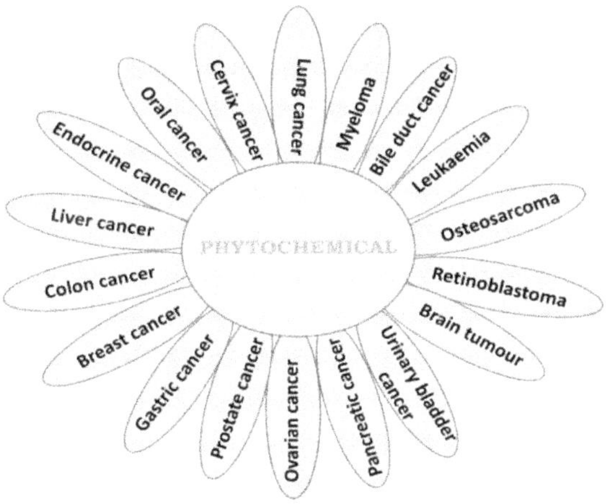

Figure 14.2. Role of phytochemicals in inhibition of different types of cancers.

necessary for disease prevention, as a single plant food product cannot provide complete protection. Daily consumption of phytochemicals in a regular human diet is essential to observe their beneficial effects [46, 47].

Several phytochemicals, such as resveratrol, curcumin, catechins, genistein, and quercetin, have been shown to effectively counteract various pathological conditions related to oxidative stress associated with aging and chronic inflammation [22, 29, 48]. Many of these phytochemicals potently inhibit breast cancer development by acting on different molecular targets which are discussed in table 14.1. The chemical structures and sources of the most widely used phytochemicals with potent anti-breast cancer properties are presented in figure 14.3.

14.5 Enhancing phytochemicals formulations for breast cancer prevention through nanotechnology

Breast cancer is a major public health concern worldwide, and the use of natural products such as phytochemicals has shown promise in preventing its development. However, the efficacy of these compounds can be limited by poor bioavailability and stability, as well as difficulty in targeting cancer cells specifically [49]. Nanophytochemicals are bioactive compounds that occur naturally in plants and have potential therapeutic effects against various diseases, including cancer. The use of nanotechnology in the formulation of phytochemical compounds can address these challenges by improving their solubility and bioavailability, enabling targeted delivery to cancer cells, and enhancing their stability in biological systems [17, 50–52]. By encapsulating drugs within these nanocarriers, targeted delivery and controlled release can be achieved, allowing for more efficient and effective treatments. Additionally, the use of nanotechnology in phytochemical formulations can also improve patient compliance by enabling convenient administration and reducing side effects [34]. Several types of nanocarrier delivery systems have been utilized in cancer treatment which can be classified into two main categories depending on their

Table 14.1. List of some dietary phytochemicals in pre-clinical trials for breast cancer treatment.

Phytochemical	Mechanism of action	Molecular targets	References
6-Shogaol (Phenyl propanoid)	BCSCs	NF-kB activation cascade	Ling *et al* [88]
Pterostilbene (polyphenol)	Apoptosis	Inhibition of CDK1 activity	Kutbi *et al* [89]
Resveratrol	Apoptosis	Cell cycle arrest	Liang *et al* [62]
Curcumin (Phyto polyphenol)	BCSCs	Modulation of cancer miRNA, NF-kB activation	Banik *et al* [90]
Genistein	Metastasis and angiogenesis	G0/G1 arrest by cell cycle transition Induction of NF-kB BCL-2 Bax	Jiang *et al* [91], Bhat *et al* [92]
Epigallocatechin-3-gallate (EGCG)	Apoptosis and cancer cell death	Induction of NF-kB and MAPKs	Musial *et al* [93]
Lycopene		NF-κB signaling	Ranjan *et al* [80]
Quercetin	Cell cycle progression and apoptosis	G2/M cell cycle arrest	Choi *et al* [94]
Artemisinin	Inhibit cell proliferation	Breast tumor site	Gharib *et al* [95]
Apigenin (flavones)	Inhibit cell proliferation and apoptosis	HER2-positive breast tumors	Scherbakov and Anndreeva [96]

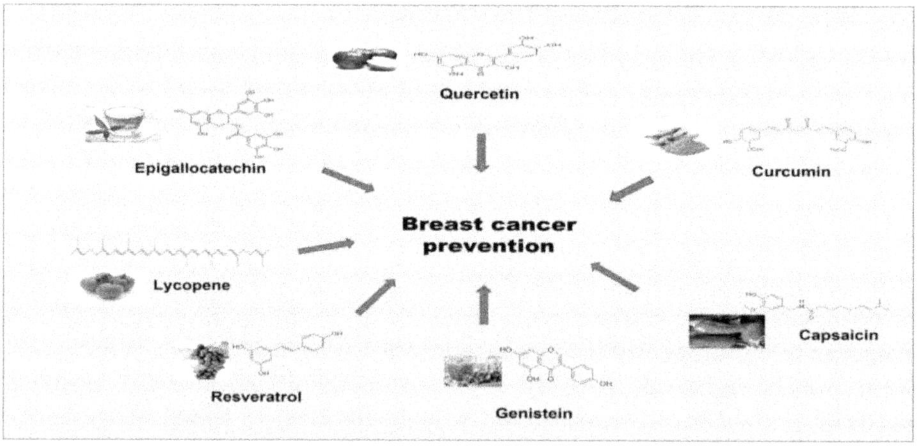

Figure 14.3. Graphical representations of structures and sources of the most commonly used phytochemicals in the prevention of human breast cancer.

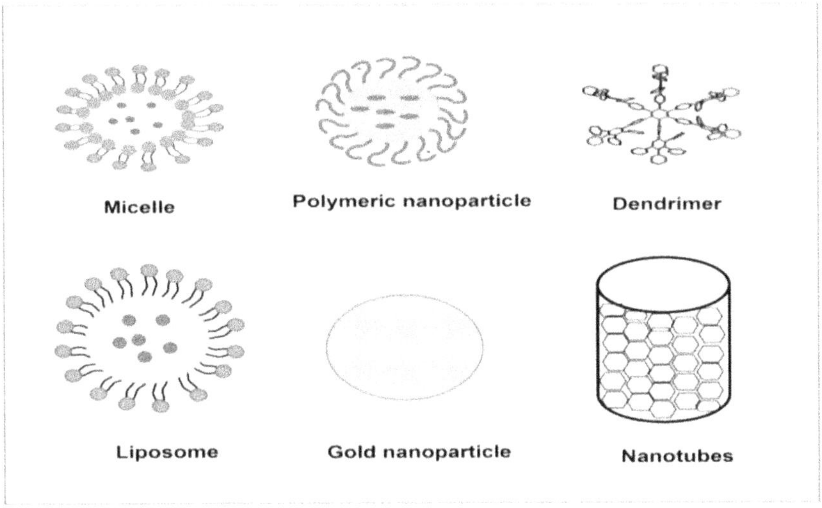

Figure 14.4. Images of the most common types of nanocarrier-based delivery systems.

physical state—solid and liquid. The solid systems include nanocrystals, lipid nanoparticles, and polymeric nanoparticles, which have a solid matrix ore, as shown in figure 14.4. The liquid systems, on the other hand, include nanoliposomes, nanoemulsions, and nanopolymersomes [18, 19, 53], which are liquid droplets or vesicles and metallic nanoparticles such as gold [53], as illustrated in figure 14.4. These nanocarrier delivery systems have unique properties and can be tailored for specific applications, depending on their physicochemical characteristics. This can lead to more effective breast cancer prevention strategies and potentially reduce the need for toxic chemotherapy drugs.

14.5.1 Nano-curcumin

The turmeric plant, scientifically known as *Curcuma longa* and belonging to the Zingiberaceae family, contains a polyphenolic compound called curcumin. This compound is synthesized from ferulic acid and is mainly found in the plant's root or rhizome. The structural formula of curcumin is [1,7-bis(4-hydroxy-3-methoxy-phenyl)-1,6-heptadiene-3,5-dione]. It has anti-bacterial, anti-inflammatory [54, 55] and anti-cancer properties [56]. Various reports have shown that curcumin can inhibit the growth and proliferation of breast cancer cells. Despite its therapeutic properties, curcumin faces a significant challenge regarding its bioavailability due to its poor solubility issues in aqueous solutions, which ultimately restricts its clinical effectiveness. To address these challenges, researchers have investigated novel drug delivery systems, including liposomes, solid dispersion, microemulsion, micelles, etc. These systems aim to enhance the bioavailability and efficacy of therapeutic agents, as well as to minimize their side effects. To address this issue, nanocarriers have been developed for curcumin delivery [57, 58].

14.5.2 Nano-resveratrol

Resveratrol (5,4′-Trihydroxystilbene) is a polyphenol compound found naturally in several plant-based foods like grapes, berries, and peanuts. Research studies have suggested that it may have the potential to offer certain health benefits due to its anti-inflammatory and antioxidant properties [17]. Studies have also investigated that resveratrol may have beneficial effects on cancer, cardiovascular disease, and neurodegenerative disorders and involve the treatment of several diseases [59]. However, more research is needed to fully understand its molecular and clinical activity. Studies have revealed that resveratrol can inhibit the growth and proliferation of breast cancer cells. More importantly, the co-administration of resveratrol with chemotherapeutic agents has been shown to decrease the associated side effects, while simultaneously enhancing the therapeutic efficacy of cancer chemotherapy. Recent studies have suggested that beta-glucan can act as a useful complementary drug carrier to increase the bioavailability of certain drugs, including resveratrol, which has potential health benefits. Furthermore, research has indicated that combining resveratrol with beta-glucan may have synergistic effects on immune reactions. Studies have investigated the potential benefits of using these compounds together in a drug delivery system, in order to enhance their therapeutic effects. However, further research is needed to fully understand the potential synergies of resveratrol and beta-glucan, as well as the safety and efficacy of such drug delivery systems in humans. The impact of these compositions on gene expression, specifically on the genes Cdc42, NF-kB2, and BcL-2, in breast cancer cells has been examined [60]. A study that has been carried out recently by Liang *et al* involved the development of a synergistic resveratrol nanoparticle system using lecithin encapsulation. The researchers utilized lecithin, which is a natural phospholipid obtained from soybeans, due to its inherent anti-tumor activity [61].

14.5.3 Nano-epigallocatechin-3-gallate

EGCG stands for Epigallocatechin-3-gallate, which is a type of polyphenol found in green tea. It has been studied for its potential health benefits, including its antioxidant, anti-inflammatory, and anti-cancer properties [62, 63]. Studies have shown that EGCG can inhibit the growth and proliferation of breast cancer cells [64]. To address the poor bioavailability and stability of EGCG, new nano-delivery systems have been investigated. In particular, solid lipid nanomolecules loaded with EGCG have shown higher potential and stability for delivery compared to non-treated EGCG [34, 68]. Narayanan *et al* developed PLGA-casein NPs that sequentially released paclitaxel and EGCG due to their core and shell structure. The NPs had increased biocompatibility and a longer circulatory lifespan and exhibited better cellular uptake by MDA-MB-231 cells. In a study using breast cancer cells, the combination therapy with functionalized NPs showed a higher rate of apoptosis and an inhibitory effect on the protein levels of NF-κB. Additionally, combination treatment including both EGFR and HER2 antibodies in breast cancer patient samples also showed significantly greater anti-tumoral activity [65]. Additionally, nanoparticles such as chitin-loaded honokiol and nanoliposomes have been developed to enhance the anti-cancer properties of EGCG [67]. These nano-delivery systems have the potential to improve the effectiveness of EGCG in cancer treatment.

14.5.4 Nano-quercetin

Quercetin (QT) is a flavonoid found in many fruit and vegetables, including apples, onions, and berries. QT has been shown to have beneficial effects against various cancer cell types. QT has cytoprotective effects that can inhibit molecules used in signaling pathways that promote carcinogeneses, such as protein kinase-C, tyrosine kinase, and phosphatidylinositol-3 kinase. In recent studies, the significance of tyrosine kinase pathways in the progression of breast cancer has been highlighted [34]. As an antioxidant polyphenol, QT can limit free radical damage. Additionally, QT has been found to inhibit lipid peroxidase, making it potentially useful as an anti-cancer agent [71]. Studies have revealed that QT can have toxic effects on various cancer cells, but its therapeutic applications have been limited due to its less solubility and bioavailability issues [51, 52, 69, 70]. To address this issue, researchers have explored different drug delivery systems, including polymeric nanoparticles, solid lipid nanoparticles (SLNs), liposomes, and micelles, to improve the bioavailability of anti-cancer agents [70]. Furthermore, the use of conjugates combining bioflavonoids and nanoparticles as targeted drug delivery systems have generated significant interest in recent times. Their data has demonstrated that QT and nanoparticle conjugation inhibit the MCF-7 cell line growth, highlighting its potential as a therapeutic agent in breast cancer treatment [72, 73]. These studies have shown that quercetin can inhibit the growth and proliferation of breast cancer cells [37].

14.5.5 Nano-genistein

Genistein is a type of phytochemical called an isoflavone, which is isolated from soybeans and soy products. It is a natural compound with a chemical structure similar to estrogen and has been examined for its potential positive impacts on health. Research suggests that genistein may have antioxidant properties and may help to reduce inflammation in the body [74]. Genistein has also been investigated for its potential to improve bone health and minimize the osteoporosis risk among postmenopausal women. It may also play a potential role in decreasing the risk of specific cancer types. such as breast and prostate cancer, by interfering with the growth of cancer cells [75–77]. While genistein is a natural compound, it can have potential side effects and interactions with certain medications, and its bioavailability is limited due to its poor solubility in water. To address this issue, researchers utilized an innovative technique called nano-spray drying to create nanoparticles loaded with a dry extract of soybean. Carboxymethyl cellulose was used as an excipient in the process [78]. The pharmacological evidence of this study revealed the low incidence of breast cancer.

14.5.6 Nano-lycopene

Lycopene is a pigment belonging to the carotenoid family, which is responsible for the characteristic color of certain fruits and vegetables, including watermelon, tomatoes, pink grapefruit, and guava. It is a non-provitamin A carotenoid, meaning it does not get converted into vitamin A in the body as beta-carotene does. Recent studies have suggested that lycopene may have health benefits, particularly in lowering the possibility of chronic diseases such as cancer and cardiovascular disease [79–81]. These benefits may be due to lycopene's antioxidant properties, which protect the cells from oxidative damage caused by free radicals [81].

Lycopene is a lipophilic molecule that is poorly soluble in water and has limited bioavailability, meaning that it is not efficiently absorbed by the body when consumed in food or supplements. Nano-encapsulation of lycopene can protect it from degradation, increase its stability, and enhance its solubility in water-based systems, making it easier for the body to absorb and utilize. Research studies have shown that nano-lycopene may have potential health benefits, such as anti-inflammatory, antioxidant, and anti-cancer properties due to their enhanced bioavailability and ability to target specific cells and tissues [82, 83]. However, more research is desirable to completely understand the potential benefits and risks of using nano-lycopene, as well as its long-term safety and efficacy in humans.

14.5.7 Nano-capsaicin

Capsaicin (trans-8-methyl-N-vanillyl-6-zonisamide) is an alkaloid compound found in chili peppers. Capsaicinoids are a type of secondary metabolite produced by these plants. The hotness or pungency of chili peppers is quantified using Scoville Heat Units (SHU), which is a measure of the extent of dilution necessary to lessen the heat of a chili extract. The concentration of capsaicin in chili pepper is directly proportional to its SHU rating. The amount of capsaicin present in different types of chili peppers can vary, ranging from 0.1% to 1.0%. It has been shown to have anti-inflammatory and anti-cancer properties [84, 85]. The anti-cancer effects of capsaicin, have been gaining more attention in recent years, particularly about its ability to combat various types of human cancers [85, 86], including breast cancer [41]. However, capsaicin has poor solubility and bioavailability, which limits its effectiveness as an anti-cancer agent. However, when capsaicin is encapsulated in nanoparticles, it is protected from degradation and delivered in a more controlled and sustained manner to the target site. A recent report has been published regarding the utilization of a nanocarrier-based drug delivery system for capsaicin. The study found that the inclusion of capsaicin-loaded alginate nanoparticles within polycaprolactone-chitosan nanofibers resulted in a notable prolongation of capsaicin release. Their release time increased from 120 h to over 500 h. Additionally, the *in vitro* analysis showed that the designed nano platform was able to effectively suppress the growth of MCF-7 human breast cells while remaining non-toxic to human dermal fibroblasts (HDF) [87].

Results from the reports on nanophytochemicals that have been studied for their anti-breast cancer properties are listed in tables 14.2 and 14.3.

Table 14.2. Nanocarrier-based delivery of phytochemicals with their mechanism of action in the treatment of breast cancer.

S. No.	Nanoformulation	Mechanism of action	References
1.	Nano-curcumin	Reduced tumor volume and induction of apoptosis breast cancer cells.	Feng *et al* [57], Mahmoudi *et al* [58]
2.	Nano-resveratrol	The combined effect of resveratrol and Beta-glucan enhances gene expression in the composition (Cdc42, NF-kB2, and BcL-2, in breast cancer cells.	Xiao *et al* [60]
3.	Nano-epigallocatechin-3-gallate (EGCG)	EGCG and NPs combination induces apoptosis and inhibitory effect on NF-κB, of breast cancer cells. EGCG-nanoethosomes reduce the volume of tumor.	Narayana *et al* [65], Narayana *et al* [65], Frias *et al* [67]
4.	Nano-quercetin (QT)	QT-SLNs induce the cytotoxic and apoptotic effects on MCF-7 breast cancer cell line.	Balakrishnan *et al* [72], Niazvand *et al* [73]
5.	Nano-genistein	Pharmacological data showed the low incidence of breast cancer.	Del Gaudio *et al* [78]
6.	Nano-lycopene	Decrease tumor proliferation, *in vitro* and *in vivo* protection.	Jain *et al* [83]
7.	Nano-capsaicin	Suppress the growth of MCF-7 human breast cells.	Ahmady *et al* [87]

14.6 Conclusions

Phytochemicals, which are natural compounds found in plants, have gained interest for their potential use in the prevention and treatment of breast cancer due to their various anti-cancer properties. Compared to conventional breast cancer treatment methods, such as chemotherapy and radiation therapy, phytochemicals have several potential advantages. The current review highlights the significant contribution of phytochemicals in the prevention and treatment of breast cancer. Studies have suggested that a diet rich in fruit and vegetables containing a diverse range of phytochemicals may aid in reducing the chances of developing different forms of cancer. Phytochemicals have been shown to have multiple mechanisms of action against breast cancer cells. They can modulate immune responses, inhibit cell proliferation, induce apoptosis, and act as antioxidant enzymes. In contrast, conventional therapies often target specific cellular pathways or molecular targets.

While phytochemicals have shown promise in the treatment of breast cancer, there are certain limitations associated with their use. One major limitation is their low bioavailability and poor solubility. Many phytochemicals are not readily absorbed by the body and may be rapidly metabolized or eliminated before they

Table 14.3. List of phytochemical-based nanoformulations used in breast cancer therapy (*in vitro and in vivo* studies analysis) [53].

Drug	Nanocarriers	Phytochemical	Size	Molecular target	References
Doxorubicin	Poly-glycerol-malic acid-dodecanedioic acid	Curcumin	~110–218 nm	Apoptosis, an increase in the uptake of the drug after conjugation	Kumari *et al* [97]
Doxorubicin	Lipid carriers	Sulforaphane/ Isothiocyanate	145 nm	Anti-cancer effects in an MCF-7 xenograft mouse model	Soni *et al* [98]
Doxorubicin	Phytosome	Quercetin	~85 nm	Anti-cancer effects in an MCF-7 xenograft mouse model	Minaei *et al* [99]
Adriamycin	Silver NPs	*Camellia sinensis*	~220 nm	Cytotoxicity increased, apoptosis, increase in uptake of drug in MCF-7	Yadav and Mendhulkar [100]

can exert their anti-cancer effects. This can limit their efficacy and require high doses to be effective, which can increase the risk of toxicity.

In addition, phytochemicals may interact with other medications, potentially reducing their effectiveness or causing adverse effects. This highlights the importance of carefully monitoring and coordinating treatment plans in patients using phytochemicals alongside conventional cancer treatments.

Finally, the complexity of the molecular mechanisms underlying the anti-cancer effects of phytochemicals makes it challenging to identify specific compounds or doses that are most effective for different types and stages of breast cancer. Further research is needed to fully understand the potential benefits and limitations of phytochemicals in breast cancer treatment.

To overcome these limitations the use of nano-based delivery systems is progressively being explored as a way to improve the effectiveness of phytochemicals in breast cancer treatment. By encapsulating the phytochemicals in nanoparticles, their solubility and stability can be improved, and they can be delivered to the target site in a more controlled and sustained manner. And these systems can help to overcome the limitations of conventional drug delivery methods. For example, they can improve the specificity of drug delivery to cancer cells, while minimizing the risk of toxicity to healthy cells. They can also help to reduce the frequency of dosing and minimize the side effects of chemotherapy. Most importantly the nano-based delivery systems can enhance the efficacy of phytochemicals by allowing for targeted drug delivery to the target site. For example, nanoparticle-based delivery systems can be designed to selectively accumulate in the tumor microenvironment and can release their cargo in response to specific triggers such as changes in pH or temperature.

Overall, the use of nano-based delivery systems for phytochemicals holds promise for the development of more effective and targeted breast cancer therapies, with reduced side effects and improved patient overall health.

Conflict of interest

The authors declare no conflict of interest.

References

[1] Sung H, Ferlay J and Siegel R L *et al* 2021 Global cancer statistics 2020: GLOBOCAN estimates of incidence and mortality worldwide for 36 cancers in 185 countries *CA Cancer J. Clin.* **71** 209–49

[2] Hong R and Xu B 2022 Breast cancer: an up-to-date review and future perspectives *Cancer Commun. (Lond.)* **42** 913–36

[3] Israel B B, Tilghman S L, Parker-Lemieux K and Payton-Stewart F 2018 Phytochemicals: current strategies for treating breast cancer *Oncol Lett.* **15** 7471–8

[4] Bridgett S, Campbell J, Lord C J and Ryan C J 2017 Cancer GD: a resource for identifying and interpreting genetic dependencies in cancer *Cell Syst.* **5** 82–86.e3

[5] Bhattacharya T, Dutta S and Akter R *et al* 2021 Role of phytonutrients in nutrigenetics and nutrigenomics perspective in curing breast cancer *Biomolecules* **11** 1176

[6] Sun Y S, Zhao Z and Yang Z N *et al* 2017 Risk factors and preventions of breast cancer *Int. J. Biol. Sci.* **13** 1387–97

[7] Maughan K L, Lutterbie M A and Ham P S 2010 Treatment of breast cancer *Am. Fam. Physician* **81** 1339–46

[8] Akram M, Iqbal M, Daniyal M and Khan A U 2017 Awareness and current knowledge of breast cancer *Biol. Res.* **50** 33

[9] Moo T A, Sanford R, Dang C and Morrow M 2018 Overview of breast cancer therapy *PET Clin.* **13** 339–54

[10] Reeder J G and Vogel V G 2008 Breast cancer prevention *Cancer Treat Res.* **141** 149–64

[11] Fisusi F A and Akala E O 2019 Drug combinations in breast cancer therapy *Pharm. Nanotechnol.* **7** 3–23

[12] Kampa M, Alexaki V I and Notas G *et al* 2004 Antiproliferative and apoptotic effects of selective phenolic acids on T47D human breast cancer cells: potential mechanisms of action *Breast Cancer Res.* **6** R63–74

[13] Rezaei-Seresht H, Cheshomi H, Falanji F, Movahedi-Motlagh F, Hashemian M and Mireskandari E 2019 Cytotoxic activity of caffeic acid and gallic acid against MCF-7 human breast cancer cells: an *in silico* and *in vitro* study *Avicenna J. Phytomed.* **9** 574–86

[14] Noolu B, Gogulothu R and Bhat M *et al* 2016 *In vivo* inhibition of proteasome activity and tumour growth by *Murraya koenigii* leaf extract in breast cancer xenografts and by its active flavonoids in breast cancer cells *Anticancer Agents Med. Chem.* **16** 1605–14

[15] Chen D, Landis-Piwowar K R, Chen M S and Dou Q P 2007 Inhibition of proteasome activity by the dietary flavonoid apigenin is associated with growth inhibition in cultured breast cancer cells and xenografts *Breast Cancer Res.* **9** R80

[16] Younas M, Hano C, Giglioli-Guivarc'h N and Abbasi B H 2018 Mechanistic evaluation of phytochemicals in breast cancer remedy: current understanding and future perspectives *RSC Adv.* **8** 29714–44

[17] Vaiserman A, Koliada A, Zayachkivska A and Lushchak O 2020 Nanodelivery of natural antioxidants: an anti-aging perspective *Front. Bioeng. Biotechnol.* **7** 447

[18] Borel T and Sabliov C M 2014 Nanodelivery of bioactive components for food applications: types of delivery systems, properties, and their effect on ADME profiles and toxicity of nanoparticles *Annu. Rev. Food Sci. Technol.* **5** 197–213

[19] Ganesan P, Ramalingam P, Karthivashan G, Ko Y T and Choi D K 2018 Recent developments in solid lipid nanoparticle and surface-modified solid lipid nanoparticle delivery systems for oral delivery of phyto-bioactive compounds in various chronic diseases *Int. J. Nanomed.* **13** 1569–83

[20] Ravindran S, Suthar J K and Rokade R *et al* 2018 Pharmacokinetics, metabolism, distribution and permeability of nanomedicine *Curr. Drug Metab.* **19** 327–34

[21] Agarwal G, Ramakant P and Forgach E R *et al* 2009 Breast cancer care in developing countries *World J. Surg.* **33** 2069–76

[22] Kapinova A, Kubatka P and Golubnitschaja O *et al* 2018 Dietary phytochemicals in breast cancer research: anticancer effects and potential utility for effective chemoprevention *Environ. Health Prev. Med.* **23** 36

[23] Liu R H 2013 Dietary bioactive compounds and their health implications *J. Food Sci.* **78** 18–28

[24] Aggarwal B B, Vijayalekshmi R V and Sung B 2009 Targeting inflammatory pathways for prevention and therapy of cancer: short-term friend, long-term foe *Clin. Cancer Res.* **15** 425–30

[25] Golubnitschaja O 2007 Cell cycle checkpoints: the role and evaluation for early diagnosis of senescence, cardiovascular, cancer, and neurodegenerative diseases *Amino Acids* **32** 359–71
[26] Cebioglu M, Schild H and Golubnitschaja O 2013 Cancer predisposition in diabetic patients: risk assessment and targeted preventive measures *New Strategies to Advance Pre/Diabetes Care: Integrative Approach by PPPM* ed M Mozaffari (Dordrecht: Springer) pp 355–70
[27] Liu R H 2004 Potential synergy of phytochemicals in cancer prevention: mechanism of action *J. Nutr.* **134** 3479S–85S
[28] Leonov A, Arlia-Ciommo A and Piano A *et al* 2015 Longevity extension by phytochemicals *Molecules* **20** 6544–72
[29] Mazurakova A, Koklesova L and Samec M *et al* 2022 Anti-breast cancer effects of phytochemicals: primary, secondary, and tertiary care *EPMA J.* **13** 315–34
[30] Cory H, Passarelli S, Szeto J, Tamez M and Mattei J 2018 The role of polyphenols in human health and food systems: a mini-review *Front. Nutr.* **5** 87
[31] Block G, Patterson B and Subar A 1992 Fruit, vegetables, and cancer prevention: a review of the epidemiological evidence *Nutr. Cancer* **18** 1–29
[32] Kubatka P, Kapinová A and Kello M *et al* 2016 Fruit peel polyphenols demonstrate substantial anti-tumour effects in the model of breast cancer *Eur. J. Nutr.* **55** 955–65
[33] Kubatka P, Kello M and Kajo K *et al* 2017 Oregano demonstrates distinct tumour-suppressive effects in the breast carcinoma model *Eur. J. Nutr.* **56** 1303–16
[34] Sindhu R K, Verma R and Salgotra T *et al* 2021 Impacting the remedial potential of nano delivery-based flavonoids for breast cancer treatment *Molecules* **26** 5163
[35] Gaudet M M, Britton J A and Kabat G C *et al* 2004 Fruits, vegetables, and micronutrients about breast cancer modified by menopause and hormone receptor status *Cancer Epidemiol. Biomarkers Prev.* **13** 1485–94
[36] Ramel F, Birtic S, Ginies C, Soubigou-Taconnat L, Triantaphylidès C and Havaux M 2012 Carotenoid oxidation products are stress signals that mediate gene responses to singlet oxygen in plants *Proc. Natl Acad. Sci. USA* **109** 5535–40
[37] Ezzati M, Yousefi B, Velaei K and Safa A 2020 A review on anti-cancer properties of quercetin in breast cancer *Life Sci.* **248** 117463
[38] Wang S, Shen P, Zhou J and Lu Y 2017 Diet phytochemicals and cutaneous carcinoma chemoprevention: a review *Pharmacol. Res.* **119** 327–46
[39] Rampogu S, Balasubramaniyam T and Lee J H 2022 Phytotherapeutic applications of alkaloids in treating breast cancer *Biomed. Pharmacother.* **155** 113760
[40] Eguchi R, Ono N, Hirai Morita A, Katsuragi T, Nakamura S, Huang M, Altaf-Ul-Amin M and Kanaya S 2019 Classification of alkaloids according to the starting substances of their biosynthetic pathways using graph convolutional neural networks *BMC Bioinf.* **20** 380
[41] Chen M, Xiao C and Jiang W *et al* 2021 Capsaicin inhibits proliferation and induces apoptosis in breast cancer by down-regulating FBI-1-mediated NF-κB pathway *Drug Des. Devel. Ther.* **15** 125–40
[42] Dhupal M and Chowdhury D 2020 Phytochemical-based nanomedicine for advanced cancer theranostics: perspectives on clinical trials to clinical use *Int. J. Nanomed.* **15** 9125–57
[43] Rosas-González V C, Téllez-Bañuelos M C and Hernández-Flores G *et al* 2020 Differential effects of alliin and allicin on apoptosis and senescence in luminal A and triple-negative breast cancer: caspase, $\Delta\Psi$m, and pro-apoptotic gene involvement *Fundam. Clin. Pharmacol.* **34** 671–86

[44] Jaiswal S, Parida S K, Murarka S and Singh P 2022 Development of S-aryl dithiocarbamate derived novel antiproliferative compound exhibiting tubulin bundling *Bioorg. Med. Chem.* **68** 116874

[45] Miller P E and Snyder D C 2012 Phytochemicals and cancer risk: a review of the epidemiological evidence *Nutr. Clin. Pract.* **27** 599–612

[46] Ginter E and Simko V 2015 Recent data on Mediterranean diet, cardiovascular disease, cancer, diabetes and life expectancy *Bratisl. Lek. Listy* **116** 346–8

[47] Hijova E and Chmelarova A 2008 The risk of cancer in relationship to diet *Bratisl. Lek. Listy* **109** 320–3

[48] Choudhari A S, Mandave P C, Deshpande M, Ranjekar P and Prakash O 2020 Corrigendum: phytochemicals in cancer treatment: from preclinical studies to clinical practice *Front. Pharmacol.* **11** 175

[49] Aqil F, Munagala R, Jeyabalan J and Vadhanam M V 2013 Bioavailability of phytochemicals and its enhancement by drug delivery systems *Cancer Lett.* **334** 133–41

[50] Salama L, Pastor E R, Stone T and Mousa S A 2020 Emerging nanopharmaceuticals and nanonutraceuticals in cancer management *Biomedicines* **8** 347

[51] Srivastava S, Somasagara R R and Hegde M *et al* 2016 Quercetin, a natural flavonoid interacts with DNA, arrests cell cycle and causes tumor regression by activating mitochondrial pathway of apoptosis *Sci. Rep.* **6** 24049

[52] Mohammed H A, Sulaiman G M and Anwar S S *et al* 2021 Quercetin against MCF7 and CAL51 breast cancer cell lines: apoptosis, gene expression and cytotoxicity of nano-quercetin *Nanomedicine (Lond.)* **16** 1937–61

[53] Ganesan K, Wang Y and Gao F *et al* 2021 Targeting engineered nanoparticles for breast cancer therapy *Pharmaceutics.* **13** 1829

[54] Deodhar S D, Sethi R and Srimal R C 1980 Preliminary study on antirheumatic activity of curcumin (diferuloyl methane) *Indian J. Med. Res.* **71** 632–4

[55] Buhrmann C, Mobasheri A and Busch F *et al* 2011 Curcumin modulates nuclear factor kappaB (NF-kappaB)-mediated inflammation in human tenocytes *in vitro*: role of the phosphatidylinositol 3-kinase/Akt pathway *J. Biol. Chem.* **286** 28556–66

[56] Thacker P C and Karunagaran D 2015 Curcumin and emodin down-regulate TGF-β signaling pathway in human cervical cancer cells *PLoS One* **10** e0120045

[57] Feng T, Wei Y, Lee R J and Zhao L 2017 Liposomal curcumin and its application in cancer *Int. J. Nanomed.* **12** 6027–44

[58] Mahmoudi R, Hassandokht F and Ardakani M T *et al* 2021 Intercalation of curcumin into liposomal chemotherapeutic agent augments apoptosis in breast cancer cells *J. Biomater. Appl.* **35** 1005–18

[59] Berman A Y, Motechin R A, Wiesenfeld M Y and Holz M K 2017 The therapeutic potential of resveratrol: a review of clinical trials *NPJ Precis. Oncol.* **1** 35

[60] Xiao Q, Zhu W and Feng W *et al* 2019 A review of resveratrol as a potent chemoprotective and synergistic agent in cancer chemotherapy *Front. Pharmacol.* **9** 1534

[61] Liang M, Guo M, Saw P E and Yao Y 2022 Fully natural lecithin encapsulated nano-resveratrol for anti-cancer therapy *Int. J. Nanomed.* **17** 2069–78

[62] Sartippour M R, Shao Z M and Heber D *et al* 2002 Green tea inhibits vascular endothelial growth factor (VEGF) induction in human breast cancer cells *J. Nutr.* **132** 2307–11

[63] Almatroodi S A, Almatroudi A, Khan A A, Alhumaydhi F A, Alsahli M A and Rahmani A H 2020 Potential therapeutic targets of epigallocatechin gallate (EGCG), the most

abundant catechin in green tea, and its role in the therapy of various types of cancer *Molecules* **25** 3146
[64] Chisholm K, Bray B J and Rosengren R J 2004 Tamoxifen and epigallocatechin gallate are synergistically cytotoxic to MDA-MB-231 human breast cancer cells *Anticancer Drugs* **15** 889–97
[65] Narayana S, Pavithran M and Viswanath A *et al* 2014 Sequentially releasing dual-drug-loaded PLGA-casein core/shell nanomedicine: design, synthesis, biocompatibility and pharmacokinetics *Acta Biomater.* **10** 2112–24
[66] Narayana S, Mony U, Vijaykumar D K, Koyakutty M, Paul-Prasanth B and Menon D 2015 Sequential release of epigallocatechin gallate and paclitaxel from PLGA-casein core/shell nanoparticles sensitizes drug-resistant breast cancer cells *Nanomedicine* **11** 1399–406
[67] Frias I, Neves A R, Pinheiro M and Reis S 2016 Design, development, and characterization of lipid nanocarriers-based epigallocatechin gallate delivery system for preventive and therapeutic supplementation *Drug Des. Devel Ther.* **10** 3519–28
[68] Granja A, Pinheiro M and Reis S 2016 Epigallocatechin gallate nanodelivery systems for cancer therapy *Nutrients* **8** 307
[69] Lamson D W and Brignall M S 2000 Antioxidants and cancer, part 3: quercetin *Altern. Med. Rev.* **5** 196–208
[70] Dhumale S S, Waghela B N and Pathak C 2015 Quercetin protects necrotic insult and promotes apoptosis by attenuating the expression of RAGE and its ligand HMGB1 in human breast adenocarcinoma cells *IUBMB Life* **67** 361–73
[71] Kim W K, Bang M H and Kim E S *et al* 2005 Quercetin decreases the expression of $ErbB_2$ and $ErbB_3$ proteins in HT-29 human colon cancer cells *J. Nutr. Biochem.* **16** 155–62
[72] Balakrishnan S, Mukherjee S and Das S *et al* 2017 Gold nanoparticles-conjugated quercetin induces apoptosis via inhibition of EGFR/PI3K/Akt-mediated pathway in breast cancer cell lines (MCF-7 and MDA-MB-231) *Cell Biochem. Funct.* **35** 217–31
[73] Niazvand F, Orazizadeh M, Khorsandi L, Abbaspour M, Mansouri E and Khodadadi A 2019 Effects of quercetin-loaded nanoparticles on MCF-7 human breast cancer cells *Medicina (Kaunas)* **55** 114
[74] Sharifi-Rad J, Quispe C and Imran M *et al* 2021 Genistein: an integrative overview of its mode of action, pharmacological properties, and health benefits *Oxid. Med. Cell Longev.* **2021** 3268136
[75] Messina M J and Loprinzi C L 2001 Soy for breast cancer survivors: a critical review of the literature *J. Nutr.* **131** 3095S–108S
[76] Chen W F, Huang M H, Tzang C H, Yang M and Wong M S 2003 Inhibitory actions of genistein in human breast cancer (MCF-7) cells *Biochim. Biophys. Acta* **1638** 187–96
[77] Schmidt S, Michna H and Diel P 2005 Combinatory effects of phytoestrogens and 17beta-estradiol on proliferation and apoptosis in MCF-7 breast cancer cells *J. Steroid Biochem. Mol. Biol.* **94** 445–9
[78] Del Gaudio P, Sansone F, Mencherini T, De Cicco F, Russo P and Aquino R P 2017 Nanospray drying as a novel tool to improve technological properties of soy isoflavone extracts *Planta Med.* **83** 426–33
[79] Rao A V and Agarwal S 2000 Role of antioxidant lycopene in cancer and heart disease *J. Am. Coll. Nutr.* **19** 563–9
[80] Ranjan A, Ramachandran S and Gupta N *et al* 2019 Role of phytochemicals in cancer prevention *Int. J. Mol. Sci.* **20** 4981

[81] Khan U M, Sevindik M and Zarrabi A *et al* 2021 Lycopene: food sources, biological activities, and human health benefits *Oxid. Med. Cell Longev.* **2021** 2713511
[82] Bano S, Ahmed F, Khan F, Chaudhary S C and Samim M 2020 Targeted delivery of thermoresponsive polymeric nanoparticle-encapsulated lycopene: *in vitro* anticancer activity and chemopreventive effect on murine skin inflammation and tumorigenesis *RSC Adv.* **10** 16637–49
[83] Jain A, Sharma G and Ghoshal G *et al* 2018 Lycopene loaded whey protein isolate nanoparticles: an innovative endeavor for enhanced bioavailability of lycopene and anticancer activity *Int. J. Pharm.* **546** 97–105
[84] Munjuluri S, Wilkerson D A, Sooch G, Chen X, White F A and Obukhov A G 2021 Capsaicin and TRPV1 channels in the cardiovascular system: the role of inflammation *Cells* **11** 18
[85] Xie Z Q, Li H X and Hou X J *et al* 2022 Capsaicin suppresses hepatocarcinogenesis by inhibiting the stemness of hepatic progenitor cells via SIRT1/SOX2 signaling pathway *Cancer Med.* **11** 4283–96
[86] Zheng J, Zhou Y, Li Y, Xu D P, Li S and Li H B 2016 Spices for prevention and treatment of cancers *Nutrients* **8** 495
[87] Ahmady A R, Solouk A, Saber-Samandari S, Akbari S, Ghanbari H and Brycki B E 2023 Capsaicin-loaded alginate nanoparticles embedded polycaprolactone-chitosan nanofibers as a controlled drug delivery nanoplatform for anticancer activity *J. Colloid Interface Sci.* **638** 616–28
[88] Ling H, Yang H, Tan S H, Chui W K and Chew E H 2010 6-Shogaol, an active constituent of ginger, inhibits breast cancer cell invasion by reducing matrix metalloproteinase-9 expression via blockade of nuclear factor-κB activation *Br. J. Pharmacol.* **161** 1763–77
[89] Kutbi H I, Kammoun A K, Farag and El-Telbany D 2021 Amelioration of pterostilbene antiproliferative, proapoptotic, and oxidant potentials in human breast cancer MCF7 cells using zein nanocomposites *Int. J. Nanomed.* **16** 3059–71
[90] Banik U, Parasuraman S, Adhikary A K and Othman N H 2017 Curcumin: the spicy modulator of breast carcinogenesis *J. Exp. Clin. Cancer Res.* **36** 98
[91] Jiang H, Fan J, Cheng L, Hu P and Liu R 2018 The anticancer activity of genistein is increased in estrogen receptor beta 1-positive breast cancer cells *Onco Targets Ther.* **11** 8153–63
[92] Bhat S S, Prasad S K and Shivamallu C *et al* 2021 Genistein: a potent anti-breast cancer agent *Curr. Issues Mol. Biol.* **43** 1502–17
[93] Musial C, Kuban-Jankowska A and Gorska-Ponikowska M 2020 Beneficial properties of green tea catechins *Int. J. Mol. Sci.* **21** 1744
[94] Choi E J, Bae S M and Ahn W S 2008 Antiproliferative effects of quercetin through cell cycle arrest and apoptosis in human breast cancer MDA-MB-453 cells *Arch. Pharm. Res.* **31** 1281–5
[95] Gharib A, Faezizadeh Z, Mesbah-Namin S A and Saravani R 2014 Preparation, characterization and *in vitro* efficacy of magnetic nanoliposomes containing the artemisinin and transferrin *DARU J. Pharmaceut. Sci.* **22** 44
[96] Scherbakov A M and Andreeva O E 2015 Apigenin inhibits growth of breast cancer cells: the role of ERα and HER2/neu *Acta Naturae* **7** 133–9
[97] Kumari M, Sharma N and Manchanda R *et al* 2021 PGMD/curcumin nanoparticles for the treatment of breast cancer *Sci. Rep.* **11** 3824

[98] Soni K, Rizwanullah M and Kohli K 2018 Development and optimization of sulforaphane-loaded nanostructured lipid carriers by the Box–Behnken design for improved oral efficacy against cancer: *in vitro*, *ex vivo* and *in vivo* assessments *Artif. Cells Nanomed. Biotechnol.* **46** 15–31
[99] Minaei A, Sabzichi M, Ramezani F, Hamishehkar H and Samadi N 2016 Co-delivery with nano-quercetin enhances doxorubicin-mediated cytotoxicity against MCF-7 cells *Mol. Biol. Rep.* **43** 99–105
[100] Yadav A and Mendhulkar V D 2018 Antiproliferative activity of *Camellia sinensis* mediated silver nanoparticles on three different human cancer cell lines *J. Cancer Res. Ther.* **14** 1316–24

www.ingramcontent.com/pod-product-compliance
Ingram Content Group UK Ltd.
Pitfield, Milton Keynes, MK11 3LW, UK
UKHW052033301026
9729IPUK00019B/217

9 780750 352536